Public Health and Nutrition

Manoranjan Pal • Md. Golam Hossain
Rashidul Alam Mahumud
Premananda Bharati
Editors

Public Health and Nutrition

The South Asian and Southeast Asian Landscape

Springer

Editors
Manoranjan Pal
Economic Research Unit
Indian Statistical Institute (ISI)
Kolkata, West Bengal, India

Md. Golam Hossain
Department of Statistics
University of Rajshahi
Rajshahi, Bangladesh

Rashidul Alam Mahumud
NHMRC Clinical Trials Centre, Faculty of Medicine and Health
The University of Sydney
Camperdown, Sydney, New South Wales, Australia

Premananda Bharati
Biological Anthropology Unit
Indian Statistical Institute (ISI)
Kolkata, West Bengal, India

ISBN 978-981-97-7889-8 ISBN 978-981-97-7890-4 (eBook)
https://doi.org/10.1007/978-981-97-7890-4

This Springer imprint is published by the registered company Springer Nature Singapore Pte Ltd.
The registered company address is: 152 Beach Road, #21-01/04 Gateway East, Singapore 189721, Singapore

Preface

The world is grappling with severe health challenges that are exacerbated by environmental degradation, sedentary lifestyles, and poor hygiene practices. The recent COVID-19 pandemic continues to cast a long shadow over us. Communicable and noncommunicable diseases are both of significant concern. This book aims to raise awareness about the health issues and offer effective strategies to address them.

Originally focused on health problems in South Asia, the overwhelming response led to the inclusion of papers from other natural and social sciences, resulting in a broader scope that encompasses the Southeast Asian region. This expansion prompted a title change to *Public Health and Nutrition: The South Asian and Southeast Asian Landscape*. It is evident in many chapters that poverty and illiteracy are closely interlinked with everyday problems, including health issues.

The editorial team, with its extensive experience and strong connections to contemporary researchers across Asia and beyond, facilitated the smooth publication of this book. We are confident that this book will significantly benefit researchers in public health and related fields.

Kolkata, West Bengal, India — Manoranjan Pal
Rajshahi, Bangladesh — Md. Golam Hossain
New South Wales, Australia — Rashidul Alam Mahumud
Kolkata, West Bengal, India — Premananda Bharati

Introduction

In the vast expanse of scholarly literature, few topics resonate as deeply and affect as profoundly the lives of millions as public health and nutrition. These two pillars of human well-being stand as bulwarks against disease, malnutrition, and societal inequities, shaping the very fabric of communities and nations. Within the intricate tapestry of global health, South and Southeast Asia emerge as a region of immense significance, grappling with a myriad of challenges and opportunities in the realms of public health and nutrition. It is within this context that our edited book, aptly titled *Public Health and Nutrition: The South Asian and Southeast Asian Landscape*, seeks to illuminate and explore the multifaceted dimensions of these critical issues.

South and Southeast Asia is home to nearly one-third of the world's population. Within this populous region lies a rich tapestry of cultures, traditions, and histories, interwoven with the complexities of modernity and globalization. Yet, amid this diversity, common threads bind the region together—challenges such as infectious diseases, maternal and child health issues, chronic noncommunicable diseases, food insecurity, and nutritional deficiencies resonate across national boundaries, transcending political and geographical divides.

The genesis of this edited book lies in the recognition of the urgent need to comprehensively examine and address the public health and nutrition challenges facing South and Southeast Asia. While the region has made significant strides in recent decades, progress has been uneven, and many communities continue to grapple with entrenched health disparities and nutritional deficiencies. Against the backdrop of rapid urbanization, environmental degradation, and shifting dietary patterns, the imperative for evidence-based interventions and policy initiatives has never been greater.

Our edited book brings together a diverse array of perspectives, expertise, and insights from leading scholars, practitioners, and policymakers across South Asia and beyond. Through a multidisciplinary lens, we aim to critically examine the determinants of health and nutrition in the region, assess the effectiveness of existing interventions, and chart a course forward toward greater equity and sustainability. By synthesizing cutting-edge research, best practices, and case studies, we seek to catalyze dialogue, inform policy discourse, and inspire action at local, national, and regional levels.

The structure of our edited book reflects the multifaceted nature of public health and nutrition in the South and Southeast Asian context. We begin by providing a comprehensive overview of the epidemiological landscape, highlighting the burden of disease and nutritional challenges facing the region. From there, we delve into the social determinants of health, exploring the intricate interplay of factors such as poverty, gender inequality, education, and cultural practices in shaping health outcomes.

Building upon this foundation, subsequent chapters delve into specific thematic areas, ranging from maternal and child health to infectious diseases, noncommunicable diseases, and mental health. We also examine the complex nexus between nutrition, food security, and sustainable agriculture, recognizing the integral role of food systems in promoting health and well-being.

Throughout this book, we emphasize the importance of contextually tailored approaches that acknowledge the diversity of South and Southeast Asia's sociocultural landscape. We highlight innovative interventions and successful case studies that have demonstrated tangible impact in improving health outcomes and reducing nutritional disparities. At the same time, we critically interrogate prevailing paradigms and explore avenues for greater collaboration, innovation, and policy coherence across sectors.

Our ultimate goal is not merely to document the challenges facing South and Southeast Asia but to catalyze transformative change toward a healthier, more equitable future for all. By harnessing the collective wisdom and expertise of our contributors, we aspire to chart a roadmap toward resilient health systems, sustainable food systems, and thriving communities across the region.

In conclusion, *Public Health and Nutrition: The South Asian and Southeast Asian Landscape* represents a timely and indispensable contribution to the scholarly discourse on global health and development. As we navigate the complexities of the twenty-first century, the insights collected from this book will serve as a beacon of hope and inspiration for policymakers, practitioners, researchers, and advocates striving to build a healthier, more prosperous future for generations to come.

Contents

About the Authors

Manoranjan Pal After obtaining B. Stat. (Hons.), M. Stat. (Econometrics and Planning), and Ph.D. from the Indian Statistical Institute (ISI), Manoranjan Pal served ISI throughout his career. He was the Head, Economic Research Unit, ISI; Professor-in-Charge, Social Sciences Division, ISI; and Member Secretary, International Statistical Education Centre (ISEC), ISI. He taught ISEC, B. Stat., MS in Quantitative Economics (MSQE), and many other courses in ISI and abroad and is still teaching the MSQE course as a Guest Faculty after superannuation from ISI. He has authored a dozen books published by Springer, McGraw Hill, Oxford University Press, and others and has also published over 150 research papers in reputable national and international journals and books. His research interests include measurement of health and nutrition status, gender bias, the empowerment of women, and the measurement of poverty, inequality, and segregation, as well as applied econometrics.

Md. Golam Hossain Dr. Hossain is doing job as a Professor in Department of Statistics, University of Rajshahi, Rajshahi-6205, Bangladesh. Besides teaching regular courses on statistics, mathematics, operations research, health statistics, and epidemiology at the graduate and postgraduate levels, he assumes the responsibility of convening the Health Research Group in the department. He has extensive experience in handling research projects, particularly in the areas of health and nutrition. He guided one postdoctoral, nine Ph.D., and many postgraduate theses. Within a short time, he has published more than 200 papers, mostly in international journals, as well as chapters in many books. His current research interests include health, nutrition, medical statistics, epidemiology, and physical anthropology.

Rashidul Alam Mahumud is an early-career academic health economist currently based at the NHMRC Clinical Trials Centre, The University of Sydney, Australia. He holds three master's degrees: an MSc from Rajshahi University, an MPH from Independent University in Bangladesh, and a Master of Cancer Sciences from the University of Melbourne, Australia. Dr. Mahumud completed his Ph.D. from the University of Southern Queensland, Australia. His areas of expertise include economic evaluation, health economics, cancer economics, clinical epidemiology, biostatistics, and public health research. Dr. Mahumud focuses his research on oncology and chronic disease management, evaluating the clinical and economic value of cancer treatments, including melanoma and skin cancer, as well as chronic disease. He has produced 140 publications, including 130 peer-reviewed articles. He serves as an editor for two Q1-ranked journals: PLoS ONE (since 2021) and Annals of Epidemiology (since 2022). He previously served as an associate editor in BMC Public Health.

Premananda Bharati is a former Professor at the Indian Statistical Institute. He has extensive teaching experience, including teaching courses in anthropology/genetics to graduate and postgraduate students at the Indian Statistical Institute and other universities, including institutions abroad. He was declared "International Man of the Year (1993/94)" in recognition of the services to Science by the International Biographical Centre, Cambridge, England. He is an examiner and paper setter in anthropology for various universities and reviews papers for several journals. He has published more than 200 papers in reputed national and international journals. He also published several books. His research interests include nutrition and health, anthropometry, and the empowerment of women and tribal communities.

Part I

Health and Nutrition

1 Acute Malnutrition and its Determinants of School Children in Rajshahi District of Bangladesh: A Statistical Analysis

Md. Reazul Karim, Md. Sabiruzzaman, Md. Ripter Hossain, Abu Sayed Md. Al Mamun, and Md. Golam Hossain

1.1 Background

Malnutrition among school children is a global public health problem, especially in low-income countries, and it has a negative impact on many facets of a child's life, including their mental, social, and spiritual well-being (Abdel Wahed et al. 2017). In underdevelopment countries, about 52.0% and 34.0–62.0%, of school-age children are stunted and underweight, respectively (Degarege et al. 2015). Malnutrition is linked to several physiological weaknesses, including immunological dysfunction, disturbance of the intestinal barrier, dysbiosis of the gut flora, and deficiencies in vital nutrients (Bourke et al. 2016). Age, gender, father's occupation, parental education, mother's nutritional knowledge, and children's nutritional status are all key risk factors for malnutrition in school-aged children between the ages of 6 and 12 years (Alredaisy and Ibrahim 2011). In addition, it was shown that inadequate household income, food insecurity, and limited access to basic water and sanitation services were the root causes of malnutrition in each student's school years (Khalid et al. 2021).

Acute malnutrition is the term used to describe rapid weight loss brought on by decreased food consumption, illness, or possibly other exogenous factors. Children with acute malnutrition have reduced immune systems, which makes them more susceptible to common childhood infections that can be fatal. The severity of this ailment can vary, and it may have long-term effects on a person's ability to grow and

M. R. Karim · M. Sabiruzzaman · M. R. Hossain · Abu Sayed Md. Al Mamun
M. G. Hossain (✉)
Health Research Group, Department of Statistics, University of Rajshahi,
Rajshahi, Bangladesh

M. Pal et al. (eds.), *Public Health and Nutrition*,
https://doi.org/10.1007/978-981-97-7890-4_1

develop. It puts them at risk for a future characterized by disease, poor academic performance, and poverty, with potential long-term effects (WHO 2021).

Several methods can be used to measure acute malnutrition. Measurement of mid-upper arm circumference (MUAC) provides a simple and reliable tool for screening nutritional status and also enables rapid assessment of large populations in epidemiological study. Usually, MUAC has functioned as a convenient substitute indicator for under-nutrition, specifically severe acute malnutrition, in infants and children under the age of 5 (Goossens et al. 2012). In recent studies, MUAC has demonstrated high accuracy in identifying malnutrition among school children in South Africa (Craig et al. 2014) and the Netherlands (Talma et al. 2019), as well as in Southeast African children and adolescents (Mramba et al. 2017) and Sri Lankan school children (Shinsugi et al. 2020).

Students between the ages of 5 and 9 are classified as experiencing severe acute malnutrition (SAM) when their mid-upper arm circumference (MUAC) measures below 135 mm, and moderate acute malnutrition (MAM) if it falls below 145 mm. For children aged 10–14, SAM is identified when their MUAC is less than 160 mm, and MAM when it is less than 185 mm. Those with MUAC measurements between 145 and 185 mm are deemed acutely malnourished in both scenarios (Kristen and Lesley 2018).

The Rajshahi district is located in north-western Bangladesh and it is known for its distinctive geography and ethnic diversity. It is primarily composed of the Barind tract and is inhabited by various ethnic minority communities (BBS 2011). A few studies have shown that schoolchildren in the high Barind tract area in Rajshahi district are particularly susceptible to acute malnutrition outcomes. As far as I am aware, there have been no studies about the affiliation between the malnutrition of school children in plain land communities. It is crucial to examine how socio-economic and other relevant factors influence the malnutrition of these children. Therefore, the purpose of this study is to determine the prevalence of acute malnutrition and the factors that contribute to it among schoolchildren in the Rajshahi district of Bangladesh.

1.2 Materials and Methods

1.2.1 Methods

The rural area of Rajshahi district was the study area, and school children aged 6–13 years were considered as population of this study. It was cross-sectional study conducted from January to June 2019.

1.2.2 Sample Size Determination

The following mathematical formula (Cochran 1963) was used to calculate sample size for this prevalence cross-sectional study:

$$n = z^2 p \frac{1-p}{d^2} \tag{1}$$

where n is the number of required samples, $z = 1.96$ for 95% confidence interval (CI), p is the proportion of malnourished children, here we considered $p = 0.323$ (the prevalence of malnourished school children has been estimated to be 32.3% (Hossain et al. 2014)), and d is the margin of error, here we considered, $d = 0.05$. Formula (1) provided that 337 was the adequate sample size for this study. To get more accurate results, we have calculated 500 samples but initially, we considered 550 samples (10% absent rate).

1.2.3 Inclusion/Exclusion Criteria

We included children in our present study who were living with his/her parents in Rajshahi district and studied grade 1–7 classes and were aged 6 to 13 years and had no severe disease.

1.2.4 Study Design and Sample Selection Procedures

Multi-stage random sampling for selecting samples from our population. After selecting the sample, we contacted school officials. The school's information was obtained from the respective education office. The households of our selected school children were also selected for gathering household-related information from the household head or his/her selected person. We scheduled training for our four field employees. We scheduled a meeting with selected school children, teachers, and parents before collecting/measuring variables. In this meeting, we discussed in detail the objective of our study and we took their written consent. The sample selection procedure has been described- in the first stage, one Upazila (Godagari) was randomly chosen from the nine Upazilas of the Rajshahi district. In the second stage, one union (Gogram) was randomly from the nine unions of the selected Upazila. In the third stage, five schools (Gogram Govt. Primary School, Gogram Adarsha Girl High School, Gogram High School, Muraripur BRAC School, and Gogram Dakhil Madrasa) were randomly selected from our selected union. In the fourth and final stage, 500 school children aged 6–13 years were randomly selected with proportional allocation from the selected schools.

1.2.5 Outcome Variable of the Study

The study focused on the nutritional status of school children, using mid-upper arm circumference (MUAC) as the dependent variable. For children aged 5–9, a mid-upper arm circumference (MUAC) below 135 mm indicates severe acute malnutrition (SAM), while a measurement less than 145 mm indicates moderate acute malnutrition (MAM). In the case of children aged 10–14, severe acute malnutrition (SAM) is diagnosed if MUAC is below 160 mm, and moderate acute malnutrition (MAM) if it is below 185 mm. Children with mid-upper arm circumference (MUAC) readings between 145 and 185 mm are considered acutely malnourished in both age groups (Kristen and Lesley 2018).

1.2.6 Independent Variables of the Study

In this study, socio-economic, demographic, anthropometric, health, and nutritional factors were considered as the independent variables. Majority of the variables were selected from previous published papers (Hossain et al. 2014; NIPORT 2020). Other variables were selected on the basis of our knowledge.

1.2.7 Questionnaire Developing and Pre-Testing

A partially structured questionnaire was utilized to collect data from the respondents. The questionnaire was developed in English based on literature reviews and was reviewed for feedback by five health sciences specialists. The questionnaire was revised and finalized after receiving the suggestions of the specialists. For clarity, the English questionnaire was translated into Bangla, the mother tongue of the selected respondents. The author and supervisor checked the meaning of both the Bangla and English versions of the questionnaire and made modifications as necessary before finalizing it. A pilot survey was conducted with 50 respondents to test the consistency and Cronbach's alpha (α) was used to assess the questionnaire's reliability, with a value of more than 0.80 indicating good internal consistency. The questionnaire was deemed reliable and was used to collect data with written agreements obtained from the selected mothers or guardians. Data entry was preceded by editing and coding.

1.2.8 Data Processing and Management

The collected data from the field was entered into the SPSS software. Daily checks were conducted to ensure accuracy and completeness in recording the responses. Missing information was identified and screened for abnormalities or outliers. Prior to data entry, editing and coding were performed. The SPSS IBM version 22 was used to analyze the data.

1.3 Statistical Analysis

Descriptive analysis was used to summarize the data set and distribution and find out the prevalence of the nutritional status of the school children. Chi-square test was applied to find the association between selected socio-economic and demographic factors and child nutritional status. Logistic regression model was used to find the effect of independent variables on dependent variable. The results of the multiple logistic regression model were presented by adjusted odds ratios (AORs) with 95% confidence interval (CI) for the effects of the associated factors. Statistical significance was accepted at $p < 0.05$.

1.4 Ethical Approval

Prior to gathering data, we had extensive conversations with our selected participants regarding the aim of our research, and we took written consent from each individual. The study was approved by the Department of Statistics, University of Rajshahi, Bangladesh. We followed all rules and regulations of the Institute of Biological Science (IBSc), University of Rajshahi, Bangladesh, and IBSc approved this study and provided an ethical clearance letter (Memo No: 37(21)/320/IAMEBBC/IBSc).

1.5 Results

The prevalence of acute malnutrition amongst school children was 24.0%, among them 4.8% and 19.2% were severe acute malnutrition and moderate acute malnutrition, respectively (Fig. 1.1). This study included 500 children below the school age range (6–13 years), with 38.4% being boys and 51.6% being girls, respectively. Furthermore, 58.6% of the children were aged 5–9 years, while 41.4% were in the 10–13 years age group (Table 1.1). We observed that 43.8% of children's fathers passed primary education and 57.2% of mothers were secondary and higher level. Most of the children's fathers' occupations were day laborers, 42.8% of children

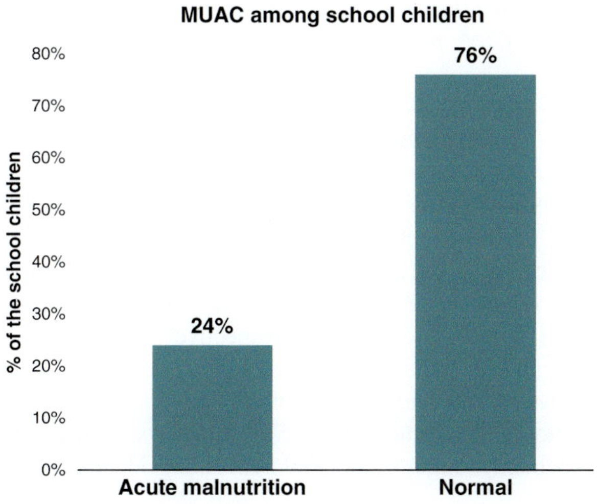

Fig. 1.1 Distribution of malnutrition status based on MUAC among school children

Table 1.1 Distribution of malnutrition status among school children by age group

Children age group	MUAC School children			Total
	SAM	MAM	Normal	
5–9 years	4 (1.4%)	31 (10.6%)	258 (88.1%)	293 (58.6%)
10–14 years	20 (9.7%)	65 (31.4%)	122 (58.9%)	207 (41.4%)
Total	24 (4.8%)	96 (19.2%)	380 (76.0%)	500 (100.0%)

living in middle families (monthly income, 7501–10,000 Bangladeshi Taka), and 40.8% of school children living in houses where hygienic latrine facilities were available. More than 63% of children intake tiffin in school period (Table 1.1). The chi-square test demonstrated that children's age ($p < 0.01$), mother's nutritional status ($p < 0.01$), household food insecurity status ($p < 0.05$), sufficient food (kcal) intake by age ($p < 0.05$), school children intake tiffin sometimes ($p < 0.05$), and mother's knowledge on nutrition ($p < 0.05$) were significantly associated factors of acute malnutrition status of school children (Table 1.2). These variables factors considered independent variables in multiple logistic regression analysis.

It was observed that the standard errors of all selected variables were less than 0.50, and there was no evidence of multicollinearity problems among independent variables in the multiple logistic regression model. After controlling the effect of other variables, the multiple logistic regression model demonstrated that older children (age, 10–13 years) had a 6.194 times higher chance of getting acute malnutrition than younger children (age, 5–9 years) (aOR = 6.194, 95% CI: 13.821–10.040; $p < 0.01$). Normal-weight nutritional status mother's school children had less chance to get acute malnutrition than underweight nutritional status mother's school children (aOR = 0.409, 95% CI: 0.205–0.814; $p < 0.05$). Overweight nutritional status mother's school children had less chance to get acute malnutrition than underweight nutritional status mother's school children (aOR = 0.387, 95% CI: 0.179–0.836; $p < 0.05$). School children who didn't intake (kcal) daily sufficient food according to their age had 2.177 times more chance of getting acute malnutrition than those who intake (kcal) sufficient food daily according to their age (aOR = 2.177, 95% CI: 1.280–3.705; $p < 0.01$) (Table 1.3).

1.6 Discussion

According to this study, there were 24.0% of school children with acute malnutrition, 24.0% of school children were identified with acute malnutrition, with 4.8% exhibiting severe acute malnutrition and 19.2% having moderate acute malnutrition. The values for severe and moderate acute malnutrition in Sudanese schoolchildren were 6.99% and 19.19%, respectively (Taha et al. 2013). Another study in Bangladesh found that wasting among school children in the Haor area was 48% (Khanam and Haque 2021) and thinness among school children was 21.6% in rural Ethiopia. This study observed that older school children were 6.20 times more at risk than younger school children. Alongside underweight mothers, school children

Table 1.2 Frequency distribution and association between nutritional status of school children and socio-demographic factors

Variable	Group	Nutritional status		χ^2-value	p-value
		Acute malnutrition	Normal nutrition		
Children's age (in years)	5–9, 293 (58.6%)	11.9%	88.1%	56.383	0.001
	10–14, 207 (41.4%)	41.1%	58.9%		
Gender of children	Boys 242 (48.4%)	24.0%	76.0%	0.001	0.987
	Girls 258 (51.6%)	24.0%	76.0%		
Father's education	Uneducated 87 (17.9%)	20.7%	79.3%	2.382	0.304
	Primary 213 (43.8%)	21.6%	78.4%		
	Secondary & higher 186 (38.3%)	27.4%	72.6%		
Mother's education	Uneducated 32 (6.4%)	21.9%	78.1%	0.545	0.762
	Primary 182 (36.4%)	25.8%	74.2%		
	Secondary & Higher 286 (57.2%)	23.1%	76.9%		
Father's occupation	Labor 351 (72.2%)	23.1%	76.9%	0.240	0.624
	Farmer & Others 135 (27.8%)	25.2%	74.8%		
Mother's nutritional status	Underweight (<18.5 kg/m^2) 52 (10.4%)	42.3%	57.7%	10.854	0.004
	Normal weight (18.5–24.99 kg/m^2) 319 (63.8%)	21.3%	78.7%		
	Overweight & obese (≥25 kg/m^2) 129(25.8%)	23.3%	76.7%		
Household average monthly income (in BDT)	<7500 Taka 151 (28.0%)	26.9%	73.1%	0.430	0.806
	7501–10,000 Taka 231 (42.8%)	24.3%	75.7%		
	≥10,000 Taka 158 (29.3%)	23.1%	76.9%		
Household food insecurity status	Food secured	28.4%	71.6%	6.653	0.036
	Moderate food insecurity	17.8%	82.2%		
	Severe food insecurity	23.2%	76.8%		
Sufficient food (kcal) intake by age	Intake require kcal 164 (32.8%)	17.7%	82.3%	5.339	0.021
	Intake not require kcal 336 (67.2%)	27.1%	72.9%		
Household having hygienic latrine	Yes 204 (40.8%)	23.0%	77.0%	0.174	0.676
	No 296 (59.2%)	24.7%	75.3%		
School tiffin intake sometimes	Yes 319 (63.8%)	27.0%	73.0%	4.231	0.040
	No 181 (36.2%)	18.8%	81.2%		
Mother's knowledge on nutrition	Poor knowledge 121 (24.2%)	31.4%	68.6%	4.799	0.028
	Good knowledge 379 (75.8%)	21.6%	78.4%)		

Table 1.3 Frequency distribution and association between nutritional status of school children and socio-demographic factors

Independent variables	Coefficient (β)	SE of (β)	*p*-value	Adjusted Odds Ratio (aOR)	95% CI of AOR
School children's age (in years)					
5–9 years®				1.00	
10–14 years	1.824	0.246	0.001	6.194	3.821–10.040
Mother's nutritional status					
Underweight (<18.5 kg/m^2)®				1.00	
Normal weight (18.5–24.99 kg/m^2)	−0.895	0.352	0.011	0.409	0.205–0.814
Overweight & obese (≥25 kg/m^2)	−0.949	0.393	0.016	0.387	0.179–0.836
Household food insecurity status					
Food secured®				1.00	
Moderate food insecurity	−0.324	0.269	0.228	0.723	0.427–1.226
Severe food insecurity	0.102	0.382	0.790	1.107	0.524–2.338
Daily sufficient food intake (kcal) of children by age					
Yes®					
No	0.778	0.271	0.004	2.177	1.280–3.705
School tiffin intake sometimes					
Yes®					
No	−0.416	0.270	0.123	0.659	0.389–1.119
Mother's knowledge on nutrition					
Poor knowledge®				1.00	
Good knowledge	0.053	0.280	0.851	1.054	0.609–1.825
Constant	−1.642	0.457	0.001	0.194	

were more suffering acute malnutrition compared to normal-weight and overweight mothers. School children who didn't intake (kcal) daily sufficient food according to their age were 2.18 times more likely to face acute malnutrition than those who intake (kcal) sufficient food by their age.

1.7 Strength and Limitation of this Study

One of the major strengths of the present study was looking at the acute malnutrition status of the school children in the Rajshahi district. We believe and hope that our findings had immense utility in reducing the prevalence of malnutrition among school children in Bangladesh. However, we had some limitations of the study. First, we could not further monitor the situation of school children's nutritional status, because we conducted a cross-sectional study. Moreover, this study was confined to a specific rural geographical area, so it was not possible to generalize the results for Bangladeshi school children. More research is required regarding the nutritional status of Bangladeshi school children.

1.8 Conclusions

The main health concern in the study area was the high prevalence of acute malnutrition among school children (ages 6–13). However, the study also observed that junior high school children more suffer the malnutrition compared to younger school children. Several factors were identified as significantly associated with acute malnutrition including the mother's nutritional status, and sufficient food intake by the age of school children.

1.9 Recommendations and Policy Implications

Based on our research, the Bangladeshi government should make an effort to address the issue of severe malnutrition among schoolchildren. The modifiable factors linked to malnutrition should receive special attention. Increased access to household income and food security for low-income schoolchildren is urgently needed to improve the nutritional status of the parents. Ensure and expand government-sponsored mid-meal programs in schools as well as initiatives to promote health, such as the provision of vitamin A supplements and routine child health checks. Additionally, it is necessary to educate and mobilize parents of low-income households regarding their children's nutritional health.

References

Abdel Wahed WY, Hassan SK, Eldessouki R (2017) Malnutrition and its associated factors among rural school children in Fayoum governorate, Egypt. J Environ Public Health 2017:4783791

Alredaisy MAS, Ibrahim SH (2011) Assessment of nutritional status of children less than 10 years old in rural western Kordafan. IIOABJ 2(4):40–49

BBS (2011) Population and Housing Census 2011 Bangladesh Bureau of Statistics (BBS). Ministry of Planning, Government of the People's Republic of Bangladesh, Dhaka

Bourke CD, Berkley JA, Prendergast AJ (2016) Immune dysfunction as a cause and consequence of malnutrition. Trends Immunol 37(6):386–398

Cochran WG (1963) Sampling Technique. 2nd Edition, John Wiley and Sons Inc., New York

Craig E, Bland R, Ndirangu J, Reilly JJ (2014) Use of mid-upper arm circumference for determining overweight and over fatness in children and adolescents. Arch Dis Child 99:763–766

Degarege D, Degarege A, Animut A (2015) Undernutrition and associated risk factors among school age children in Addis Ababa, Ethiopia. BMC Public Health 15(1):1–9

Goossens S, Bekele Y, Yun O, Harczi G, Ouannes M, Shepherd S (2012) Mid-upper arm circumference based nutrition programming: evidence for a new approach in regions with high burden of acute malnutrition. PLoS ONE 7:e49320

Hossain MG, Islam MS, Hoque KE, Islam MA, Mamun ASMA, Kamruzzaman M, Saw A (2014) Prevalence of underweight and effect of nutritional status on academic performance of primary school children in chapainawabganj district, Bangladesh. Malaysian Journal of Nutrition, 20(1):71–81

Khalid FAK, Eldirdery MME, ElGasim MEOE, Elhaj MAEE, Desogi MAAD, Mukhtar MMM (2021) Prevalence of malnutrition in school aged children. Kassala state, Sudan

Khanam SJ, Haque MA (2021) Prevalence and determinants of malnutrition among primary school going children in the haor areas of Kishoreganj district of Bangladesh. Heliyon 7:9

Kristen C, Lesley O (2018) Guide to anthropometry: a practical tool for program planners, managers, and implementers. Food and Nutrition Technical Assistance III, Washington, DC. Project (FANTA)/ FHI 360

Mramba L, Ngari M, Mwangome M, Muchai L, Bauni E, Walker AS, Gibb DM, Fegan G, Berkley JA (2017) A growth reference for mid upper arm circumference for age among school age children and adolescents, and validation for mortality: growth curve construction and longitudinal cohort study. Br Med J 358:j3423

National Institute of Population Research and Training (NIPORT), and ICF. 2020. Bangladesh Demographic and Health Survey 2017–18. Dhaka, Bangladesh, and Rockville, Maryland, USA: NIPORT and ICF

Shinsugi C, Gunasekara D, Takimoto H (2020) Use of mid-upper arm circumference (MUAC) to predict malnutrition among Sri Lankan schoolchildren. Nutrients 12(1):168

Taha HM, Elrasheed AA, Hassan HM, Arshad K (2013) Anthropometric parameters of malnutrition in children 5-15 years old in Khartoum state, Sudan. J Public Health Epidemiol 5(8):313–318

Talma H, van Dommelen P, Schweizer JJ, Bakker B, Kist-van Holthe JE, Chinapaw JMM, Hirasing RA (2019) Is mid-upper armcircumference in Dutch children useful in identifying obesity? Arch Dis Child 104:159–165

World Health Organization (2021) Microbial safety of lipid-based ready-to-use foods for management of moderate acute malnutrition and severe acute malnutrition–second report. Food & Agriculture Org

Assessment of Nutritional Status Using Anthropometric Index and its Associated Factors Among Under-Five Children in India: A Cross-Sectional Study from the National Family Health Survey-V (2019–2021)

2

Sreeparna Banerjee, Manoranjan Pal, Subir Biswas, Susmita Bharati, Premananda Bharati, and Suman Chakrabarty

2.1 Introduction

Child undernutrition is the major public health concern in many developing countries such as in India. It also continues to be one of the principal causes of ill-health and premature mortality and morbidity along with delayed mental and motor development during these childhood days (Dasgupta et al. 2014; Lahiri and Lahiri 2020). India is having the highest number of global childhood undernutrition (Black et al. 2013). Global Nutrition report (2021) reveals that universally 14.6 percent newborn of all live births (25 million children) have low birth weight. The Indian Government has encouraged the global recommendations for optimal infant and young child feeding (IYCF) suggesting an early initiation of breastfeeding, exclusive breastfeeding for the first 6 months of life and child feed thereafter with continued

S. Banerjee (✉) · S. Biswas
Department of Anthropology, West Bengal State University, Barasat, India

M. Pal
Economic Research Unit, Indian Statistical Institute (ISI), Kolkata, West Bengal, India

S. Bharati
Sociological Research Unit, Indian Statistical Institute, Kolkata, India

P. Bharati
Biological Anthropology Unit, Indian Statistical Institute (ISI), Kolkata, West Bengal, India

S. Chakrabarty
Department of Anthropology, Mrinalini Datta Mahavidyapith, Birati, Kolkata, India

M. Pal et al. (eds.), *Public Health and Nutrition*,
https://doi.org/10.1007/978-981-97-7890-4_2

breastfeeding up to 2 years (Food and Nutrition Board 2004). An organized review on under-five child malnutrition in the Indian context gives an outline of some potential child undernutrition determinants as low family income, place of residence, gender difference, poor feeding practices, low maternal educational, and so on (Bharati et al. 2009; Sahu et al. 2015).

Svedberg (2000), Nandy et al. (2005) and Nandy and Miranda (2008) developed a Composite Index of Anthropometric Failure (CIAF) which promotes six anthropometric indices of undernutrition status using the conventional nutritional index (Svedberg 2000; Nandy et al. 2005; Nandy and Miranda 2008; Islam and Biswas 2020). They argued that anthropometric indicators of stunting, wasting and underweight provides a comprehensive picture of the overall burden of undernutrition among young children in a population. The CIAF, however, provides a more detailed picture of the relationship between ill health and undernutrition. It can also be used to examine the relationship between different forms of undernutrition and poverty (Nandy and Svedberg 2012).

A handful of schemes initiated by the Government of India among them ICDS are the most outstanding schemes on child and maternal health issues. The range of services provided by ICDS scheme includes supplementary nutrition, immunization, health checkups, referral services, nutrition and health education, and preschool education (Kapil and Pradhan 1999). The burden of undernutrition among under-five children has not changed much even though various intervention programs are in operation in India. Dietary changing patterns are also affecting the nutritional status of under five children resulting in increased prevalence of adult noncommunicable diseases such as obesity, diabetes, hypertension, and coronary heart disease (Sahu et al. 2015).

There are several studies done on composite index of anthropometric failure by various research studies to find out overall dimensions of undernourishment among preschool children (Biswas et al. 2009; Mukhopadhyay and Biswas 2011; Titoria et al. 2019; Ghritlahre and Das 2021; Lahiri and Lahiri 2020). Children who experienced multiple anthropometric failure or malnutrition are more likely to have higher morbidity rates and these children also have shown a greater risk of early death (McDOnald et al. 2013). The present study aims to assess undernutrition using CIAF and its determinants on under-five children in India. The study also tries to explore the influence of mother's health status with child nutrition status.

2.2 Materials

It is a cross-sectional study and uses descriptive statistics. The data for the present study was availed from the recent National Family Health Survey (NFHS-V) in India conducted by International Institute for Population Sciences (IIPS) during 2019–2021 covering all the states and UT. The participants in this study are mothers aged 15–49 years with children aged less than 59 months currently residing in India.

Table 2.1 Categories of anthropometric failures in under-five-year children

Group		Description of the level	Wasting	Stunting	Underweight
1	No failure	Normal WAZ, HAZ and WHZ	No	No	No
2	Stunting only	HAZ < – 2 SD, other two normal	No	Yes	No
3	Wasting only	WAZ < – 2 SD, other two normal	Yes	No	No
4	Underweight only	WHZ < – 2 SD, other two normal	No	No	Yes
5	Wasting & stunting	WHZ & HAZ < −2SD, normal WAZ	Yes	Yes	No
6	Stunting & underwt	HAZ & WAZ < −2SD, normal WHZ	No	Yes	Yes
7	Wasting & underwt	WHZ & WAZ < −2SD, normal HAZ	Yes	No	Yes
8	Wasting, stunting & underweight	WHZ, HAZ and WAZ < – 2 SD	Yes	Yes	Yes
Composite index of anthropometric (failure) CIAF= (2) + (3) + (4) + (5) + (6) + (7) + (8)					

Note: No children are usually found in the group "Wasting and stunting only"

2.3 Methods

Anthropometric measurements were performed using conventional Indices, i.e., weight-for-age, height/length-for-age, and weight-for-height/length. In addition, CIAF combines three indices of weight-for-age, height-for-age, and weight-for-height to determine the nutritional status of under-five children. The categories of undernutrition were based on different anthropometric failures, no failure, and CIAF. The categories are shown in Table 2.1.

2.4 Mother and Child Characteristics

Mother's and child characteristics were measured by direct interviews, using a structured questionnaire. Mother's age during childbirth was categorized as 11–20 and 21–49 years, height of mother was categorized as short if the height was less than 150.9 cm or tall, if more than or equal to 151.0 cm. Mother's education was categorized as (1) No education, (2) Primary educated, (3) Secondary educated, and (4) higher secondary and above educated. Mother's employment status was grouped into (1) not working and (2) working status. Mother's BMI status was grouped into (1) Underweight, (2) Normal, and (3) Overweight, mother's anemic status was categorized into (1) anemic and (2) not anemic. Gestational period of mother was categorized as (1) Less than 9 months and (2) more than or equal to 9 months; Religion was categorized as (1) Hindu, (2) Muslim, (3) Christian and (4) others; Caste was categorized as (1) Scheduled caste (SC), (2) Scheduled Tribe (ST), (3) OBC (Other Backward Classes) and (4) general; geographical region was categorized as (1)

North (Jammu & Kashmir, Himachal Pradesh, Punjab, Uttarakhand, Haryana, Delhi, Rajasthan), (2) Central (Uttar Pradesh, Chhattisgarh, Madhya Pradesh), (3) East (Bihar, West Bengal, Jharkhand, Odisha), (4) West (Gujarat, Maharashtra, Goa), (5) South (Andhra Pradesh, Karnataka, Kerala, Tamil Nadu, Telangana), (6) North-East (Sikkim, Arunachal Pradesh, Nagaland, Manipur, Mizoram, Tripura, Meghalaya), and (7) UT (Chandigarh, Dadra and Nagar Haveli and Daman and Diu, Lakshadweep, Puducherry, Andaman and Nicobar Island). Wealth Index of the household was categorized as (1) Poor and (2) Rich. The age of the child was categorized as (1) less than or equal to 24 months and (2) 25–59 months. Sex of the child was categorized into (1) girl and (2) boy. Child's dietary pattern was also taken into consideration for analyzing the nutritional status of children.

2.5 Data Analysis

All the categorical variables (socio-economic and demographic variables) were summarized using frequency distribution tables. Pearson Chi-Square tests were used to analyze the association of child age and sex with nutritional status of the child. Binary logistic regression was performed to analyze the dominant factors associated with malnutrition based on stunting, underweight, wasting, and CIAF of the child under 5 years. A 95% confidence level and a value of $p < 0.05$ were considered statistically significant.

2.6 Results

Table 2.2 shows the prevalence of anthropometric failure—overall prevalence of undernutrition based on CIAF- in toddlers under-5 years was 49.1 percent. The prevalence for wasting only (4.52%), wasting and underweight (8.15%), wasting, underweight and stunting (3.93%), underweight and stunting (16.63%), stunting only (9.97%), and underweight only (5.90%). In contrast, the frequency of other forms of undernutrition based on conventional anthropometric indices, namely, underweight, stunting, and wasting was 33.2%, 28.5%, and 15.5%, respectively.

The result pointed out that toddlers aged less than 24 months who experienced stunting only, wasting only, wasting and underweight only were 10.6%, 6.6%, and 8.3%, respectively. This was higher than toddlers of age group 25–59 months, i.e., 9.6%, 3.2%, and 8.1%. Underweight only, stunting and underweight only; stunting, underweight and wasting was higher among toddlers aged 25–59 months than toddlers aged less than 24 months. Pearson chi-square values showed a significant relationship of nutritional status with age of the toddlers (p-value = 0.000). The table also revealed that the percentage of no failure in girls is higher than in boys. The percentages of stunting only, wasting only, wasting and underweight only, and all failure (stunting, wasting, and underweight) in boys were higher compared to girls. The proportion of children in the age range less than or equal to 24 months who experienced wasting (16.5%) was higher compared to children aged 25–59 months.

Table 2.2 Classification of nutritional status of under-five children: NFHS-5 data (2019–2021)

	Age (0–24 months)		Age (25–59 months)		*p*-value	Boys		Girls		Total		
5 (valid%)	*N*	%	*N*	%		*N*	%	*N*	%	*N*	%	*p*-value
No failure (1)	41,032	52.76	59,182	49.69	*p*-value = 0.000	51,559	50.65	48,655	51.2	100,214	50.9	*p*-value = 0.000
S only (2)	8219	10.57	11,394	9.57		10,353	10.18	9260	9.73	19,613	9.97	
W only (3)	5103	6.56	3806	3.20		4667	4.59	4242	4.46	8909	4.52	
U only (4)	3353	4.31	8236	6.92		5673	5.58	5916	6.22	11,589	5.90	
S & W only (5)	0	0	0	0		0	0	0	0	0	0	
S & U only (6)	10,774	13.85	21,967	18.44		16,775	16.48	15,966	16.78	32,741	16.63	
W & U only (7)	6414	8.25	9647	8.10		8504	8.35	7557	7.94	16,061	8.15	
S, W & U (8)	2878	3.70	4865	4.08		4246	4.17	3497	3.67	7743	3.93	
Total	77,773	100.00	119,097	100.00		101,777	100	95,093	100	196,870	100	
Composite index of anthropometric (failure) CIAF = [(2) + (3) + (4) + (5) + (6) + (7) + (8)]												
CIAF	36,741	47.24	59,915	50.31		50,218	49.3	46,438	48.8	96,656	49.1	
Nutritional status based on conventional (single) anthropometric index												
Weight-for-age												
Severely underwt (<-3SD)	9196	10.5	14,012	11.3	*p*-value = 0.000	7934	7.5	7812	8.0	15,746	7.7	*p*-value = 0.001
Underwt (-3SD to <-2SD)	12,675	14.5	24,214	19.6		27,264	25.6	25,124	25.4	52,388	25.5	
Normal weight (-2SD to +1SD)	54,437	62.4	79,529	64.2		63,495	59.7	58,595	59.3	122,090	59.5	
Risk of overwt (> + 1SD)	10,864	12.6	6062	4.9		7705	7.2	7249	7.3	14,954	7.3	
Total	87,172	100.00	123,817	100.00		106,398	100.00	9,338,780	100.0	205,178	100.00	
Length/height-for-age												

(continued)

Table 2.2 (continued)

5 (valid%)	Age (0–24 months)		Age (25–59 months)		*p*-value	Boys		Girls		Total		*p*-value
	N	%	*N*	%		*N*	%	*N*	%	*N*	%	
Severely stunted (<−3 SD)	9196	10.6	14,012	11.3	*p*-value = 0.000	12,094	11.1	11,114	10.9	23,208	11.0	*p*-value = 0.005
Stunted (−3 SD to <−2 SD)	12,675	14.5	24,214	19.6		19,280	17.7	17,609	17.3	36,889	17.5	
Normal (−2 SD to 3SD)	54,437	62.4	79,529	64.2		69,104	63.4	64,862	63.6	133,966	63.5	
Tall (>3 SD)	10,864	12.5	6062	4.9		8595	7.8	8331	8.2	16,926	8.0	
Total	87,172	100	123,817	100		109,073	100	101,916	100	210,989	100	
Weight-for-length/height												
Severely wasted (<−3 SD)	3565	4.1	4321	3.5	*p*-value = 0.000	4387	4.0	3499	3.4	7886	3.7	*p*-value = 0.000
Wasted (−3 SD to <−2 SD)	10,835	12.4	14,011	11.3		13,042	12.0	11,804	11.6	24,846	11.8	
Normal (−2 SD to +1 SD)	55,495	63.6	95,155	76.7		77,715	71.2	72,935	71.5	150,650	71.4	
Risk of overwt (>1 SD to 2 SD)	5034	5.9	3795	3.1		4350	4.0	4479	4.4	8829	4.1	
Overweight (>2 SD to 3SD)	2033	2.3	1261	1.0		1640	1.5	1654	1.6	3294	1.6	
Obese (>3 SD)	10,233	11.7	5392	4.4		8006	7.3	7619	7.5	15,625	7.4	
Total	87,195	100	123,935	100		109,140	100	101,990	100	211,130	100	

Source: National Family Health Survey-5 (2019–2021)
S stunting, *W* Wasting, *U* Underweight

The proportions of stunting and wasting were higher among children aged 25–59 months than children less than 24 months. Pearson Chi-square test shows a significant difference in nutritional status with respect to child age and sex.

Table 2.3 depicts the relationship of mother and child characteristics based on anthropometric failure (overall prevalence of undernutrition using CIAF) and other undernutrition with socio-economic and demographic factors. The percentages of anthropometric failure (CIAF) were higher for mothers aged 11–20 years. Similarly, the percentages for stunting, underweight, and wasting in children under five were higher among children of younger mothers (aged 11–20 years). The percentages of children under five who experienced anthropometric failure (57.4%), stunting (38.9%), wasting (17.5%), and underweight (42.1%) were higher for short height mothers than that of tall mothers (42.6%, 24.0%, 16.0%, and 28.7%, respectively). Similarly, the percentages of CIAF, stunting, wasting, and underweight were higher among mothers who have no education. Mothers with better educational attainment showed a decrease in percentage of CIAF, stunting, wasting, and underweight. The percentages of children under five suffering from anthropometric failure (CIAF) 51.1%, stunting (32.5), wasting (17%), and underweight (36.8%) were higher for employed mothers compared to mothers who were not employed. The result also showed that percentages of children under five suffering from anthropometric failure (CIAF), stunting, wasting, and underweight were higher for mothers who were underweight or suffering from anemia. Gestational period of childbearing of mother also played an important role in the assessment of children nutritional status. The percentages of children suffering from CIAF, stunting, wasting, and underweight were higher among children whose mothers experienced less than 9 months of gestational period. Regarding religion, Muslim children showed higher percentages of CIAF, stunting, wasting, and underweight than other religious groups of children. The lowest percentages of CIAF, stunting, wasting, and underweight were found among children belonging to 'others' religious groups. The percentages of anthropometric failure (CIAF), stunting, wasting, and underweight were higher among children belonging to SC than ST and OBC.

The study also explored that the percentage of multiple undernutrition (based on CIAF) was higher in Western region than in other regions. The percentage of Stunting was high in Eastern region. Wasting and underweight were higher in Western region also. It was observed that the prevalence of CIAF was highest in Bihar (60.8%), followed by Gujarat (59.5%). The Bihar state belongs to Eastern region, whereas Gujarat belongs to Western region. Between the Eastern and Western regions, the states like Bihar, Jharkhand, Gujarat, and Maharashtra experienced very high percentages of CIAF. Jharkhand had more than 50 percent children undernourished (56.3%). States like Meghalaya, Assam in North-Eastern region had more than 50 percent of children with CIAF. The lowest percentages of CIAF were in Chandigarh (UT), Punjab, and Jammu and Kashmir, which belong to northern region.

Regarding wealth index, the percentages of under-five children suffering from CIAF, stunting, wasting, and underweight were higher in families with poor wealth

Table 2.3 Mother and child characteristic based on anthropometric failures (overall prevalence of undernutrition using CIAF) and other undernutrition

	CIAF	Stunting	Wasting	Underweight
Mother's age during childbirth				
11–20	47,885 (53.1)	30,800 (34.2)	15,556 (17.2)	34,787 (38.6)
21–49	48,771 (45.7)	29,297 (27.5)	17,176 (16.1)	33,347 (31.2)
Total	96,656 (49.1)	60,097 (30.5)	32,732 (16.6)	68,134 (34.6)
Pearson Chi sq	1073.66**	1037.0**	46.7**	1162.0**
Height				
Short	49,714 (57.4)	33,671 (38.9)	15,140 (17.5)	36,492 (42.1)
Tall	46,932 (42.6)	26,420 (24.0)	17,589 (16.0)	31,636 (28.7)
Total	96,646 (49.1)	60,091 (30.5)	32,729 (16.6)	68,128 (34.6)
Pearson Chi sq	4243.7**	5067.5**	79.5**	3852.8**
Educational attainment				
No education	25,268 (59.6)	17,054 (40.2)	8106 (19.1)	18,812 (44.4)
Primary	14,089 (55.4)	9270 (36.4)	4415 (17.3)	10,184 (40.0)
Secondary	47,809 (46.8)	28,659 (28.1)	16,554 (16.2)	33,252 (32.6)
Higher	9490 (35.2)	5114 (19.0)	3657 (13.6)	5886 (21.8)
Total	96,656 (49.1)	60,097 (30.5)	32,732 (16.6)	68,134 (34.6)
Pearson Chi sq	4569.2**	4290.9**	389.6**	4250.6**
Working status				
Unemployed	92,814 (49.0)	57,653 (30.4)	31,452 (16.6)	65,367 (34.5)
Employed	3842 (51.1)	2444 (32.5)	1280 (17.0)	2767 (36.8)
Total	96,656 (49.1)	60,097 (30.5)	32,732 (16.6)	68,134 (34.6)
Pearson Chi sq	12.2**	14.1**	0.814	16.3**
Mother's BMI status				
Underweight	21,403 (61.1)	13,409 (38.3)	7601 (21.7)	16,871 (48.2)
Normal	60,334 (49.2)	37,493 (30.6)	20,391 (16.6)	41,739 (34.0)
Overweight	12,985 (36.6)	7987 (22.5)	4073 (11.5)	8159 (23.0)
Total	94,722 (49.1)	58,889 (30.5)	32,065 (16.6)	66,769 (34.6)
Pearson Chi sq	4216.2**	2058.4**	1322.4**	4960.5**
Mother's anemic status				
Anemia	58,284 (50.8)	36,572 (31.9)	19,524 (17.0)	41,752 (36.4)
Not anemia	36,934 (46.7)	22,619 (28.6)	12,729 (16.1)	25,368 (32.1)
Total	95,218 (49.1)	59,191 (30.5)	32,253 (16.6)	67,120 (34.6)
Pearson Chi sq	308.0**	232.9**	27.5**	379.4**
Pregnancy duration				
Less than 9 months	7685 (55.9)	5103 (37.1)	2343 (17.0)	5667 (41.2)
9 months or more	88,971 (48.6)	54,994 (30.0)	30,389 (16.6)	62,467 (34.1)
Total	96,656 (49.1)	60,097 (30.5)	32,732 (16.6)	68,134 (34.6)
Pearson Chi sq	276.1**	304.6**	1.9	287.4**
Religion				
Hindu	71,959 (49.8)	44,400 (30.7)	24,640 (17.0)	51,998 (36.0)
Muslim	14,091 (51.1)	8554 (31.0)	4996 (18.1)	9725 (35.3)

(continued)

Table 2.3 (continued)

	CIAF	Stunting	Wasting	Underweight
Christian	7430 (44.6)	5094 (30.6)	2121 (12.7)	4433 (26.6)
Others	3176 (39.0)	2049 (25.2)	975 (12.0)	1978 (24.3)
Total	96,656 (49.1)	60,097 (30.5)	32,732 (16.6)	68,134 (34.6)
Pearson Chi sq	538.7**	116.4**	371.9**	978.8**
Caste				
SC	21,251 (52.7)	13,623 (33.8)	6871 (17.0)	15,481 (38.4)
ST	20,648 (51.3)	13,476 (33.5)	6784 (16.8)	14,202 (35.3)
OBC	37,184 (49.6)	22,680 (30.2)	12,847 (17.1)	26,642 (35.5)
General	12,386 (40.1)	7253 (23.5)	4339 (14.0)	8219 (26.6)
Total	91,469 (49.1)	57,032 (30.6)	30,841 (16.5)	64,544 (34.6)
Pearson Chi sq	1304.8**	1098.6**	169.0**	1170.2**
Region				
North	14,301 (39.7)	8692 (24.1)	4748 (13.2)	9315 (25.9)
Central	25,903 (51.7)	16,791 (33.5)	8033 (16.0)	18,488 (36.9)
East	21,583 (56.0)	13,308 (34.5)	7753 (20.1)	16,484 (42.8)
West	9497 (57.5)	5462 (33.1)	3896 (23.6)	7153 (43.3)
South	10,627 (45.9)	6166 (26.6)	3699 (16.0)	7590 (32.8)
North-East	13,653 (45.6)	9.16 (30.1)	4216 (14.1)	8372 (28.0)
Others (UT)	1092 (42.1)	662 (25.5)	387 (14.9)	732 (28.2)
Total	96,656 (49.1)	60,097 (30.5)	32,732 (16.6)	68,134 (34.6)
Pearson Chi sq	2894.6**	1439.8**	1392.2**	3681.8**
Wealth Index				
Poor	74,202 (53.9)	47,643 (34.6)	24,414 (17.7)	53,731 (39.0)
Rich	22,454 (37.9)	12,454 (21.0)	8318 (14.0)	14,403 (24.3)
Total	96,656 (49.1)	60,097 (30.5)	32,732 (16.6)	68,134 (34.6)
Pearson Chi sq	4220.2**	3591.8**	402.0**	3949.6**
Child age				
Less than 24	36,741 (47.2)	21,871 (28.1)	14,400 (18.5)	23,419 (30.1)
25–60	59,915 (50.3)	38,226 (32.1)	18,332 (15.4)	44,715 (37.5)
Total	96,656 (49.1)	60,097 (30.5)	32,732 (16.6)	68,134 (34.6)
Pearson Chi sq	4072.5**	3105.1**	197.9**	6153.9**
Sex of the child				
Boy	50,218 (49.3)	31,374 (30.8)	17,429 (17.1)	35,198 (34.6)
Girl	46,438 (48.8)	28,723 (30.2)	15,303 (16.1)	32,936 (34.6)
Total	96,656 (49.1)	60,097 (30.5)	32,732 (16.6)	68,134 (34.6)
Pearson Chi sq	5.05*	8.9**	37.8**	0.059

Source: National Family Health Survey-5 (2019–2021)
*$p < 0.05$
**$p < 0.01$

index than in families with not so poor wealth index. The prevalence of CIAF, stunting, and underweight were higher among children aged 25–59 months than less than 24 months children. The prevalence of wasting was higher among less than or equal to 24-month children than 25-to-59-month children. Boys experienced higher percentages of CIAF, stunting, and wasting than girls. The percentages of underweight were the same among boys and girls.

The percentages of CIAF have been computed for combinations of Breastfed, semisolid-fed, and solid-food-fed children. Breastfed children have been found to perform better than semisolid-fed and solid-food-fed children as shown in Table 2.4.

The occurrences of CIAF in children with respect to specific combinations of food intake patterns (ever breastfeeding, semisolid, and solid food intake) were computed as shown in Table 2.5.

It showed categorized list of different food intake patterns of children under five. Combinations of food intake were divided into eight categories shown row wise. The children who had never taken breastmilk, solid and semisolid food were in the first row. Subsequently, children who had never taken breastfed and solid food but taken semisolid food were put in the next row and so on. The percentage of CIAF was the highest in the group of children who were given only breastmilk and solid food then followed by children who were only solid food, and so on.

Taking the last column of Table 2.5, the average percentage of CIAF children who were breastfed was computed as (36.98 + 44.95 + 56.35 + 51.52)/4 = 47.45 and the average of CIAF who were not breastfed was (49.19 + 47.92 + 55.33 + 49.50)/4 = 50.48. The difference of the two percentages, i.e. (average of "percentages not breastfed" minus average of "percentages breastfed" was 3.03). Similar differences were found for Semi-Solid-food-fed and Solid-food-fed children as shown in Table 2.6. Breastfed children were found to perform better than semisolid-fed and solid-food-fed children, because this value (3.03) was higher than −8.41 and 0.99.

The results of binary logistic regression of CIAF, stunting, wasting, and underweight of under-five children on socio-demographic variables are given in Table 2.7. It showed that mothers who married at a later age of 21–49 years were 0.946 and

Table 2.4 Percentages of CIAF among children in India by different food intake patterns

	Among ever-breast-fed children	Among semisolid-fed children	Among solid-fed children
CIAF	48.0%	50.7%	52.8%

Source: National Family Health Survey-v (2019–2021)

Table 2.5 Calculations toward computations of exclusive changes in the percentages of CIAF for combination of ever breastfed, solid food, and semisolid food: children of less than 59 months

EverBF	Solid	Semisolid	Value	Total	CIAF	Total	% of CIAF
No	No	No	1	2389	785	1596	49.19
No	No	Yes	2	1110	380	793	47.92
No	Yes	No	3	831	322	582	55.33
No	Yes	Yes	4	3346	1233	2491	49.50
Yes	No	No	5	28,282	8303	22,450	36.98
Yes	No	Yes	6	9236	3528	7848	44.95
Yes	Yes	No	7	11,887	5899	10,469	56.35
Yes	Yes	Yes	8	35,433	15,964	30,989	51.52
		Total		92,514	36,414	77,218	47.16

Source: National Family Health Survey- v (2019–2021)
BF breastfed

Table 2.6 Average effects of ever breastfed, solid and semisolid food of less than or equal to 59-month children on CIAF

	No	Yes	No-Yes
Ever breast fed	50.48	47.45	3.03
Solid fed	44.76	53.17	−8.41
Semisolid fed	49.46	48.47	0.99

Source: National Family Health Survey- v (2019–2021)
BF breastfed

Table 2.7 Results of binary logistic regression of CIAF, stunting, wasting, and underweight of under-five children on socio-demographic variables

	CIAF, AOR (95% CI)	Stunting, AOR (95% CI)	Wasting, AOR (95% CI)	Underweight, AOR (95% CI)
Mother's age during childbirth: 11–20®				
21–49	0.994 (0.962–1.026)	0.946 (0.913–0.980)**	1.039 (0.998–1.082)	0.958 (0.925–0.993)*
Height: Short®				
Tall	0.659 (0.638–0.680)**	0.611 (0.590–0.632)**	0.940 (0.903–0.979)**	0.623 (0.602–0.645)**
Educational attainment: No education®				
Primary	0.892 (0.843–0.944)**	0.901 (0.849–0.956)**	0.921 (0.860–0.987)**	0.910 (0.858–0.965)**
Secondary	0.746 (0.715–0.778)**	0.740 (0.708–0.774)**	0.868 (0.824–0.913)**	0.727 (0.695–0.760)**
Higher	0.637 (0.600–0.677)**	0.629 (0.589–0.673)**	0.811 (0.751–0.875)**	0.591 (0.552–0.632)**
Working status: Unemployed®				
Employed	1.043 (0.956–1.139)	1.109 (1.010–1.217)*	0.997 (0.894–1.112)	1.034 (0.940–1.136)
Mother's BMI status: Underweight®				
Normal	0.662 (0.637–0.689)**	0.769 (0.737–0.801)**	0.750 (0.716–0.786)**	0.592 (0.568–0.616)**
Overweight	0.501 (0.475–0.529)**	0.629 (0.592–0.668)**	0.583 (00544–0.625)**	0.420 (0.395–0.447)**
Mother's anemic status: Anemia®				
Not anemic	0.946 (0.916–0.976)**	0.951 (0.918–0.985)**	0.993 (0.954–1.034)	0.958 (0.925–0.992)*
Pregnancy duration: Less than 9 months®				
9 months or more	0.642 (0.598–0.688)**	0.615 (0.574–0.659)**	0.871 (0.803–0.945)**	0.629 (0.586–0.674)**
Religion: Hindu®				
Muslim	1.162 (1.104–1.224)**	1.133 (1.071–1.200)**	1.064 (0.998–1.135)	1.116 (1.055–1.182)**
Christian	0.823 (0.760–0.890)**	0.901 (0.826–0.983)*	0.812 (0.731–0.902)**	0.764 (0.698–0.837)**
Others	0.817 (0.750–0.890)**	0.939 (0.854–1.034)	0.776 (0.690–0.872)**	0.812 (0.734–0.897)**

(continued)

Table 2.7 (continued)

	CIAF, AOR (95% CI)	Stunting, AOR (95% CI)	Wasting, AOR (95% CI)	Underweight, AOR (95% CI)
Caste: SC®				
ST	0.994 (0.943–1.048)	0.972 (0.919–1.028)	1.041 (0.976–1.110)	0.989 (0.930–1.040)
OBC	0.896 (0.859–0.934)**	0.882 (0.843–0.922)**	0.970 (0.921–1.022)	0.869 (0.831–0.908)**
General	0.777 (0.737–0.820)**	0.807 (0.760–0.857)**	0.877 (0.819–0.940)**	0.730 (0.687–0.776)**
Region:North®				
Central	1.189 (1.131–1.250)**	1.151 (1.088–1.218)**	1.104 (1.035–1.177)**	1.221 (1.154–1.292)**
East	1.209 (1.145–1.276)**	1.038 (0.977–1.102)	1.287 (1.202–1.378)**	1.245 (1.173–1.322)**
West	1.621 (1.515–1.734)**	1.364 (1.267–1.468)**	1.543 (1.423–1.674)**	1.612 (1.498–1.735)**
South	1.188 (1.119–1.261)**	1.107 (1.035–1.184)**	1.136 (1.052–1.227)**	1.230 (1.149–1.316)**
North-East	0.882 (0.821–0.949)**	0.947 (0.873–1.027)	0.890 (0.808–0.981)*	0.760 (0.699–0.827)
Others (UT)	1.245 (1.076–1.442)**	1.230 (1.044–1.449)*	1.149 (0.950–1.390)	1.326 (1.125–1.564)**
Wealth Index: Poor®				
Rich	0.767 (0.737–0.799)**	0.778 (0.744–0.815)**	0.858 (0.814–0.904)**	0.713 (0.681–0.747)**
Child age:0–24 months®				
25–60	1.375 (1.273–1.484)**	1.551 (1.430–1.682)**	0.725 (0.653–0.806)**	1.892 (1.744–2.053)**
Sex of the child: Boy®				
Girl	0.875 (0.848–0.902)**	0.852 (0.823–0.881)**	0.907 (0.873–0.943)**	0.887 (0.858–0.918)**
Everbreastfed: No®				
Yes	1.061 (0.986–1.142)	1.014 (0.936–1.098)	0.987 (0.896–1.087)	1.138 (1.049–1.235)**
Solidfed: No®				
Yes	1.613 (1.556–1.672)**	1.613 (1.549–1.678)**	1.303 (1.245–1.364)**	1.906 (1.831–1.985)**
Semisolid fed: No®				
Yes	1.161 (1.121–1.204)**	1.156 (1.111–1.202)**	1.040 (0.995–1.088)	1.182 (1.137–1.230)**

N.B: *AOR* Adjusted Odds Ratio, *CI* Confidence Interval, *R* Reference category
**: 1% level of significance ($p < 0.01$); *: 5% level of significance ($p < 0.05$)

0.958 times less likely to have stunted and underweight children, respectively, compared to early wed mothers at 11–20 years. And it was statistically significant at 1% level and 5% levels, respectively. It was also seen that tall mothers were less likely to have undernourished children. In addition, educational attainment of mothers also showed positive influence toward reducing both CIAF and conventional index.

And it is significant at 1% level. Mothers' employment status did not show clear picture. Children whose mothers were normal, overweight, or non-anemic had less risk for CIAF, stunting, wasting, and underweight than underweight and anemic mother. The chances of CIAF, stunting, wasting, and underweight were less among children of mothers who had gestational period more than 9 months than among mothers with less gestational period.

Religion also had significant effect on nutritional status of children showing adverse effects among Muslim children.

Children belonging to OBC and general category were 0.91 times and 0.76 times less likely to have CIAF than SC children. The study also revealed that children in the middle belt, i.e., in Western, Central, and Easter regions, were very much adversely affected nutritionally.

2.7 Discussion

In the present study, it is seen that nearly half (49.1%) of children under 5 years of age experienced CIAF. However, component wise the prevalence were 9.97% for stunting only, 4.52% for wasting only, 5.90% for underweight only, 16.63% for stunting and underweight only, 8.15% for wasting and underweight only and 3.93% for stunting, wasting and underweight only. Meanwhile, based on conventional anthropometric indices, one-third of children under five were underweight (33.2%), nearly one-third were stunted (28.5%) and almost one-sixth (15.5%) of the children experienced wasting.

Research conducted by Fenta et al. (2021) and Boregowda et al. (2015) reported that the high prevalence of anthropometric failure using CIAF, and other kinds of undernutrition as measured by conventional anthropometric indices was associated with socio-demographic variables as well as characteristics pertaining to food intake, sanitation conditions and clean-living behavior. Another impressive study conducted by Islam and Biswas (2020) in Bangladesh reported a higher prevalence of children experiencing stunting and underweight only (18.2%). Lower prevalence of combinations of wasting and underweight (5.5%), combination of wasting, underweight and stunting (5.7%) were observed. Similar study conducted by Permatasari and Chadirin (2022) found that 42.1% children experienced CIAF, which was a little less than our figure.

The results of the present study indicated that there were 13 factors associated with the occurrence of CIAF in children under 5 years, namely, mother's height, educational status of mother, BMI, anemia status, gestational period of childbearing, religion, caste, geographic region, wealth index, age, and sex of the child. Addo et al. (2013) opined that a mother's height was the dominant factor that caused child growth failure. The size of the uterus, which is supposed to be proportional to height, might matter.

Seboka et al. (2021) found that children in the older age group had a higher risk of undernutrition than the younger age which conforms to our finding (see also Erismann et al. 2017; Mzumara et al. 2018). Mzumara et al. (2018) also found that anthropometric failure and other undernutrition were higher among boys compared to girls.

Exclusive breastfeeding of babies up to the first six months plays an important role in increasing the baby's immunity (Fatimah et al. 2021). Our findings confirmed the same. Moreover, the percentages of CIAF computed for combinations of breastfed, semisolid-fed, and solid-food-fed children also led to the same result. Breastfed children were found to perform better than semisolid-fed and solid-food-fed children.

Mother's educational status plays an important role to the children's long-term and short-term anthropometric status (Burchi 2012). It was found that children with illiterate mothers were 2 times more likely to be moderately and severely stunted than with their counterparts (Fenta et al. 2020). Mother's health status also has dominant influence on toddler's anthropometric failure based on CIAF. Several studies found links between maternal BMI and child stunting (Casapía et al. 2007; Huntsman and White 2007). We found that anemic mother contributed to a greater risk of multiple anthropometric failure of children. Longer gestation period is associated with reduced morbidity and mortality (Espel et al. 2014).

Maternal age during childbirth plays an important role in determining the child health status. In our study, we found that children of younger mothers were more likely to be stunted and/or underweight. CIAF and wasting showed no significant relationship with maternal age during childbirth.

Wealth index of the family is also a dominant factor for CIAF and other undernutrition in children under five. Children belonging to rich wealth index were less likely to be CIAF, stunted, wasted, and underweight as the odds were 0.767, 0.778, 0.858, and 0.713, respectively. Similar findings were also observed in the study of Chowdhury et al. (2018) in Bangladesh. Low-income level is associated with low-education levels (Kumar and Paswan 2021).

In India, SCs and STs have close link with infant and child mortality (Bora et al. 2019; Sabharwal et al. 2014). In our study we clearly observed that SC and ST toddlers were more likely to experience stunting, wasting, underweight, and CIAF compared to those of general category.

Geographic regions also had association with child health. In our study, we found that the middle belt, i.e., Western, Central, and Eastern regions were more prone CIAF and other undernutrition.

2.8 Conclusion

Various factors including better health status of mother, better wealth index, child age (less than 24moths vs 25–59 months), upper caste, religion (Hindu), and feeding practices of children influence the nutritional status of children. These results can serve as a basis for determining appropriate interventions to prevent early undernutrition of children.

References

Addo OY, Stein AD, Fall CH, Gigante DP, Guntupalli AM, Horta BL (2013) Maternal height and child growth patterns. J Pediatr 163(2):549–554.e1

Bharati P, Bharati S, Pal M, Chakraborty S, Som S, Gupta R (2009) Growth and nutritional status of pre-school children in India: rural-urban and gender differences. Coll Anthropol 33(1):7–21

Biswas S, Bose K, Mukhopadhyay A, Bhadra M (2009) Prevalence of undernutrition among pre-school children of Chapra, Nadia District, West Bengal, India, measured by composite index of anthropometric failure (CIAF). Anthropol Anz 67(3):269–279

Black RE, Victora CG, Walker SP, Bhutta ZA, Christian P, Onis DPM (2013) Maternal and child undernutrition and overweight in low-income and middle-income countries. Lancet 392(9890):427–451

Bora JK, Raushan R, Lutz W (2019) The persistent influence of caste on under five mortality: factors that explain the caste-based gap in high focus Indian states. PLoS One 14(8):e0211086

Boregowda GS, Soni GP, Jain K, Agrawal S (2015) Assessment of undernutrition using composite index of anthropometric failure (CIAF) amongst toddlers residing in urban slums of Raipur city, Chhattisgarh, India. J Clin Diagn Res 9(7):LC04-6

Burchi F (2012) Whose education affects a child's nutritional status? From parents to household education. Demogr Res 23(27):681–704

Casapía M, Joseph SA, Núñez C, Rahme E, Gyorkos TW (2007) Parasite and maternal risk factors for malnutrition in preschool-age children in Belen, Peru using the new WHO child growth standards. Br J Nutr 98:1259–1266

Chowdhury TR, Chakrabarty S, Rakib M, Saltmarsh S, Davis KA (2018) Socioeconomic risk factors for early childhood underweight in Bangladesh. Glob Health 14(1):1–12

Dasgupta A, Parthasarathi R, Prabhakar RV, Biswas R, Geethanjali A (2014) Assessment of undernutrition with composite index of anthropometric dailure (CIAF) among under-five children in a rural area of West Bengal. Indian J Community Health 26(2):132–138

Erismann S, Knoblauch A, Diagbouga S, Odermatt P, Gerold J, Shrestha A, Tarnagda G, Savadogo B, Schindler C, Utzinger J (2017) Prevalence and risk factors of undernutrition among schoolchildren in the Plateau Central and Centre-Ouest regions of Burkina Faso. Infect Dis Poverty 6:1–14

Espel EV, Glynn LM, Sandman CA, Davis EP (2014) Longer gestation among children born full term influences cognitive and motor development. PLoS One 9(11):e113758

Fatimah MMN, Febriani ADB, Hatta M, Permatasari TAE, Hidayati E et al (2021) Effect of breast-feeding on children's health and its relationship to NRAMP1 expression: a cross-sectional study. Ann Med Surg 71:103017

Fenta HM, Workie DL, Zike DT, Taye BW, Swain PK (2020) Determinants of stunting among under-five years children in Ethiopia from the 2016 Ethiopia demographic and health survey: application of ordinal logistic regression model using complex sampling designs. Clin Epidemiol Glob Health 8(2):404–413

Fenta HM, Zewotir T, Muluneh EK (2021) Disparities in childhood composite index of anthropometric failure prevalence and determinants across Ethiopian administrative zones. PLoS One 16(9):1–17

Food and Nutrition Board (2004) Dietary reference intakes for vitamins. National Academy of Sciences, Washington DC

Ghritlahre M, Das S (2021) Composite index of anthropometric failure among 2-5 years Anganwadi children Bilaspur, Chhattisgarh, India. Journal of the department of anthropology university of North Bengal 17(1):271–282

Global Nutrition report (2021) A world free from malnutrition: an assessment of progress towards the global nutrition targets. Cesare M, Ghosh S, Osendarp S, Mozaffarian D (ed)

Huntsman AC, White NG (2007) Modernization in Bali, Indonesia and the influence of socio-economic factors on the nutritional status of preschool children in 1989/1990: an anthropometric study. Ann Hum Biol 34:411–424

Islam MS, Biswas T (2020) Prevalence and correlates of the composite index of anthropometric failure among children under 5 years old in Bangladesh. Matern Child Nutr 16(2):1–12

Kapil U, Pradhan R (1999) Integrated child development services scheme (ICDS) and its impact on nutritional status of children in India and recent initiatives. Indian J Public Health 43(1):21–25

Kumar R, Paswan B (2021) Changes in socio-economic inequality in nutritional status among children in EAG states, India. Public Health Nutr 24(6):1304–1317

Lahiri S, Lahiri SK (2020) Assessment of undernutrition by composite index of anthropometric failure among under five children in a slum of Kolkata, West Bengal. Int J Commun Med Public Health 7(4):1422–1426

McDOnald CM, Olofin I, Flaxman S, Fawzi WW, Spiegelman D, Caulfield LE, Black RE, Ezzati M, Danaei G (2013) The effect of multiple anthropometric deficits on child mortality: meta-analysis of individual data in 10 prospective studied from developing countries. Am J Clin Nutr 97(4):896–901

Mukhopadhyay DK, Biswas AB (2011) Food security and anthropometric failure among tribal children in Bankura, West Bengal. Indian Pediatr 48(4):311–314

Mzumara B, Bwembya P, Halwindi H, Mugode R, Banda J (2018) Factors associated with stunting among children below five years of age in Zambia: evidence from the 2014 Zambia demographc and health survey. BMC Nutr 51(4):1–8

Nandy S, Miranda JJ (2008) Overlooking undernutrition? using a composite index of anthropometric failure to assess how underweight misses and misleads the assessment of undernutrition in young children. Soc Sci Med 66(9):1963–1966. https://doi.org/10.1016/j.socscimed.2008.01.021

Nandy S, Svedberg P (2012) The composite index of anthropometric failure (CIAF): an alternative indicator for malnutrition in young children. Handbook of anthropometry: physical measures 127 of human form in health and disease. V.R. Preedy (ed)

Nandy S, Irving M, Gordon D, Subramanian S, Smith GD (2005) Poverty, child undernutrition and morbidity: new evidence from India. Bull World Health Organ 83:210–216. PMID: 15798845

Permatasari TAE, Chadirin Y (2022) Assessment of undernutrition using the composite index of anthropometric failure (CIAF) and its determinants: a cross-sectional study in the rural area of the Bogor District in Indonesia. BMC Nutr 133:1–20

Sabharwal NS, Mishra VK, Naik AK, Holmes R, Hagen-Zanker J (2014) How does social protection contribute to social inclusion in India: Evidence from the national health insurance programme (RSBY) in Maharashtra and Uttar Pradesh. Report of Overseas Development Institute, http://cdn-odi-production.s3-website-eu-west-1.amazonaws.com/media/documents/8938.pdf

Sahu SK, Kumar SG, Bhat BV, Premarajan KC, Sarkar S, Roy G, Joseph N (2015) Malnutrition among inder-five children in India and strategies for control. J Nat Sci Biol Med 6(1):18–23

Seboka BT, Hailegebreal S, Yehualashet DE, Demeke AD (2021) Tracking progress in anthropometric failure among under-five children in Ethiopia: a geospatial and multilevel analysis. Arch Public Health 79(1):1–17

Svedberg P (2000) Poverty and undernutrition: theory, measurement and policy. Oxford India Paperbacks, New Delhi. https://doi.org/10.1093/0198292686.001.0001

Titoria R, Ponnusamy P, Mehra S (2019) Identification of undernutrition in under five children: Z score or a composite index of anthropometric failure. Int J Commun Med Public Health 6(7):3150–3155

Factors Associated with Maternal and Child Health Services in Bangladesh

3

Mst. Nadira Parvin, Md. Nazrul Islam Mandal, and Md. Mosiur Rahman

Abbreviations

AABF	Age-appropriate breastfeeding
CCI	Composite coverage index
CoC	Continuum of care
CI	Confidence interval
FP	Family planning
GoB	Government of Bangladesh
MCH	Maternal and child health
MNCH	Maternal, Newborn and Child Health
MMR	Maternal mortality rates
NGOs	Non-Government organizations
PNC	Prenatal care
SBA	Skilled birth attendants
SES	Socio-economic status
UNFPA	United Nations Population Fund
UNICEF	United Nation's International Children's Emergency Funds
WB	World Bank
WI	Wealth index

M. N. Parvin (✉)
Department of Epidemiology, Faculty of Public Health, Bangladesh University of Health Sciences, Dhaka, Bangladesh

Department of Population Science and Human Resource Development, University of Rajshahi, Rajshahi, Bangladesh
e-mail: nadiraepi@buhs.ac.bd

M. N. I. Mandal · M. M. Rahman
Department of Population Science and Human Resource Development, University of Rajshahi, Rajshahi, Bangladesh

M. Pal et al. (eds.), *Public Health and Nutrition*,
https://doi.org/10.1007/978-981-97-7890-4_3

3.1 Introduction

Preconception and prenatal care are crucial foundations for best maternal and child health (MCH) outcomes among women of reproductive age. Preconception and prenatal care are essential for naming and managing potential health risks or complications before and during pregnancy (Hurst et al. 2015). The MCH refers to the support and services given to women throughout pregnancy, childbirth, and the motherhood period (Kerber 2007). The MCH is vital during labor and delivery to ensure the mother receives the right and prompt care to minimize risks to her and the newborn's health (Lalonde et al. 2019). During childbirth, trained healthcare providers, such as skilled birth attendants (SBA), obstetricians, midwives, and nurses, provide care and support for pain management and monitoring of any signs of complications (WHO 2018). Postpartum care is crucial for ensuring the maternal and the child's health and wellbeing, including physical recovery, breastfeeding support, and mental health support (Alsabi et al. 2022). Postpartum care includes breastfeeding, checking postpartum depression, and providing follow-up care for any complications or health conditions arising during pregnancy or delivery. Follow-up care is also an essential part of the MCH for mothers, such as regular check-ups and screening (Aune et al. 2023). The MCH service is essential for ensuring overall maternal and child health worldwide. Access to MCH services socio-economic status (SES) is an essential factor. People with lower SES tend to have less entry to quality healthcare services and may need help to afford the costs associated with maternal and child health services. They are more likely to experience a lack of transportation, information, and cultural barriers. MCH outcomes are also worse among women with lower levels of education (Sarker et al. 2016). Only about 44% of women in Bangladesh have a basic knowledge of maternal health. Many women may lack awareness on the risks linked to pregnancy and childbirth and the crucial importance of looking for prompt and appropriate care. The lower SES populations need more education and awareness about maternal health and health outcomes (Das et al. 2017). The women might also be more likely to give birth at home and have less access to prenatal care, which can raise the threat of maternal and newborn death. To enhance maternal and child health results for all populations, it is essential to ensure the continuum of care (CoC) for mothers is thorough and practical by addressing the socioeconomic determinants of health, including SES (Khan et al. 2020a, b). In Bangladesh, individuals living in impoverished conditions, especially in rural regions, often face restricted access to healthcare services of high quality and demonstrate lower utilization rates. According to the United Nations International Children's Emergency Funds (UNICEF), Bangladesh's economically marginalized mothers have higher maternal mortality rates (MMR) than their more advantaged counterparts. Women with reduced SES are more likely to experience inadequate prenatal care and choose home deliveries, increasing maternal and neonatal mortality risks. Additionally, the lack of access to SBA poses an extra hurdle to the CoC for mothers in Bangladesh, with only about 55% of deliveries attended by SBAs. It means that many mothers are not receiving the proper care during delivery, which can lead to increased maternal and neonatal mortality. Another issue is the limited access to emergency obstetric care, which is essential for managing complications during pregnancy and childbirth (Panciera et al. 2016). Additionally, cultural barriers also affect the CoC for mothers in Bangladesh. For example, traditional beliefs and practices may discourage women from seeking care during pregnancy or childbirth and limit their access to information and services. Another critical aspect of the CoC for mothers in Bangladesh is the absence of comprehensive prenatal care (PNC) (Khan et al. 2020a, b). Only approximately 30% of mothers in Bangladesh undergo PNC within two days after delivery, and only about 42% do so by two weeks (Sheba et al. 2022). Approximately 63% of women obtained PNC from any provider between 24 and 42 days after giving birth. More than 48% of them obtained it from professionals with medical training (Sheba et al. 2022). After giving birth, many mothers do not receive the proper care and help, which raises morbidity and mortality rates for both mothers and newborns. A prominent issue in Bangladesh is the lack of easily available family planning (FP) facilities. Around 30% of married women in the country use modern contraceptive methods, reflecting a large gap in meeting the demand for FP services (Fan and Koski 2022). The inequalities of SES remain a significant problem in Bangladesh. Inequalities in income, education, and health contribute to socioeconomic inequality (Islam et al. 2020). Over 40% of Bangladesh's population, based on World Bank (WB) data, is estimated to fall below the daily international poverty level of US$1.90 (Saber 2021). Income inequality is also a significant issue, with the top 20% of earners taking home nearly 60% of all national income. It leaves the bottom 80% of earners with just 40% of the national income, often insufficient to cover basic needs (Mahembe and Odhiambo 2018). For instance, the Government of Bangladesh (GoB) has put in place measures to boost access to emergency obstetric care and the quantity of qualified birth attendants. The non-Government organizations (NGOs) are crucial to the provision of MCH care in the nation. Bangladesh must lower the MMR to under 70 per 100,000 live births by 2030 in order to meet Sustainable Development Goal (SDG) Target 3.1. (Bhowmik et al. 2020). Therefore, if Bangladesh is to achieve the MMR target of the SDGs, it is essential to accelerate efforts toward reducing maternal and child mortality.

3.2 Data and Methods

Data Source and Study Design This investigation employed a cross-sectional design using data from Bangladesh Demographic and Health Survey (BDHS). A nationally representative household-based survey was conducted in 2017–2018 (BDHS, 2020). The BDHS surveyed ever-married women of reproductive age (15–49 years) who had given birth to a child within the three years preceding the survey. This study focused on ever-married women who delivered a child within the 3 years preceding the survey. One of the CoC's components chose nonpregnant women to gauge the prevalence of contemporary contraception use. This analysis excluded mothers with children outside 12–23-month age ranges from the calculation of child vaccine coverage. In Bangladesh, all four recommended immunizations are typically completed by 12 months.

Outcome Measures The primary outcome of interest was the CoC for Maternal, Newborn and Child Health (MNCH) services. The CoC was evaluated using the composite coverage index (CCI) rather than focusing on how each MCH care was used. The following criteria were used to choose the indicators that were used to measure CCI:

1. They were advised by international standards (Kerber 2007).
2. They were related to important outcomes for health (Paulson et al. 2021).

Using the seven crucial MCH interventions—pregnancies, delivery, PNC, and FP—the CoC was divided into its four stages. (1) maternal care (ANC > 4), (2) SBA; (3) PNC for new moms within two days of giving birth; and (4) Age-appropriate breastfeeding (AABF), (5) PNC within two days of birth for a neonate, (6) Immunization (BCG, DPT, PL, MSL), and (7) FP.

The level of CoC for maternal health is calculated with the following formula (Sakuma et al. 2019):

$$\text{CCI for maternal health} = \frac{1}{3}\left(\text{ANC} \geq 4 + \text{SBA} + \text{PNCM}\right).$$

The level of CCI for child health is calculated with the following formula (Sakuma et al. 2019):

$$\text{CCI for child health} = \frac{1}{3}\left(\frac{1\text{AABF} + \text{PNCN} + \left(\text{BCG} + 2\text{DPT3} + 2\text{PL} + \text{MSL}\right)}{6}\right).$$

All stages and indicators within each stage were assigned equal weights. The resulting scores are then categorized into terciles (thirds) and leveled as low, middle, and high CCI.

Socioeconomic Status (SES) The wealth index (WI) was used in this study as an indicator for SES. The WI for this survey was created using information on family assets, including possession of lasting items, house characteristics, and building objects (Khan et al. 2021a, b). Using principal part analysis, a weight (factor score) was assigned to each asset. Each household was then given a score for each asset. The sample was then split into residents' terciles with each home placed in the low, medium, or rich tercile. Women were then rated according to the overall score of the household in which they lived.

Dependent Variable The CoC for maternal and child health services assessed by CCI.

Independent Variables Age, education, husband's education, decision-making autonomy on own health care, respondents' employment, mass media exposure, parity, pregnancy intended, number of household members, place of residence, offspring sex, SES, maternal health, Post natal care of new born within two days of giving birth (PNCN), one dosage of *Bacillus Calmette–Guérin* (BCG), three dosages of Diphtheria Pertussis Tetanus (DPT), three dosages of Poliomyelitis vaccine (PL), one dosage of Measles vaccine (MSL), Age appropriate breast feeding (AABF), and current use of modern contraceptive.

Statistical Analyses This study examined the backdrop characteristics of the sample using descriptive statistics. Along the continuum, descriptive data on the use rate of essential MNCH services throughout the reproductive life cycle of women was also provided. We used three regression-based techniques, relative index of inequality (RII), slope index of inequality (SII), and adjusted odds ratio (AOR), to measure several aspects of SES discrepancies in the CCI scores. STATA version 14.1 software was used to extract, clean, record, and analyze the data. Weighting was used in the analysis to correct for unequal selection probabilities brought on by the BDHS data sampling strategy. The RII is a regression-based index that evaluates CCI scores over the entire socioeconomic allocation in the research population to assess the size of SES as a source of inequality. According to Zou's advice, the study used a modified Poisson approach to calculate RII. The low SES group has lower CCI scores than the wealthy group when $RII < 1$ (Tatulashvili et al. 2020). Similar to the SII, the RII has a similar interpretation. Applying adjusted ordinal logistic analysis and low CCI scores as the reference level, the relationship concerning the SES and the CCI scores low, medium, and high was examined. The estimated odds ratios and performed a significance test using the 95% confidence intervals (CIs) to assess the strength of the association. The significance level was set at $p < 0.05$ for all analyses.

$$\textbf{Model 1}: y_1 = \beta_{10} + \beta_{11}x_1 + \beta_{12}x_2 + \beta_{13}x_3 + \beta_{14}x_4 + \beta_{15}x_5 + \beta_{16}x_6 + \beta_{17}x_7 + \beta_{18}x_8 + \beta_{19}\ x_9 + \beta_{110}x_{10} + \beta_{111}x_{11}.$$

$$\text{Here, } \mathrm{y}_1 = \text{CCI for maternal Health} = \begin{cases} 1, & \text{low;} \\ 2, & \text{middle;} \\ 3, & \text{high.} \end{cases}$$

$$\mathrm{y}_2 = \text{CCI for child Health} = \begin{cases} 1, & \text{low;} \\ 2, & \text{middle;} \\ 3, & \text{high.} \end{cases}$$

3.3 Results

Table 3.1 shows the bivariate analysis that several significant variations between maternal CCI score and other covariates. Especially women who were aged 25–34 years ($p < 0.014$) had secondary and higher secondary levels of education, mass media exposure, one parity, intended pregnancy, who were lived in urban places, and rich SES ($p = 0.000$) were more likely to represent high maternal CCI score than others.

Table 3.2 shows bivariate analysis that several significant variations between children CCI score and other covariates. Especially women who were aged 15–24 years ($p < 0.020$) had secondary and higher secondary levels of education, mass media exposure, one parity, intended pregnancy, who was lived in urban places ($p < 0.005$), and rich SES ($p = 0.000$), were more likely to represent high child CCI score than others.

Inequality figures out SES and the CoC for maternal health are summarized in Table 3.3. A rise from the low to the high in SES distribution is associated with a 72% rise in high CCI scores, according to RII 1.72. The SII implies that the one-unit change from the low to the high of the SES unit is accompanied with a 0.52 unit increase in the high CCI scores.

Table 3.4 details the socioeconomic status (SES) disparities in child health continuum of care (CoC) completion. Results show a significant association between SES and high CCI scores. Women in the highest SES category have a 75% greater likelihood of achieving high CCI scores compared to those in the lowest category (RII = 1.75). Additionally, the slope index of inequality (SII) says that a one-unit increase in SES is associated with a 0.45 unit increase in the probability of achieving high CCI scores.

The results of the ordinal logistic regression model assessing the relationship between CCI scores, SES the CoC for maternal health and other considerations are shown in Table 3.5. Compared to the low SES group, participants in the high SES group were 2.50 times (95% CI 1.74–3.60) more likely to have higher CCI scores. For the reason that the proportional odds assumption was upheld, the results produced by modeling medium CCI scores against low CCI values were interpreted similarly. Education and access to mass media also appeared as significant factors. Women with a secondary or higher secondary education, as well as those exposed to mass media at least once a week, proved a greater likelihood of achieving high CCI scores compared to their counterparts. Compared to participants who lived in an urban location and had an intended pregnancy were 1.61 (95% CI: 1.23–2.11) and 1.62 (95% CI: 1.24–2.13) times more likely to have high CCI scores. Compared to one parity woman, ≥3 parity women were associated with a decreased odd of higher CCI scores.

The findings of the ordinal logistic regression model evaluating the correlation between CCI scores, SES the CoC for child health, and added factors are shown in Table 3.6. Compared to the low SES group, participants in the middle SES group were 1.38 times (95% CI 0.98–1.93) and the high SES group was 2.03 times (95% CI 1.42–2.90) high CCI scores. As the proportional odds assumption was upheld, the results produced by modeling medium CCI scores against low CCI values were

Table 3.1 Bivariate analysis of maternal CCI score and other covariates

Factors	Maternal CCI score, percentage (%)[a]			Total	*p*-values
	Low	Middle	High		
Respondents age (in years)					
15–24	30.3	38.6	31.1	100.0	0.014
25–34	35.8	31.5	32.6	100.0	
35–49	33.9	42.9	23.2	100.0	
Level of education					
No education	58.9	33.3	7.8	100.0	0.000
Primary	47.9	39.4	12.6	100.0	
Secondary	30.7	37.1	32.1	100.0	
Higher	7.3	28.7	64.0	100.0	
Decision-making autonomy, own healthcare					
No	36.6	31.3	32.0	100.0	0.039
Yes	31.4	37.9	30.8	100.0	
Respondent employed					
No	28.9	36.4	34.7	100.0	0.000
Yes	39.5	35.4	25.2	100.0	
Mass media exposure					
No	52.2	32.4	15.4	100.0	0.000
Yes	23.8	37.7	38.5	100.0	
Parity (tercile)					
1	21.9	37.4	40.6	100.0	0.000
2	32.8	37.6	29.7	100.0	
≥3	46.1	32.5	21.4	100.0	
Pregnancy intended					
No	43.4	36.0	20.6	100.0	0.000
Yes	29.8	36.0	34.2	100.0	
Number of household member (tercile)					
1–4	30.9	39.2	29.9	100.0	0.180
5–6	35.0	35.6	29.4	100.0	
≥7	32.4	33.3	34.3	100.0	
Place of residence					
Rural	37.2	37.4	25.4	100.0	0.000
Urban	20.7	32.4	46.8	100.0	
Offspring sex					
Female	34.0	35.9	30.1	100.0	0.550
Male	31.7	36.2	32.2	100.0	
SES					
Poor	49.9	36.3	13.8	100.0	0.000
Middle	34.0	40.7	25.3	100.0	
Rich	14.6	30.8	54.5	100.0	

Note: *SES* socio-economic status, *CCI* composite coverage index, *CI* confidence interval
[a]Percentages are weighted

Table 3.2 Bivariate analysis of child CCI score and other covariates

Factors	Child CCI score, percentage (%) [a]			Total	*p*-value
	Low	Middle	High		
Respondents age in years					
15–24	53.2	4.2	42.6	100.0	0.020*
25–34	58.1	3.4	38.6	100.0	
35–49	66.7	0.0	33.3	100.0	
Level of education					
No education	80.0	2.2	17.8	100.0	0.000*
Primary	73.2	3.2	23.6	100.0	
Secondary	54.8	3.1	42.1	100.0	
Higher	26.2	5.6	68.2	100.0	
Decision-making autonomy, own healthcare					
No	57.7	4.4	37.9	100.0	0.354
Yes	55.4	3.3	41.2	100.0	
Respondent employed					
No	51.8	4.2	44.1	100.0	0.000*
Yes	63.3	2.6	34.2	100.0	
Mass media exposure					
No	70.3	3.6	26.1	100.0	0.000*
Yes	49.4	3.6	47.0	100.0	
Parity (Tercile)					
1	43.4	3.7	52.8	100.0	0.000*
2	57.9	4.9	37.3	100.0	
≥3	69.4	1.9	28.7	100.0	
Pregnancy intended					
No	67.7	2.6	29.7	100.0	0.000*
Yes	52.8	3.8	43.4	100.0	
Number of household member (tercile)					
1–4	54.6	4.3	41.2	100.0	0.446
5–6	58.9	3.2	37.9	100.0	
≥7	54.7	3.1	42.2	100.0	
Place of residence					
Rural	58.3	3.8	37.9	100.0	0.005*
Urban	49.8	3.2	47.1	100.0	
Offspring sex					
Female	57.2	3.0	39.8	100.0	0.421
Male	55.1	4.1	40.8	100.0	
SES					
Poor	71.4	3.4	25.2	100.0	0.000*
Middle	57.7	3.0	39.3	100.0	
Rich	39.3	4.5	56.2	100.0	

Note: *SES* socio-economic status, *CI* Confidence interval, $p \leq 0.05$ at 95% CI, *significant
[a]Percentages are weighted

Table 3.3 Socioeconomic disparities in continuum of care completion for maternal health: Bangladesh 2017–18 (n = 1527)

	Relative index of inequality (RII)		Slope index of inequality (SII)	
Inequality measure	RR (95% CI)	*p*-value	ß (95% CI)	*p*-value
SES	1.72 (1.41–2.11)	<0.001	0.52 (0.31–0.74)	<0.001

Note: *SES* socio-economic status, *CI* confidence interval, *RR* risk ratio, ß = coefficient

Table 3.4 SES and the CoC completion: Bangladesh Demographic and Health Survey 2017–18 (n = 1527)

	Relative index of inequality (RII)		Slope index of inequality (SII)	
Inequality measure	RR (95% CI)	*p*-value	ß (95% CI)	*p*-value
SES	1.75 (1.32–2.32)	<0.001	0.45 (0.23–0.68)	<0.001

Note: *SES* socio-economic status, *CI* confidence interval; *RR* risk ratio, ß coefficient

Table 3.5 Ordinal logistic regression models for the association between SES and the CoC for maternal health and other covariates (n = 1527)

	CCI scores for maternal health	
Characteristics	AOR (95% CI)	*p*-values
Age (in years) (ref = 15–24)		
25–34	1.42 (1.03–1.96)	0.032
35–49	1.78 (1.03–3.15)	0.040
Education (ref = no education)		
Primary	1.55 (0.93–2.61)	0.094
Secondary	2.91 (1.78–4.75)	<0.001
Higher	7.38 (4.12–13.2)	<0.001
Decision-making autonomy, own health care (ref = no)		
Yes	1.21 (0.95–1.55)	0.128
Respondent employed (ref = no)		
Yes	0.92 (0.72–1.17)	0.497
Mass media exposure (ref = no)		
Yes	1.83 (1.39–2.42)	<0.001
Parity (ref = 1)		
2	0.64 (0.47–0.0.87)	0.005
≥3	0.51 (0.33–0.78)	0.002
Pregnancy intended (ref = no)		
Yes	1.62 (1.24–2.13)	<0.001
No. household member (ref = 2–4)		
5–6	1.07 (0.80–1.43)	0.638
≥7	1.01 (0.73–1.36)	0.995
Place of residence (ref = rural)		
Urban	1.61 (1.23–2.11)	0.001
Offspring sex (ref = female)		
Male	1.16 (0.91–1.46)	0.218
SES (ref = low)		
Middle	1.25 (0.93–1.68)	0.132
High	2.50 (1.74–3.60)	<0.001

Note: *SES* socio-economic status, *CI* confidence interval, *AOR* adjusted odds ratio

Table 3.6 Ordinal logistic regression models for the association between SES and the CoC for child health and other covariates ($n = 1527$)[a]

Characteristics	CCI scores for child health	
	AOR (95% CI)	*P*-value
Age, years (ref = 15–24)		
25–34	1.27 (0.92–1.76)	0.151
35–49	1.25 (0.70–2.23)	0.442
Education (ref = no education)		
Primary	1.33 (0.70–2.55)	0.386
Secondary	2.37 (1.29–4.39)	0.006
Higher	5.11 (2.56–10.2)	<0.001
Decision-making autonomy, own health care (ref = no)		
Yes	1.27 (0.97–1.65)	0.080
Respondent employed (ref = no)		
Yes	0.85 (0.65–1.10)	0.215
Mass media exposure (ref = no)		
Yes	1.44 (1.07–1.92)	0.015
Parity (ref = 1)		
2	0.57 (0.41–0.0.80)	0.001
≥3	0.49 (0.31–0.75)	0.001
Pregnancy intended (ref = no)		
Yes	1.49 (1.12–1.99)	0.006
No. household member (ref = 2–4)		
5–6	0.98 (0.72–1.34)	0.907
≥7	0.89 (0.65–1.20)	0.441
Place of residence (ref = rural)		
Urban	0.96 (0.71–1.28)	0.761
Offspring sex (ref = female)		
Male	1.07 (0.85–1.36)	0.555
SES (ref = low)		
Middle	1.38 (0.98–1.93)	0.062
High	2.03 (1.42–2.90)	<0.001

Note: *SES* socio-economic status, *CI* confidence interval, *AOR* adjusted odds ratio
[a]**All table formats are adapted from** Parvin et al. (2022)

interpreted equally. In terms of other factors, women with higher secondary education and women exposed to mass media were affected by their peers to have high CCI scores. Compared to participants who had an intended pregnancy were 1.49 (95% CI 1.12–1.99) times increase the chance to have high CCI scores. Compared to one parity, women 2, ≥3 parity women were associated with a decreased odd of higher CCI scores.

3.4 Discussion

This study explores maternal and child health coverage and the CoC achievement based on SES. According to the data, women who live in poverty are less likely to obtain all MCH interventions and complete CoC throughout their lives with the exception of contemporary family planning techniques. The rate of CoC for MNCH shown in this study is in line with comparable trends seen in other Gambia and Ghana-based analyses (Oh et al. 2020; Shibanuma et al. 2018). Study revealed that roughly 72% of women made independent healthcare decisions. Only 5.8% of women claimed to have no formal education, while 13.1% of women claimed that their spouses or partners shared same lack of education. A large majority of respondents (68.1%) said they were exposed to the media at least once a week. This study explores how media exposure affects the CoC for using maternal health services (Chaka 2022). The study summarizes inequality measures related to socio-economic status (SES) and the CoC for child health. An increase in SES distribution from low to high is associated with a 75% growth in high CCI scores, as written down by an RII of 1.75. The SII also reveals that a one-unit adjustment from the low to high SES group is associated with a 0.45-unit improvement in high CCI scores. Furthermore, the findings from the ordinal logistic regression model shed light on the relationship between CCI scores, SES, the CoC for child health, and other factors. Compared to the low SES group, participants in the high SES group were 2.03 times (95% CI 1.42–2.90) more probable to have higher CCI scores. The proportional odds assumption was upheld, allowing for the interpretation of results that model medium CCI scores against low CCI values similarly. Amongst other factors, women with higher secondary education and those subjected to mass media were likelier than their peers to have high CCI scores. Additionally, participants with intended pregnancies were 1.49 (95% CI 1.12–1.99) times more likely to have high CCI scores than those with unintended pregnancies. In contrast, women with two or more earlier pregnancies (≥3 parity) showed reduced odds of having higher CCI scores than women with only one last pregnancy. In addition to the AOR, we utilized RII and SII estimations to assess socio-economic inequalities in the CoC for maternal health care. These indices are considered more vigorous measures of socio-economic inequality, delivering a complete interpretation of disparities.

3.5 Conclusion

This study stands for the first exploration of national survey data in Bangladesh to investigate the association between the CoC for maternal and child health care across women's reproductive life cycle and SES. It implies that socio-economic considerations have a meaningful impact on whether the CoC for maternal and child health care services is completed. After taking into account other socio-demographic factors, it was shown that women with secondary or higher secondary education, frequent exposure to media, urban domicile, intentional pregnancies, and one parity were much more likely to have high CCI scores. To increase the CoC achievement rate for maternal and child health, it is necessary to take into account additional socio-demographic parameters in addition to SES.

Acknowledgments The authors' express their gratitude to the authority of DHS and National Institute of Population Research and Training (NIPORT) for providing the dataset.

Author's Contributions M.R. and M.N.P. conceived the idea, conducted statistical analyses, and drafted the manuscript. N.I.M. provided valuable feedback on the statistical analyses and the draft manuscript. All authors have read and approved the final manuscript.

Competing Interests No copeting interests were declared by the authors.

Data Availability Bangladesh Demographic and Health Survey (BDHS), 2017–2018.

Funding None.

References

Alsabi RNS, Zaimi AF, Sivalingam T, Ishak NN, Alimuddin AS, Dasrilsyah RA, Jamil AAM (2022) Improving knowledge, attitudes and beliefs: a cross-sectional study of postpartum depression awareness among social support networks during COVID-19 pandemic in Malaysia. BMC Womens Health 22(1):221

Aune I, Haugen K, Holst-Jenson M, Lund-Tyvoll I (2023) Women's experiences of continuity of care from student midwives–a qualitative study from Norway. Sex Reprod Healthc 100814

Bhowmik J, Biswas RK, Ananna N (2020) Women's education and coverage of skilled birth attendance: an assessment of sustainable development goal 3.1 in the South and Southeast Asian Region. PLoS One 15(4):231489

Chaka EE (2022) Multilevel analysis of continuation of maternal healthcare services utilization and its associated factors in Ethiopia: a cross-sectional study. PLOS Glob Public Health 2(5):517

Das S, Mia MN, Hanifi SMA, Hoque S, Bhuiya A (2017) Health literacy in a community with low levels of education: findings from Chakaria, a rural area of Bangladesh. BMC Public Health 17:1–10

Demographic, B. Health Survey (BDHS) 2017-18: Key Indicators Report.

Fan S, Koski A (2022) The health consequences of child marriage: a systematic review of the evidence. BMC Public Health 22(1):1–17

Hurst TE, Semrau K, Gawande A, Hirschhorn LR (2015) Demand-side interventions for maternal care: evidence of more use, not better outcomes. BMC Pregnancy Childbirth 15(1):1–14

Islam MR, Rahman MS, Rahman MM, Nomura S, De Silva A, Lanerolle P, Rahman MM (2020) Reducing childhood malnutrition in Bangladesh: the importance of addressing socio-economic inequalities. Public Health Nutr 23(1):72–82

Kerber KJ (2007) The continuum of care of maternal, newborn and child health: coverage, co-coverage and equity analysis from demographic and health surveys. University of Cape Town

Khan MN, Harris ML, Loxton D (2020a) Assessing the effect of pregnancy intention at conception on the continuum of care in maternal healthcare services use in Bangladesh: evidence from a nationally representative cross-sectional survey. PLoS One 15(11):242729

Khan MN, Kumar P, Rahman MM, Islam Mondal MN, Islam MM (2020b) Inequalities in utilization of maternal reproductive health Care Services in Urban Bangladesh: a population-based study. SAGE Open 10:1

Khan JR, Hossain M, Gupta RD (2021a) Household cooking fuels associated with elevated blood pressure among adult women: a national-wide assessment in Bangladesh. Environ Sci Pollut Res 28(47):67814–67821

Khan JR, Sultana A, Islam M, Biswas RK (2021b) A negative association between prevalence of diabetes and urban residential area greenness detected in nationwide assessment of urban Bangladesh. Sci Rep 11(1):1–9

Lalonde A, Herschderfer K, Pascali-Bonaro D, Hanson C, Fuchtner C, Visser GH (2019) The international childbirth initiative: 12 steps to safe and respectful MotherBaby–family maternity care. Int J Gynecol Obstet 146(1):65–73

Mahembe E, Odhiambo NM (2018) The dynamics of extreme poverty in developing countries. Studia Universitatis "Vasile Goldis" Arad-Economics Series 28(2):18–35

Oh J, Moon J, Choi JW, Kim K (2020) Factors associated with the continuum of care for maternal, newborn and child health in The Gambia: a cross-sectional study using Demographic and Health Survey 2013. BMJ Open 10(11):36516

Panciera R, Khan A, Rizvi SJR, Ahmed S, Ahmed T, Islam R, Adams AM (2016) The influence of travel time on emergency obstetric care seeking behavior in the urban poor of Bangladesh: a GIS study. BMC Pregnancy Childbirth 16(1):1–13

Parvin N, Rahman M, Islam MJ, Haque SE, Sarkar P, Mondal MNI (2022) Socioeconomic inequalities in the continuum of care across women's reproductive life cycle in Bangladesh. Sci Rep 12(1):15618

Paulson KR, Kamath AM, Alam T, Bienhoff K, Abady GG, Abbas J, Abd-Elsalam SM (2021) Global, regional, and national progress towards Sustainable Development Goal 3.2 for neonatal and child health: all-cause and cause-specific mortality findings from the Global Burden of Disease Study 2019. Lancet 398(10303):870–905

Saber N (2021). Poverty reduction in Bangladesh through cash tranfser programs (Master's thesis, OsloMet-Storbyuniversitetet).

Sakuma S, Yasuoka J, Phongluxa K, Jimba M (2019) Determinants of continuum of care for maternal, newborn, and child health services in rural Khammouane, Lao PDR. PloS One 14(4):e0215635

Sarker BK, Rahman M, Rahman T, Hossain J, Reichenbach L, Mitra DK (2016) Reasons for preference of home delivery with traditional birth attendants (TBAs) in rural Bangladesh: a qualitative exploration. PLoS One 11:1

Sheba IT, Sarker AR, Tasnim A (2022) Factors Associated with Post-Natal Care Utilization among the Women of Reproductive age Group: Evidence from Bangladesh Demographic and Health Survey 2017–18. Health Services Research and Managerial Epidemiology, 9, 23333928221136393

Shibanuma A, Yeji F, Okawa S, Mahama E, Kikuchi K, Narh C, Owusu-Agyei S (2018) The coverage of continuum of care in maternal, newborn and child health: a cross-sectional study of woman-child pairs in Ghana. BMJ Glob Health 3:4

Tatulashvili S, Fagherazzi G, Dow C, Cohen R, Fosse S, Bihan H (2020) Socioeconomic inequalities and type 2 diabetes complications: a systematic review. Diabetes Metab 46(2):89–99

WHO (2018) Definition of skilled health personnel providing care during childbirth: the 2018 joint statement by WHO, UNFPA, UNICEF, ICM, ICN, FIGO and IPA

Further Reading

Islam N, Islam MT, Yoshimura Y (2014). Practices and determinants of delivery by skilled birth attendants inBangladesh. Reproductive health, 11, 1–7.

Islam RM, Khan MN, Oldroyd JC, Rana J, Magliago DJ, Chowdhury EK, Hossain MB (2021) Prevalence of diabetes and prediabetes among Bangladeshi adults and associated factors: evidence from the Demographic and Health Survey, 2017–18. medRxiv

Khan MN, Harris ML, Shifti DM, Laar AS, Loxton D (2019) Effects of unintended pregnancy on maternal healthcare services utilization in low-and lower-middle-income countries: systematic review and meta-analysis. Int J Public Health 64:743–754

Misu F, Alam K (2023). Comparison of inequality in utilization of maternal healthcare services between Bangladesh and Pakistan: evidence from the demographic health survey 2017–2018. Reproductive health, 20(1),43.

Sarker BK, Rahman M, Rahman T, Rahman T, Khalil JJ, Hasan M, Mridha MK (2020a) Status of the WHO recommended timing and frequency of antenatal care visits in Northern Bangladesh. PLoS One 15:11

Sarker M, Saha A, Matin M, Mehjabeen S, Tamim MA, Sharkey AB, Shahabuddin ASM (2020b) Effective maternal, newborn and child health programming among Rohingya refugees in Cox's Bazar, Bangladesh: implementation challenges and potential solutions. PLoS One 15:3

Wasting Among Under-Five Children from 1990 to 2020: A Systematic Review and Meta-Analysis

4

Md. Ismail Hossain, Md. Nurul Islam, Md. Abu Syed Md. Al Mamun, Ripter Hossain, Premananda Bharati, and Md. Golam Hossain

4.1 Introduction

The nutritional status of children under the age of five is assessed using three key indicators: (a) height-for-age (stunting), (b) weight-for-age (underweight), and (c) weight-for-height (wasting) (WHO 2010). Wasting, which measures acute malnutrition using both height and weight, is particularly crucial for global child nutrition assessments. Surveys on the nutritional status of under-five children have been conducted since the 1970s, but comparing their findings is challenging due to varied methodologies and contexts across regions. Over the decades, there has been some progress in reducing childhood malnutrition. For instance, the prevalence decreased from 47% in 1980 to 33% in 2000 in developing countries. However, trends vary significantly across regions. Stunting increased in East Africa but declined in Southeast Asia, South Central Asia, and South America. North Africa and the Caribbean have seen slight improvements, while West Africa and Central America have shown limited progress. These disparities highlight the complex nature of childhood malnutrition and the need for targeted interventions based on regional contexts. Despite these declines, childhood malnutrition remains a major public health concern, with stunting rates rising in some countries and remaining high in others (WHO 2010). It is found that children born at home through traditional delivery

M. I. Hossain · M. N. Islam · Md. Abu Syed Md. Al Mamun · R. Hossain
Health Research Group, Department of Statistics, University of Rajshahi, Rajshahi, Bangladesh

P. Bharati
Biological Anthropology Unit, Indian Statistical Institute (ISI), Kolkata, West Bengal, India

M. G. Hossain (✉)
Department of Statistics, University of Rajshahi, Rajshahi, Bangladesh

M. Pal et al. (eds.), *Public Health and Nutrition*, https://doi.org/10.1007/978-981-97-7890-4_4

methods are more likely to be stunted compared to those born in hospitals (Rahman and Chowdhury 2007). Mothers' acute malnutrition is an important predictor for their children growth, and shorter birth intervals are linked to higher rates of malnutrition among children (Rayhan and Khan 2006). According to the WHO report, a combined stunting and wasting rate exceeding 30% indicates a critical state of malnutrition in a particular population, and chronic malnutrition significantly impacts on health and mortality of preschool children and affects a nation's future productivity (WHO 2010). A study in Dhaka city, involving 380 randomly selected under-five children, found that 39.5%, 25%, and 14% were stunted, severely stunted, and moderately stunted, respectively, also found that socioeconomic and demographic factors such as parental education, maternal employment and nutrition knowledge, maternal height, family education level, normal birth weight, frequent meals (>6 times in a day), and fewer episodes of fever in the past six months were associated with better child nutrition (Jesmin et al. 2011). The study aimed to meet the Millennium Development Goal of reducing undernutrition prevalence to 34% by 2015, requiring targeted government interventions (Jesmin et al. 2011). It was also reported that economic difficulties and lack of information contribute to a cycle of malnutrition, where malnourished mothers give birth to malnourished children, who then continue the cycle into adulthood (Jesmin et al. 2011). Now it is important to estimate the pool prevalence and common risk factors of wasting among under-five children globally.

Therefore, the authors of this study aimed to assess the overall prevalence of wasting among children under the age of five and investigate the factors contributing to wasting through a systematic review and meta-analysis.

4.2 Methods

A systematic review and meta-analysis were conducted to determine the pool prevalence of wasting of children under-five children from 1990 to 2020. Authors of the current study searched the required published paper on wasting of under-five children using search engines such as PubMed, Endnote, Elsevier, Eric, MEDLINE, Cochrane Library, and EMBASE databases using combinations of search terms. Key terms "child" and "wasting" were used for searching in each database to identify observational studies published in English during the specific period. From an initial pool of 623 English papers (600 from PubMed and the rest from other databases), the researchers selected only articles that focused on wasting of under-five children in worldwide and were available in full text. Duplicate papers, case-control studies, and clinical trials were excluded from the study. Two individuals, a computer science graduate and a specialist, conducted the searches and analyses separately. A checklist was prepared to assess the final set of articles, which included details like titles, authors, study settings, sample sizes, subject ages, sex, and wasting percentages. Finally, 12 papers were selected in the present study. The flow chart for selecting procedure is given below:

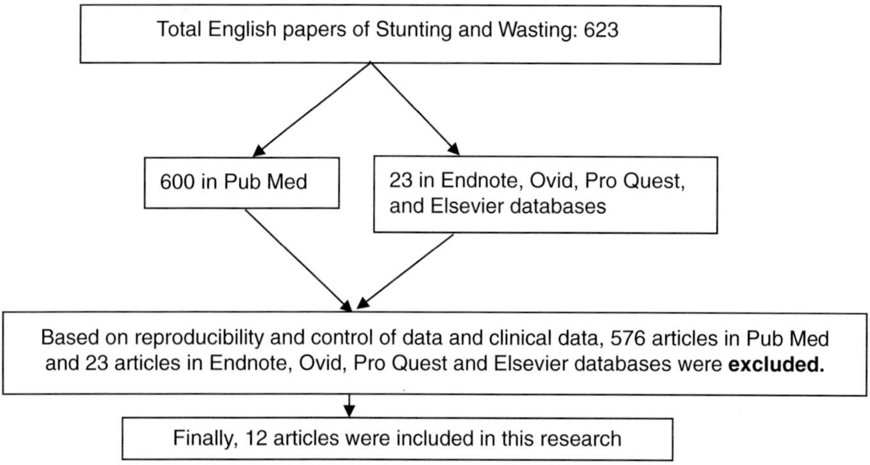

Statistical Methods Stata software (version 11) was used for Statistical analysis. The pooled prevalence was estimated using fixed effects, and risk factors for wasting were examined by considering the 95% confidence intervals (CI) in each case. A fixed-effects model was used to combine the effect sizes, considering both sampling error and differences between studies, using the inverse variance method. The effect sizes from all eligible studies were combined using this method because it assumes a distribution of effects, leading to differences among study results. The χ^2 test, the Q statistic, and the I^2 statistic were utilized to check the heterogeneity among studies, and when I^2 was greater than 60%, possible sources of heterogeneity were investigated based on the definitions used for children's nutritional status. The results were presented in tables and forest plots, showing the pool prevalence rates, effect sizes, and 95% CIs for each study, along with the overall estimate.

4.3 Results and Discussion

Prevalence of Wasting In this study, a systematic review and meta-analysis were conducted on 12 papers published in English, focusing on the prevalence rates of wasting among children under the age of five. Table 4.1 summarizes data from these studies, revealing a wide range in wasting prevalence, from 5.3% reported by Boah and Azupogo (2019) to 30% by Neel and Alvarez (1991). The meta-analysis aimed to determine the pooled prevalence estimate of wasting across these studies, yielding an overall estimate of 8.88% (95% CI: −3.03, 20.78). Notably, the heterogeneity between the studies was very low ($I^2 = 0.00\%$, $p = 1000$), indicating consistency in the findings (Fig. 4.1).

The analysis of global data revealed a significant increase in the number of children affected by wasting over the past three decades, albeit with varying trends among countries. Developed nations initially saw an increase starting in the 1970s,

Table 4.1 Overview of research on wasting in children under five

Author(s)	Year	Sample	Wasting (%)	Risk factors
Neel & Alvarez	1991	148,000	30	Fetal growth restriction
Haidar et al.	2005	200	9	Maternal behaviors
Gewa and Yandell	2012	2720	10.1	Household wealth index
Yang et al.	2012	336	11.31	Maternal behaviors
Christian et al.	2013	60,206	3.4	Fetal growth restriction
Rahman and Alam	2015	6506	16	Maternal behaviors
Victora et al.	2015	306	26.5	Fetal growth restriction
Abdulahi et al.	2017	610	7.9	Child age
Wasihun et al.	2018	394	7.2	Child age
Boah & Azupogo	2019	174	5.3	Household wealth index
Tekile, Woya, & Basha	2019	1851	8	Household wealth index
Gebru et al.	2019	39,585	15	Child age

which has since slowed in recent years. Conversely, the study's findings suggest that wasting continues to be a growing concern in the developing world, where nearly two-thirds of all wasted children reside. This underscores the persistent challenges and disparities in addressing childhood malnutrition globally, necessitating targeted interventions tailored to regional contexts and ongoing monitoring to mitigate the impact on child health and development.

Risk Factor for Wasting Our study reviewed 12 research papers to investigate the factors contributing to wasting among children under the age of five. We specifically examined four primary factors: fetal growth, maternal behaviors, child's age, and household socioeconomic status. Through our analysis, we calculated pooled hazard ratios, which ranged significantly from 6.97 to 14.37, indicating strong associations between these factors and the risk of wasting.

Children from poorer households and those with fetal growth issues exhibited the highest risk of wasting according to our findings. This underscores the critical role of socioeconomic status and early developmental factors in shaping nutritional outcomes during childhood. Across the studies we reviewed, there were varying results on how each factor—fetal growth, maternal behaviors such as nutrition during pregnancy and breastfeeding practices, and the age of the child—contributes to wasting (see Fig. 4.2).

Studies have consistently pointed to fetal growth restriction as a leading factor contributing to childhood wasting, highlighting how inadequate intrauterine development can heighten vulnerability to nutritional deficiencies early in life. Maternal behaviors, such as poor feeding practices and limited access to nutritious foods, have also been identified as significant contributors to the risk of wasting among young children. Moreover, younger children are particularly susceptible due to their increased susceptibility to infections and challenges in meeting nutritional needs. These findings highlight the complex interplay of biological, behavioral, and socioeconomic factors influencing childhood wasting. Addressing these multifaceted

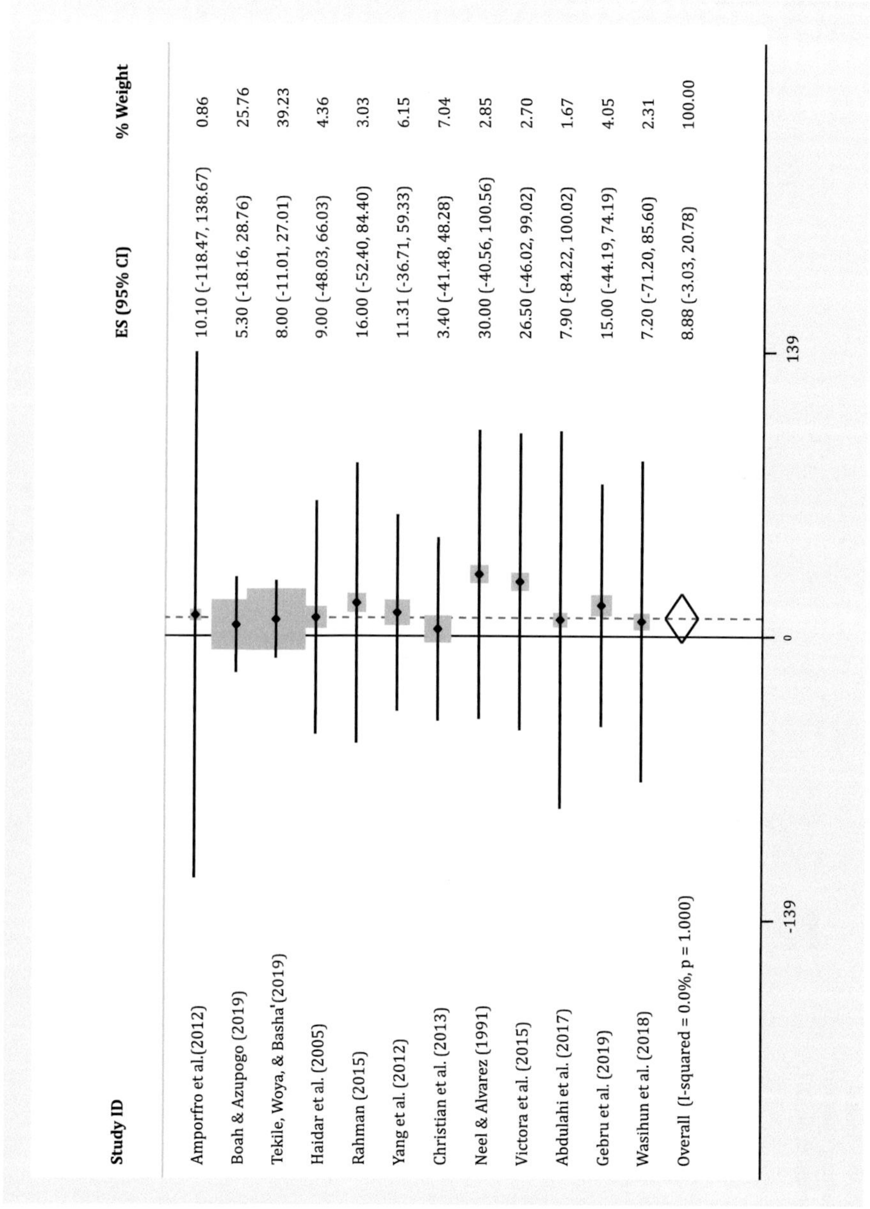

Fig. 4.1 Prevalence of effect size and 95% CI of wasting children. (**Source:** Hossain et al. 2023)

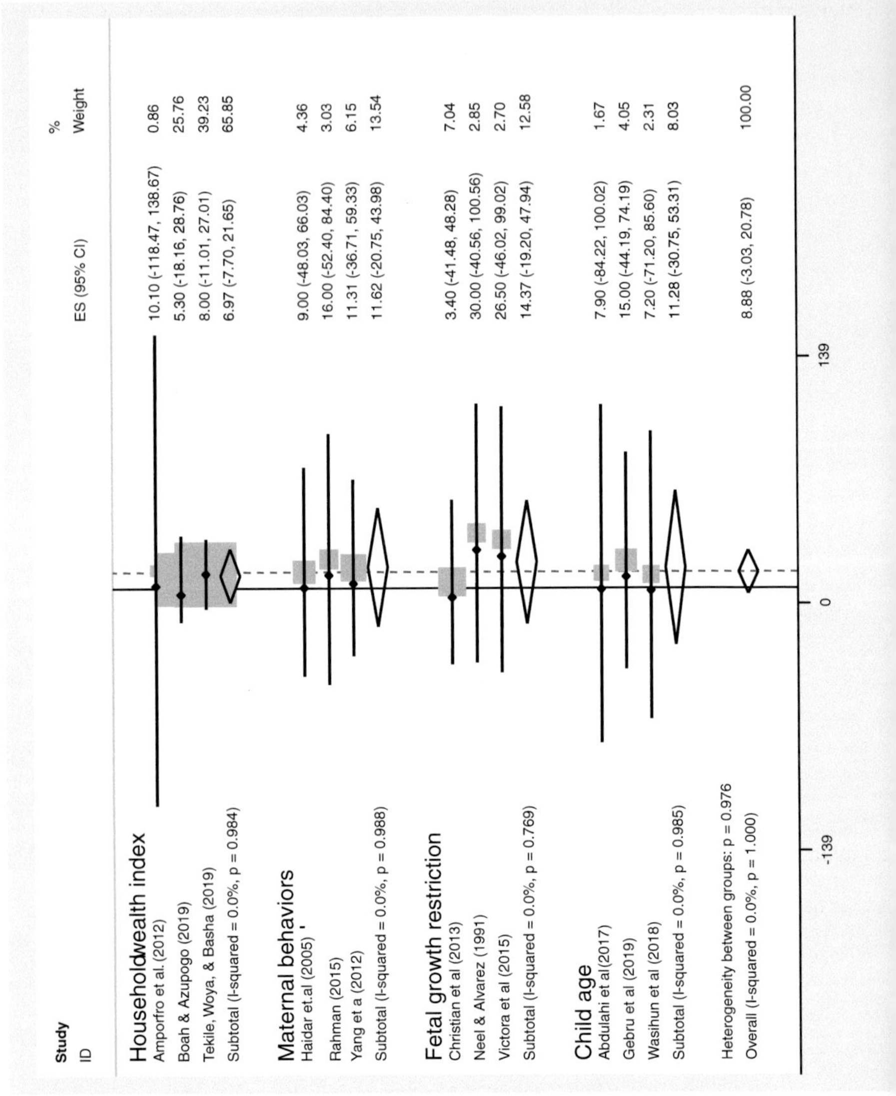

Fig. 4.2 Risk factors and 95% CI of wasting children. (**Source:** Hossain et al. 2023)

determinants is essential for developing targeted interventions that effectively reduce wasting prevalence and promote improved overall health outcomes for children worldwide.

4.4 Conclusion

This study conducted a systematic review and meta-analysis to determine the pool prevalence and common factors of wasting among under-five children in worldwide from 1990 to 2020. We used Q and I^2 statistics to compare findings across studies and created a Forest plot to show the prevalence and factors contributing to wasting. The pooled hazard ratios for risk factors, such as household wealth and fetal growth problems, ranged from 6.97 to 14.37. Studies showed varying results regarding how fetal growth issues, maternal behavior, and a child's age contribute to wasting. The study suggests that achieving target levels of reducing wasting will be challenging without substantial efforts and further research. To improve child health globally, especially in developing countries, strong leadership is necessary to ensure access to nutritious food, healthcare, and improved socio-economic and educational conditions. It's crucial to implement effective health policies, educate families about wasting, and encourage lifestyle changes to reduce sickness and death associated with wasting.

References

Abdulahi A, Shab-Bidar S, Rezaei S, Djafarian K (2017) Nutritional status of under five children in Ethiopia: a systematic review and meta-analysis. Ethiop J Health Sci 27(2):175–188. https://doi.org/10.4314/ejhs.v27i2.10

Boah M, Azupogo F (2019) The epidemiology of undernutrition and its determinants in children under five years in Ghana. 14(7):e0219665. https://doi.org/10.1371/journal.pone.0219665

Christian P, Lee SE, Donahue Angel M, Adair LS, Arifeen SE, Ashorn P, Black RE (2013) Risk of childhood undernutrition related to small-for-gestational age and preterm birth in low- and middle-income countries. Int J Epidemiol 42(5):1340–1355. https://doi.org/10.1093/ije/dyt109

Gebru TT, Abady GG, Teklu FG, Tesfamichael YA, Bitow MT, Tekola KB et al (2019) Assessment of wasting and associated factors among under five children of Wukro town, Tigray regional, North Ethiopia: a cross sectional study. Pan Afr Med J 33:330. https://doi.org/10.11604/pamj.2019.33.330.18808

Gewa CA, Yandell N (2012) Undernutrition among Kenyan children: contribution of child, maternal and household factors. Public Health Nutrition. 15(6):1029–1038. https://doi.org/10.1017/S136898001100245X

Haidar J, Abate G, Kogi-Makau W, Sorensen P (2005) Risk factors for child under-nutrition with a human rights edge in rural villages of North Wollo, Ethiopia. East African Medical Journal 82:625–630

Hossain MI, Islam MN, Mamun MASA, Bharati P, Hossain MG (2023) Prevalence and risk factors of undernutrition among under-five children from 1990–2020: a systematic review and meta-analysis. Int J Stat Sci 23(1):71–80

Jesmin A et al (2011) Prevalence and determinants of chronic malnutrition among preschool children: a cross-sectional study in Dhaka City, Bangladesh. J Health Popul Nutr 29(5):494

Neel NR, Alvarez JO (1991) Maternal risk factors for low birth weight and intrauterine growth retardation in a Guatemalan population. Bull Pan Am Health Organ 25(2):152–165

Rahman MH, Alam SS (2015) Nutritional status of children in slums of dhaka, Bangladesh. J Nutr Food Sci 5:425. https://doi.org/10.4172/2155-9600.1000425

Rahman A, Chowdhury S (2007) Determinants of chronic malnutrition among preschool children in Bangladesh. J Biosoc Sci 39(2):161

Rayhan MI, Khan MSH (2006) Factors causing malnutrition among under five children in Bangladesh. Pak J Nutr 5(6):558–562

Tekile AK, Woya AA, Basha GW (2019) Prevalence of malnutrition and associated factors among under-five children in Ethiopia: evidence from the 2016 Ethiopia Demographic and Health Survey. BMC Res Notes 12(1):391. https://doi.org/10.1186/s13104-019-4444-4

Victora CG, Villar J, Barros FC, Ismail LC, Chumlea C, Papageorghiou AT et al (2015) Anthropometric characterization of impaired fetal growth: risk factors for and prognosis of newborns with stunting or wasting. JAMA Pediatr 169(7):e151431. https://doi.org/10.1001/jamapediatrics.2015.1431

Wasihun AG, Dejene TA, Teferi M, Marugán J, Negash L, Yemane D, McGuigan KG (2018) Risk factors for diarrhoea and malnutrition among children under the age of 5 years in the Tigray region of Northern Ethiopia. PLoS One 13(11):e0207743. https://doi.org/10.1371/journal.pone.0207743

WHO (2010) Nutrition landscape information system (NLIS) country profile indicators: interpretation guide. World Health Organization, Geneva

Yang W, Li X, Li Y, Zhang S, Liu L, Wang X, Li W (2012) Anemia, malnutrition and their correlations with sociodemographic characteristics and feeding practices among infants aged 0–18 months in rural areas of Shaanxi province in northwestern China: a cross-sectional study. BMC Public Health12:1127. https://doi.org/10.1186/1471-2458-12-1127

Undernutrition Among Infants Through Composite Index of Anthropometric Failures

5

Susmita Bharati, Manoranjan Pal, and Premananda Bharati

5.1 Introduction

Like other developing countries, undernutrition among under-five children is a major public health problem in many countries, especially in south-Asian countries (Talukder 2017). Available data on under-five children suggests that globally, the percentage of stunted children is more than the percentages of underweight and wasted children combined (WHO 2015). In India, 62 million children were stunted (UNICEF 2013). Undernourished children are mainly found in low-income and lower-middle-income countries (Romieu et al. 2017; Victora et al. 2021). Among them, the first worst-ranked country in the world for child malnutrition is Yemen, it ranks 1 for underweight and 2 for stunting (UNICEF 2014). Indonesia has a very high prevalence in South-east Asia where the percentage of stunted children is 30.8 percent while in Cambodia, the percentage is more than in Indonesia (IFPRI 2016). In West Java provinces, the percentage of stunting is 31.1%, 13.2% underweight, and 8.4% wasting. In India, the latest Family Health Survey (NFHS-5, 2019–21) says that there are 32.1% underweight among under-five children, 19.3% wasted, and 35.5% stunted (IIPS and ICF 2021). In particular, the percentage of underweight and stunted children in the capital of India, i.e., Delhi, are 21.2% and 30%, respectively.

S. Bharati (✉)
Sociological Research Unit, Social Sciences Division, Indian Statistical Institute, Kolkata, West Bengal, India

M. Pal
Economic Research Unit, Social Sciences Division, Indian Statistical Institute (ISI), Kolkata, West Bengal, India

P. Bharati
Biological Anthropology Unit, Biological Sciences Division, Indian Statistical Institute (ISI), Kolkata, West Bengal, India

M. Pal et al. (eds.), *Public Health and Nutrition*,
https://doi.org/10.1007/978-981-97-7890-4_5

Undernutrition is the single contributory factor for the burden of child mortality and is responsible for half of the child death (Lopez et al. 2006; Rice et al. 2000). WHO (2010) sets the critical limits for stunting as 40% and wasting at 15% (WHO 2010). India is the most significant country which carries a huge burden of undernourished children with high spatial heterogenic variations. Various factors are responsible for undernutrition among infants and under-five children. Among 6–23 months children, inappropriate complementary feeding practices, breast feeding, socio-demographic conditions, and hygienic condition of food are also responsible for undernutrition.

Anthropometric indices, namely, stunting (low height for age), wasting (low weight for height), and underweight (low weight for age) are the three conventional indicators that are used to detect child undernutrition in a population (WHO 2006). For example, both current and chronic malnutrition are reflected by the weight-for-age index, only chronic malnutrition is reflected by the height/length-for-age index. The low weight-for-height/length index, which is termed as wasting, represents acute malnutrition. Thus, a low weight-for-age index indicates general nutritional problems and is rightly termed as underweight. The children who suffer from frequent illness for a long time suffer from chronic malnutrition which is mainly caused by prolonged poverty, lack of exclusive breastfeeding, lack of timely introduction of complementary foods, etc. (Titaley et al. 2019; Permatasari et al. 2018; Permatasari and Sudiartini 2020). It may also be caused by infectious diseases such as tuberculosis, prolonged diarrhea and acute respiratory infections (ARI) (Titaley et al. 2019; Shabariah et al. 2021; Fatimah et al. 2021; Permatasari et al. 2021). In general, it is necessary to consider all three indices to arrive at a conclusion on the status of health of a child and not only the indices for which there are low values, and it is a must for looking at the status of health in a community (Ministry of Health RI 2020). This is precisely the reason why a single index is called for. In 2000, Svedberg developed single figure for the overall estimated undernourishment among under five children in a population through composite Index of Anthropometric Failure (CIAF) (Svedberg 2000). In India, Nandy et al. (2005), however, used this concept first in India.

Considering the above idea, this study has the following objectives as follows:

1. To assess the burden of undernutrition among infants in a community through a single measure "CIAF" to detect the multiple arthrometric undernutrition.
2. To assess the individual undernutrition through conventional three types of undernutrition like underweight, stunting, and wasting and its comparison with the CIAF method.
3. To find the relationship between total burden of undernutrition as measured by CIAF with different socio-economic variables.

5.2 Methods

5.2.1 The Variables in the Analysis

Our main outcome of the study is to assess the total burden of undernutrition among infants through CIAF method and its comparison with conventional method. Both conventional and CIAF methods have been used for assessing the different categories of undernutrition like underweight, stunted, and wasted. So, the outcome variable of this study was stunting, wasting and underweight. That is why, we have used both processes for assessing the undernutrition among infants. And "z-score" was computed from the data on weight, height, and age of the infants for assessing the undernutrition, namely, weight-for-age, height-for-age, and weight-for-height indices have been considered.

According to WHO (2006), the cut off point of each z-score is taken as "−2." This means that a child is declared underweight, stunted or wasted if the value of the corresponding nutrition index is less than −2. For estimation of Z-score, given the age of child, the median of the reference population of that age is subtracted from the observed score and then the difference is divided by the standard deviation of the reference population of that age. More precisely, the following formula is used.

$$Z-\text{score} = \frac{(\text{observed value}) - \begin{pmatrix} \text{median of the reference population} \\ \text{of the same age that of the child} \end{pmatrix}}{\begin{matrix} \text{SD of the reference population} \\ \text{of the same age as that of the child} \end{matrix}}.$$

If the value is less than −2, the child is at the below-normal level, if it is between −2 and less than +2, the child is normal and if the value is +2 or more then the child is above the above average level (WHO 2006). Both below −2 value and above +2 value are not good for the health of the child.

For this study, unit-level data has been extracted from National Family Health Survey of 2019–21 (NFHS-5) data (IIPS and ICF 2021). The children aged 0–11 months have been considered in our study. After eliminating outliers and unobserved data, the sample size of the actual dataset is 32,875.

Svedberg (2000) proposed some categories by taking various combinations of stunting, wasting, and underweight of children depending on the presence and absence of these three forms of malnutrition. Nandy et al. (2005) further extended it to make the groups exhaustive.[1] The groups are described in Table 5.1. Table 5.1 also contains the group representing the absence of any of these three forms of malnutrition. The composite group of anthropological failures refers to the union of these six groups symbolized as B, C, D, E, F, and Y in the table, whereas the symbol A refers to the group of "No failure" (NF). The Composite Index of Anthropological Failures (CIAF) is defined as the sum of the percentages of children in groups B, C,

[1] In fact, there are seven categories. But no children are found in the category "stunting and wasting only".

Table 5.1 The Components of the composite index of anthropometric failure among under-five children

Group	Description	Wasting	Stunting	Underweight
A	No failure	No	No	No
B	Wasting only	Yes	No	No
C	Wasting and Underweight	Yes	No	Yes
D	Wasting, Stunting, and Underweight	Yes	Yes	Yes
E	Stunting and Underweight	No	Yes	Yes
F	Stunting only	No	Yes	No
Y	Underweight only	No	No	Yes

Note: No failure (NF) = A; Anthropometric failure (AF) = Sum of B, C, D, E, F, Y
Source: Kundu et al. (2023)

D, E, F, and Y, which is same as the percentage of children in the composite group of anthropological failures, because the groups are mutually exclusive.

5.3 Independent Variables

Socio-demographic variables are the independent variables which consist of place of residence, sex of the infant, mother's educational status and age, religion, mother's nutritional status, wealth index, birthweight of the infants, and different zones. Place of residence is taken as "rural" and "urban." Sex of infant is boy and girl. Similarly, for mother's educational status, the categories are illiterate, primary (up to class IV standard), secondary (class V to class X standard), and XI and onwards (i.e., above X standard). It was further reduced to only three groups, the first two groups being combined to illiterate or up to primary standard, Secondary and Higher. Mother's age has been grouped into three categories such as 15–19 years, 20–29 years, and 30 and above. We have taken the major four religious groups, namely, Hindu, Muslim, Christian, and rest of all other groups have put in the group 'others. So, religion has four categories. Mother's nutritional status has been grouped into two categories as undernourished and other through BMI. The variable "Wealth index" was created by (Rutstein 1999) and it is composed of 33 household assets like toilet facility, flooring, roofing, material of exterior walls, number of household members per sleeping room, ownership of pressure cooker, television, mobile telephone, car, etc. It represents the standard of living of the household. They further grouped this index into five categories, each category representing one-fifth of the sample population. These are in fact quintile groups in increasing order like poorest, poorer, medium, richer, and richest. Then again five groups have been merged into three categories such as poor (poorest and poorer), medium, and rich (richer and richest). Birthweight is grouped into three categories such as very low <1500 g), low (<2500 g), and normal and above (>2500 g) and lastly, all the states and Union territories in India have been grouped into six zones like North-East, East, Central, West, North, and South.

5.3.1 Statistical Analysis

It is necessary to see how the socio-economic variables explain the variation of CIAF. CIAF takes value 1 if any of these three anthropometric health indices show z-value less than −2; otherwise, it takes the value 0. Thus, a binary logistic regression is called for. Once the regression is carried out and the odd for each explanatory variable is found, we can interpret the result. Assuming that the explanatory variable is binary, the odd greater than one indicates that the present category (i.e., the category taking value 1) has more probability to make the CIAF to be 1 than the reference category of the explanatory variable. In the case of continuous explanatory variable, if the value of it increases, then there is more chance to become the CIAF to be one. If the odd is less than one, then the interpretations are just the opposite. Naturally, the value of odd as 1 signifies that there is no difference of the influence of the categorical variable between the reference and the present category (or no influence of the continuous explanatory variable) on CIAF.

The p-values 0.01 and 0.05 were considered for deciding the significance in regression or chi-square analysis. The Statistical Package for the Social Sciences (SPSS, version 25.0) was used to analyze the data.

5.4 Ethical Approval

This study is done using the secondary data of NFHS-5 of Demographic and Health Surveys (DHS), and it was obtained through online registration in accordance with their guidelines. The International Institute for Population Sciences (IIPS) in India, a nodal organization of the host nation, and the ICF Institutional Review Board (IRB) have reviewed and approved it. Therefore, the DHS data, which was used in our analysis, is ethically acceptable.

5.5 Results

Out of total 32,875 infants, 52.6% do not have any failure, i.e., they belong to the group of "No failure" (NF). The rest of the infants suffer from at least on the failures as follows (Table 5.2): Wasting only—11.8%, Wasting and Underweight only—9.0%, Wasting, Stunting, and Underweight—2.9%, Stunting and Underweight only—9.2%, Stunting only—12.2% and underweight only—2.3%. So, percentage of anthropometric failure is 47.4% and no failure is 52.6%.

Table 5.3 depicts that among infants in India, in conventional method, the percentage of underweight, stunting, and wasting are 23.4, 24.3, and 23.7 percent, respectively. The increments of mean values between any two subsequent age groups are significant when 't' test has been done. A positive change has been seen for each pair of subsequent age groups and the maximum increment is seen from 0 to 1 and 1 to 2 months age group for both height and weight. In case of CIAF, highest anthropometric failure (AF) is seen from 0 to 1 and 1 to 2 months age group and

Table 5.2 The distribution of children to different components of CIAF

Groups	Composite index of anthropometric failure (CIAF), N = 100 (32,875)
A No failure	52.6 (17,293)
B Wasting only	11.8 (3870)
C Wasting and underweight	9.0 (2963)
D Wasting, stunting, and underweight	2.9 (957)
E Stunting and underweight	9.2 (3006)
F Stunting only	12.2 (4015)
G Underweight only	2.3 (771)
Sum (B to G) = Anthropometric failure	47.4 (15,582)

Table 5.3 Age group-wise percentage distribution of nutritional status of infants through conventional method and CIAF method among infants in India

		Nutritional status				
		Conventional method			CIAF	
Age (months)	N	Underweight	Stunted	Wasted	No Failure	Anthropometric failure
00	1881	18.8	23.9	29.2	48.4	51.6
01	2581	25.7	27.5	26.3	45.2	54.8
02	2851	27.3	25.6	26.9	46.2	53.8
03	2849	24.2	22.6	25.7	51.3	48.7
04	3024	24.8	21.5	26.2	52.9	47.1
05	2768	22.7	22.1	22.7	55.0	45.0
06	2896	21.5	22.6	22.9	56.0	44.0
07	2755	20.9	23.4	19.6	57.4	42.6
08	2699	22.7	23.6	21.8	55.1	44.9
09	2899	23.0	23.6	22.5	55.6	44.4
10	2800	22.4	26.6	21.1	54.1	45.9
11	2875	25.6	28.4	22.2	52.1	47.9
Total	32,875	23.4	24.3	23.7	52.6	47.4

then it is quite decreasing up to 7 months and after that it increased a little up to 11 months.

Through the incidence of undernutrition by socio-economic characteristics among infants in India (Table 5.4), the result shows that undernutrition among infants is negatively related with urban locality and prevalence of undernutrition among boys is more than girls. Mother's education is inversely related with undernutrition, i.e.; the highest percentages are seen among the children of illiterate and primary educated mothers. Mother's age is always inversely related. Religion wise, Hindu and Muslim mothers have more percentage of CIAF infants than other religious groups. Mother's health is always positively related with infant's health. Wealth index of the family and birth weight of the infants are directly related with better nutritional status of the infants. Zone-wise effects on infants' undernutrition

Table 5.4 Relationship between undernutrition (CIAF) and different socio-demographic variables among infants in India

Dependent variables	*N*	CIAF		
		Yes	No	Chi-square
Place of residence				
Urban	6360	43.4	56.6	49.455
Rural	26,515	48.3	51.7	df = 1 sig. 0.000
Sex of the children				
Boy	16,659	50.3	49.7	115.769
Girl	16,216	44.4	55.6	df = 1 sig. 0.000
Mother's education				
Illiterate and primary	9109	52.7	47.3	218.711
Secondary	18,184	46.9	53.1	df = 2
Higher	5582	40.3	59.7	sig. 0.000
Mother's age				
15–19	2141	53.8	46.2	38.344
20–29	24,599	47.1	52.9	df = 2
30 and above	6135	46.5	53.5	sig. 0.000
Religion				
Hindu	24,866	48.4	51.6	136.300
Muslim	4306	49.1	50.9	df = 3
Christian	2439	38.2	61.8	sig. 0.000
Others	1264	38.8	61.2	
Mother's BMI				215.299
Undernourished	6411	55.6	44.4	df = 1
Other	26,464	45.4	54.6	sig. 0.000
Wealth Index				
Poorest/poorer	15,569	52.5	47.5	358.889
Middle	6790	46.0	54.0	df = 2
Richer/Richest	10,516	40.7	59.3	sig. 0.000
Birth-weight				
(<1500 g)	587	68.5	31.5	440.776
(<2500 g)	5162	58.7	41.3	df = 2
(2500 or above)	27,126	44.8	55.2	sig. 0.000
Zone				
North-east	4408	40.9	59.1	280.760
East	6354	52.9	47.1	df = 5
Central	8460	49.5	50.5	sig. 0.000
West	2940	53.4	46.6	
North	6203	42.7	57.3	
South	4510	44.5	55.5	

"sig. 0.000" means significant at 0.001 level

show that the lowest occurrence is seen in North-east zone and the highest is seen in West zone then it is followed by East and Central zones. All these results are statistically significant at 1% level.

Table 5.5 expresses the relationship between undernutrition with socio-economy through categorical logistic regression. The result shows that in urban areas, infants are suffering less than rural areas. Boys are suffering more than girls and the result

Table 5.5 Results of categorical logistic regressions of CIAF on the independent variables

Dependent variables	OR	95% CI	*p*-value
Place of residence			
Urban®	1.00		
Rural	1.003	0.943–1.063	0.914
Sex of the children			
Boy®	1.00		
Girl	0.764	0.731–0.798	0.000
Mother's education			
Illiterate and primary®	1.00		
Secondary	0.896	0.848–0.947	0.000
Higher	0.810	0.749–0.876	0.000
Mother's age			
15–19®	1.00		
20–29	0.853	0.778–0.935	0.001
30 and above	0.900	0.811–0.998	0.045
Religion			
Hindu®	1.00		
Muslim	1.008	1.018–1.164	0.013
Christian	0.796	0.716–0.885	0.000
Others	0.809	0.716–0.913	0.001
Mother's BMI			
Undernourished®	1.00		
Other	0.772	0.729–0.818	0.000
Wealth Index			
Poorest/poorer®	1.00		
Middle	0.817	0.768–0.869	0.000
Richer/Richest	0.695	0.652–0.742	0.000
Birth-weight-			
Very Low (<1500 g) ®	1.00		
Low (<2500 g)	0.644	0.536–0.775	0.000
Normal (2500 or above)	0.384	0.322–0.459	0.000
Zone			
North-east®	1.00		
East	1.350	1.231–1.479	0.000
Central	1.253	1.145–1.372	0.000
West	1.592	1.428–1.775	0.000
North	1.102	1.001–1.213	0.047
South	1.231	1.115–1.360	0.000
Constant	**3.641**		

® Reference category; *p*-value = 0.000 means significant at 0.001 level

is statistically significant. Infants' undernutrition is directly related with mother's education and age. By religion, Hindus and Muslims have more percentages of undernutrition than Christians and other categories. Mother's health status, wealth index of the family and birth weight of the infants are directly related with undernutrition and all these results are statistically significant. Zone-wise effect on undernutrition is same as previous cross tables and the result is statistically significant.

5.6 Discussion

It is seen that in India, out of total 32,875 infants, the percentage of undernutrition through CIAF is 47.4% considering all the seven types of combinations. On the other hand, through conventional method, the percentages of underweight, stunting and wasting are 23.4, 24.3, and 23.7, respectively. In both types of undernutrition, maximum undernutrition is seen from 0 to 2 months though in case of arthrometric failure, total percentage of undernutrition is more than the conventional methods. Through the relationship between undernutrition and socio-economy, it is seen that undernutrition is negatively related with urban locality. Boys are more undernourished than girls. Zone-wise effect shows that the lowest occurrence of undernutrition is seen in North-east zone, the highest is in West zone and then it is followed by East and Central zones. Undernourished mother and low birth weight of infants are positively related with undernutrition.

Thus, in India, childhood undernutrition is a major public health problem, and the prevalence varies over regions, socio-economic groups, gender and economically challenged groups. Most precisely, it is seen that half of the undernutrition cases are found in the six states namely Bihar, Chhattisgarh, Jharkhand, Madhya Pradesh, Rajasthan, and Uttar Pradesh (SDG-2) (United Nations 2018).

Previously, conventional method with three indicators were used uniformly to understand the under-five nutritional status. But if we compare it with CIAF method, we see that conventional method has some limitations because those three types denote different facets of undernutrition, but they are mutually co-existing (Nandy and Svedberg 2012). The first limitation is that underweight is always the sum of both acute and chronic undernutrition, but it fails to distinguish between them. Another limitation is that underweight never identifies the sum of those children who are affected by both stunted and wasted. So, this method is not sufficient to estimate the extent of anthropometric failure. The third limitation is that the percentage of undernutrition through any of the conventional methods is always less than that of CIAF, which takes the union of different types of undernutrition. If the percentage of undernutrition is high in any of the conventional criterion, then the overall percentage through CIAF will also be high. That is why, it is regarded that conventional method is not sufficient to measure the overall prevalence of undernutrition. So, to overcome this situation, for the estimation of undernourished children in a population, CIAF method is going to be popular as it provides a single figure. So far, for the last 10–15 years, the assessment of undernutrition among under-five children through CIAF has been done outside India (Khan and Jamal 2009; Berger et al. 2008; Lekprichakul et al. 2010) as well as in many parts of India (Das and Bose 2009; Biswas et al. 2018; Mukhopadhyay and Biswas 2011; Brahmbhatt et al. 2013; Dasgupta et al. 2014; Anjum et al. 2012).

So finally, it can be said that there are some shortcomings of CIAF (Bhattacharya 2006) because it cannot be interpreted as the individual rate of contribution of stunting, wasting or underweight. CIAF is a measure that can be used to see the united impact of the three conventional measures, i.e., stunting, wasting, and underweight, on health and mortality. The different components of CIAF may help clinicians understand the interaction effects of the conventional measures on morbidity and mortality of children.

References

Anjum F, Pandit MI, Mir AA, Bhat IA (2012) Z score and CIAF—A comprehensive measure of magnitude of under nutrition in a rural school going population of Kashmir, India. Glob J Med Public Health 1:46–49

Berger MR, Field-Gardner C, Wagle A, Hollenbeck CB (2008) Prevalence of malnutrition in human immunodeficiency virus/acquired immunodeficiency syndrome orphans in the Nyanza province of Kenya: a comparison of conventional indexes with a composite index of anthropometric failure. J Am Diet Assoc 108:1014–1017

Bhattacharya AK (2006) Composite index of anthropometric failure (CIAF) classification: is it more useful? Bull WHO 86:335

Biswas S, Giri SP, Bose K (2018) Assessment of nutritional status by composite index of Anthropometric failure (CIAF): a study among preschool children of Sagar Block, South 24 Parganas District, West Bengal, India. Anthropol Rev 81:269–277

Brahmbhatt KR, Hameed S, Naik PM, Prasanna KS, Jayram S (2013) Role of new anthropometric indices, validity of MUAC and Weech's formula in detecting under-nutrition among under-five children in Karnataka. Int J Biomed Adv Res 3:896–900

Das S, Bose K (2009) Report on "anthropometric failure" among rural 2-6 years old Indian Bauri caste children of West Bengal. Anthropol Rev 72:81–88

Dasgupta A, Parthasarathi R, Prabhakar VR, Biswas R, Geethanjali A (2014) Assessment of under-nutrition with composite index of anthropometric failure (CIAF) among under-five children in a rural area of West Bengal. Indian J Community Health 26:132–138

Fatimah MMN, Febriani ADB, Hatta M, Permatasari TAE, Hidayati E, Hamidah EH, Akaputra R, Turrahmi H, Anggraini RP (2021) Effect of breastfeeding on children's health and its relationship to NRAMP1 expression: a cross-sectional study. Ann Med Surg 71:103017

IFPRI (International Food Policy Research Institute) (2016) Global Nutrition Report (2016) From Promise to Impact: Ending Malnutrition by 2030. Washington, DC. IFPRI

IIPS and ICF (2021) National Family Health Survey (NFHS-5), 2019–21: India. IIPS, Mumbai

Khan REA, Jamal WN (2009) Determinants of under-nutrition of primary school-age children: a case Study of urban bahawalpur. Paper presented at: ISOSS 2009. Proceedings of the 5th International Conference on statistical sciences, mathematics, statistics and applications. 23–25; Lahore, Pakistan

Kundu RN, Borah J, Bharati S, Bharati P (2023) Regional distribution of the anthropometric failure among under-five children and its determinants, India. Ethiop J Health Sci 33(3):479–490

Lekprichakul T, Umetsu C, and Yamauchi T (2010) Child growth as a measure of household resilience: a re-examination of child nutrition situation using new growth reference standard. Vulnerability and Resilience of social-ecological systems, FR3 Project report. Kyoto: Research Institute for Humanity and Nature 98

Lopez AD, Mathers CD, Ezzati M, Jamison DT, Murray CJ (2006) Global and regional burden of disease and risk factors, 2001: systematic analysis of population health data. Lancet 367:1747–1757

Ministry of Health RI (2020) Regulation of the minister of health of the Republic of Indonesia Number 2 of 2020 about child anthropometry standards

Mukhopadhyay DK, Biswas AB (2011) Food security and anthropometric failure among tribal children in Bankura, West Bengal. Indian Pediatr 48:311–314

Nandy S, Svedberg P (2012) The composite index of anthropometric failure (CIAF): an alternative indicator of malnutrition in young children. In: Preedy V (ed) Handbook of anthropometry: physical measures of human form in health and diseases. Springer, London, pp 127–137

Nandy S, Irving M, Gordon D, Subramanian SV, Smith GD (2005) Poverty, child under-[9] nutrition and morbidity: new evidence from India. Bull World Health Organ 83:210–216

Permatasari TAE, Sudiartini NW (2020) Do health workers play a role in exclusive breastfeeding among working mothers in industrial area? J Nutr Sci Vitaminol (Tokyo) 66(Supplement):S94–S98

Permatasari TAE, Sartika RAD, Achadi EL, Purwono U, Irawati A, Ocviyanti D, Martha E (2018) Exclusive breastfeeding intention among pregnant women. Kesmas 12:134–141

Permatasari TAE, Rizqiya F, Kusumaningati W, Suryaalamsah II, Hermi-wahyoeni Z (2021) The effect of nutrition and reproductive health education of pregnant women in Indonesia using quasi experimental study. BMC Pregnancy Childbirth 21:1–15

Rice AL, Sacco L, Hyder A, Black RE (2000) Malnutrition as an underlying cause of childhood deaths associated with infectious diseases in developing countries. Bull World Health Organ 78:1207–1221

Romieu I, Dossus L, Barquera S, Blottière HM, Franks PW, Gunter M, Hwalla N, Hursting SD, Leitzmann M, Margetts B, Nishida C, Potischman N, Seidell J, Stepien M, Wang Y, Westerterp K, Winichagoon P, Wiseman M, Willett WC (2017) IARC Working Group on Energy Balance and Obesity Cancer Causes Control. 28: 247–258

Rutstein S (1999) Wealth versus expenditure: comparison between the DHS wealth index and household expenditures in your departments of Guatemala. ORC Macro, Calverton, Maryland

Shabariah R, Hatta M, Idris I, Santoso A, Patellongi I, Permatasari TAE, Islam FAA (2021) Comparison TLR2 and TLR4 serum levels in children with pulmonary and extrapulmonary tuberculosis with and without a Bacillus Calmette-Guérin (BCG) scar. J Clin Tuberc Other Mycobact Dis 25:100272

Svedberg P (2000) Oxford India Paperbacks; New Delhi: 2000. Poverty and undernutrition: theory, measurement and policy. [Citation date: 21/01/2020]

Talukder A (2017) Factors associated with malnutrition among under-five children: Illustration using Bangladesh demographic and health survey, 2014 Data. Children, 4:1–8. https://doi.org/10.3390/children4100088

Titaley CR, Ariawan I, Hapsari D, Muasyaroh A, Dibley MJ (2019) Determinants of the stunting of children under two years old in Indonesia: a multilevel analysis of the 2013 Indonesia basic health survey. Nutrients 11:1106

UNICEF (2013) Improving child nutrition: the achievable imperative for global progress. New York. 1–14

UNICEF (2014) Republic of Yemen (Ministry of Planning and International Cooperation) & UNICEF, Situation analysis of children in Yemen 2014. (https://www.unicef.org/media/files/Yemen_Situation_Analysis_report_-_English_Final.pdf, Accessed 27 August 2018)

United Nations (2018) Ending poverty and hunger for all persons with disabilities 9Goals 1 and 2). UN: https://www.un.org/development/desa/disabilities/envision2030-goal2.html)

Victora CG, Christian P, Vidaletti LP, Gatica-Domínguez G, Menon P, Black RE (2021) Revisiting maternal and child undernutrition in low-income and middle-income countries: variable progress towards an unfinished agenda. Lancet 397:1388–1399

WHO (2006) WHO Child Growth Standards: length/height-for-age, weight-for-age, weight-for-length, weight-for-height and body mass index-for-age: methods and development

WHO (2010) Nutrition Landscape Information System country profile indicators: interpretation guide. http://apps.who.int/iris/bitstream/handle/10665/44397/9789241599955_eng.pdf?sequence=1&isAllowed=y, Accessed 27 August 2018)
WHO (2015) Millennium development goals to SDGs, sustainable development goals

Zonal Distribution and Determinants of Stunting, Wasting, Underweight, and Thinness among the Indian Under-Five Children: Findings from NFHS-5

6

Ramendra Nath Kundu, Arna Chatterjee, Susmita Bharati, Manoranjan Pal, Md. Golam Hossain, and Premananda Bharati

6.1 Introduction

Undernutrition accounts for over half of all deaths among children under the age of five worldwide, making it a serious public health concern (UNICEF 2021). Child undernutrition is the inability to meet a child's requirements for physiological function, growth, and the ability to respond to illness as a result of an insufficient diet (Griffiths et al. 2001; Jain et al. 2020; Wells et al. 2019). It impairs the immune system and raises the risk of childhood mortality and morbidity, including increased infection severity, drug toxicity, risk of tuberculosis, and anemia in children (Padmapriyadarsini et al. 2016; Reddy et al. 2021; Tandoh et al. 2021; UNICEF 2021). In 2017, UNICEF, WHO, and World Bank Group jointly assumed that 155 million children under the age of five are chronically undernourished (UNICEF/

R. N. Kundu
Department of Anthropology, West Bengal State University, Barasat, West Bengal, India

A. Chatterjee
Anthropological Survey of India, SRC, Mysuru, India

S. Bharati
Sociological Research Unit, Indian Statistical Institute, Kolkata, West Bengal, India

M. Pal
Economic Research Unit, Indian Statistical Institute (ISI), Kolkata, West Bengal, India

M. G. Hossain (✉)
Department of Statistics, University of Rajshahi, Rajshahi, Bangladesh

P. Bharati
Biological Anthropology Unit, Indian Statistical Institute (ISI),
Kolkata, West Bengal, India

M. Pal et al. (eds.), *Public Health and Nutrition*,
https://doi.org/10.1007/978-981-97-7890-4_6

WHO/WBG 2017; WHO 2017). In 2021, the same joint venture estimated that globally 149.2 million under-five children were suffering from stunting and 45.5 million from wasting (UNICEF/WHO/WBG 2021). Stunting is diminishing globally, with some exceptions in Africa, but wasting is more prevalent in Southern Asia. Asia is home to more than three-quarters of children suffering from severe wasting (UNICEF/WHO/WBG 2021). Child undernutrition is a major public health burden in developing nations, accounting for around 45 percent of children dying before their fifth birthday, mostly in low- and middle-income countries (Pike et al. 2021; Victora et al. 2021; WHO 2021).

India contains about one-fifth of the world's population and is one of the fastest-growing nations in terms of economic, educational, and technical development, but still confronting undernutrition, disease, poverty, poor sanitation, maternal health, and low education (Bishwajit et al. 2014; Narayan et al. 2019; Pandit et al. 2021). Undernutrition was widespread across the country, with children in the Northeast were suffering, which was geographically an integral part of the Indo-Burma biodiversity (Singh et al. 2015). Stunting was most common in Meghalaya and Assam, while Arunachal Pradesh and Sikkim were experiencing an increase in stunting and wasting (Meitei 2020). In the East, West Bengal suffered most from stunting and underweight, while stunting was most prevalent in Bihar, and children in Orissa were particularly suffering from wasting (Pati et al. 2018; Roshania et al. 2022; Stiller et al. 2020). Maharashtra is the richest state in India, yet had a high prevalence of stunting, wasting, and underweight among under-five children, especially in the urban sector. In Gujarat, children also suffered from severe underweight . Both Maharashtra and Gujarat belong to West zone (Ghosh and Varerkar 2019; Matariya et al. 2016; Murarkar et al. 2020). Underweight and wasting rates among children have increased in Delhi, the country's capital, as well as in Madhya Pradesh (Wachs 2008; Yirga et al. 2019).

According to previous studies, the primary factors of child undernutrition were maternal health and education, food scarcity, and poverty (Wachs 2008; Yirga et al. 2019). Therefore, the Government of India launched numerous initiatives under the National Health Mission (NHM) to accomplish the Sustainable Development Goals (SDGs), the most notable of which was Janani Shishu Suraksha Karyakram (JSSK) in 2011, Reproductive, Maternal, Newborn, Child and Adolescent Health (RMNCH+A) in 2013, Rashtriya Bal Swasthya Karyakram (RBSK) in 2013, and India Newborn Action Plan (INAP) in 2014, which are still ongoing (NHM 2011, 2013a, b, 2014). But still, the progress of the nutritional status of children was not very encouraging as it is reflected by the findings of the present study. The nutritional status of children, however, depends on many things some of which were beyond the purview of these action plans.

The current study is to compare child (under-five) undernutrition, which included stunting, wasting, underweight, and thinness among all the zones of India. The study also intended to determine the effect of child health and demographic, maternal, and socio-demographic factors on child undernutrition.

6.2 Methods

Data Source The unit-level data were obtained from the National Family Health Survey 2019 to 2021, a systematic household survey conducted in India that emphasizes child and mother health, mortality and sociodemographic characteristics. The NFHS adhered to the guidelines of the Demographic and Health Surveys (DHS) Program, which included standardized field methodology, sampling designs, and data management. In order to comprehend child undernutrition in various zones of India, the NFHS data was selected. As a nodal body in the country, the International Institute for Population Sciences (IIPS) has conducted the survey in compliance with the DHS Program's standards. Out of the 2,834,297 recorded household members, 221,364 children under the age of five were taken into account in the statistical analysis; the flow chart in Fig. 6.1 demonstrates the data inclusion and exclusion criteria. Invalid samples were excluded from the analysis, which included a range of incomplete and extraneous data, such as height, weight, and age beyond reasonable limits, and missing anthropometric measurements.

Division of Zone in India India has 28 States and 8 Union Territories (UTs), which were classified into six zones in NFHS-5 based on geographical location, namely, Central, East, North, Northeast, South and West. The most populous state Uttar Pradesh along with Madhya Pradesh, and Chhattisgarh, were included in the Central Zone. The states, Bihar, Jharkhand, Odisha, and West Bengal comprise

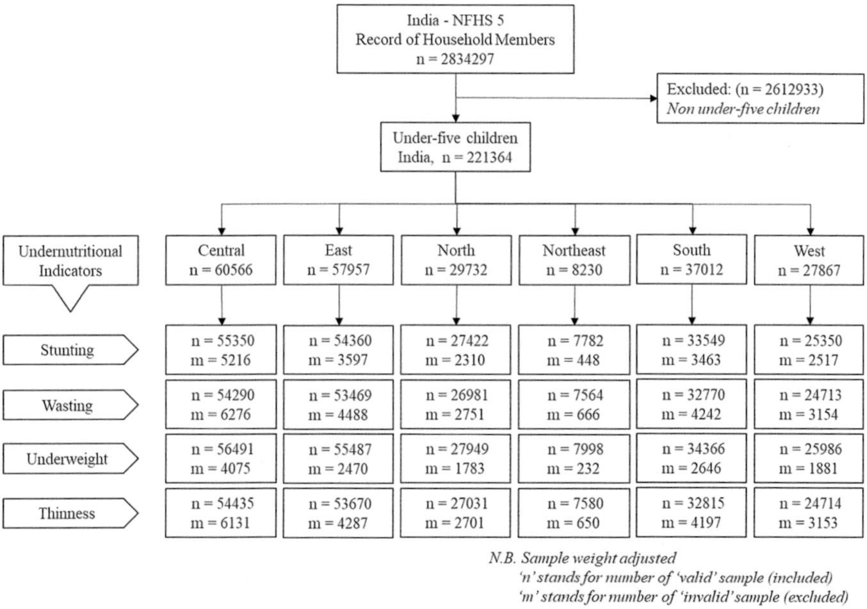

Fig. 6.1 Sample determination of under-five children in India for this study

the East zone, with West Bengal and Orissa situated on the Eastern Indian coast (Mukhopadhyay and Karisiddaiah 2014). The North Zone includes four states, namely, Haryana, Himachal Pradesh, Punjab, and Rajasthan, and four UTs, namely, Chandigarh, Jammu and Kashmir, and Ladakh with the capital Delhi. The Himalayas, Tibetan Plateau, and a desert called "Thor" are all part of the area (Kar 2014). The Northeast zone consists of eight states, namely, Arunachal Pradesh, Assam, Manipur, Meghalaya, Mizoram, Nagaland, Sikkim, and Tripura, characterized by unique geography and ethnic diversity. The South zone consists of the five states of Andhra Pradesh, Karnataka, Kerala, Tamil Nadu, and Telangana, and three UTs of Andaman and Nicobar Islands, Lakshadweep, and Puducherry. The three states of Goa, Gujarat, and Maharashtra and the UTs of Dadra & Nagar Haveli and Daman & Diu are all part of the west zone.

Indicators of Child Undernutrition Four indicators were considered to measure undernutrition of under-five children, namely, stunting, wasting, underweight, and thinness. Each of these indicators denotes inadequate and poor nutrition, with distinct impacts on health. A child is considered to be stunted if their height is too short for their age. This results in a child being more frequently afflicted by infections during the first 1000 days of life, as well as impaired cognitive and physical development (WHO 2014). Wasting refers to children who have less weight for their height as a result of inadequate nourishment. Particularly when the wasting is severe, it impairs the immune system, leading to long-term developmental problems and increasing the chance of death (UNICEF/WHO/WBG 2021). Underweight refers to children who have too little weight for their age. Thinness is defined as a low BMI for the age of a child (Cameron 2007). Both underweight and thinness have a detrimental effect on health, resulting in poor academic performance as well as mental and physical deterioration.

6.3 Study Variables

Outcome Variable Stunting, wasting, underweight, and thinness were the outcome variables, considered as the indicator of undernutrition among under-five Indian children. The z-score was taken into account while determining indicators of child undernutrition. The World Health Organization's standard z-score was used to estimate the sample's z-score, which classified undernutrition as having a z-score less than -2SD (WHO 2006). Stunting was defined as a z-score less than -2SD in height-for-age, while wasting in weight-for-height, underweight in weight-for-age, and thinness in BMI-for-age. Children, who met the criteria for sufficient height, weight, and BMI (z-score ≥ -2SD) comparatively, were deemed to be in a non-undernourished category. The data on child nutrition was analyzed using a dichotomous category, with a z-score of <-2SD considered for target groups and ≥ -2SD for reference groups.

Explanatory Variables The study examined potential predictors of stunting, wasting, underweight, and thinness in children, such as child health and demographics, maternal and sociodemographic factors. Explanatory variables were categorized directly by utilizing or modified from previously published studies, while the meaning remained the same. The child health-and-demographic factors include anemia in children (anemic, non-anemic), gender of the children (boy, girl), and parents alive (alive, not alive) (Islam et al. 2021; Teferi and Teshome 2021; Tesfaw and Fenta 2021). The maternal factors include birth order (1st & 2nd, 3rd & more) and mother's education (non-educated, primary, secondary, higher) (Aboagye et al. 2021; Geda et al. 2021). Maternal education in this context refers to the mother's formal educational credentials. The variables of socio-demographic factors include residence (rural, urban), social category (ST, SC, OBC, general), family type (nuclear, non-nuclear), and wealth index (poor, middle, rich) (Blankenship et al. 2020; Hasan et al. 2020; Soni et al. 2022; Tesema et al. 2021). Here, ST stands for scheduled tribe, SC for scheduled caste, and OBC for other backward classes.

Statistical Analysis The descriptive analysis involves mean and standard deviation for quantitative variables that were used to evaluate z-score distribution, as well as frequency distribution and percentage for categorical variables. The ANOVA test was used to compare the variations in the mean z-score of the nutritional indicator across the zones. The Pearson's Chi-square (χ^2) test was used to examine the association between two categorical variables, including undernutrition indicators and explanatory variables. Binary logistic regression was used to determine the explanatory factors that contribute to child undernutrition. In the regression, undernutrition was coded as "1," while its counterpart, non-undernutrition, was coded as "0." A multicollinearity test was performed before the selection of the independent variables, and the tests suggest that the variance inflation factor (VIF) was under 5 (Berhe et al. 2021; Cheng et al. 2022). Statistical significance was examined using a 95% confidence interval, and $p < 0.05$ was considered significant. The Omnibus Chi-square was used to determine whether the data fit properly into the logistic regression model. The Statistical Package for the Social Sciences (SPSS, version 25.0) was used for statistical analysis.

6.4 Results

The study included a total of 221,365 under-five children, with a mean age of 29.55 months (SD 17.42). These differed by zone, North 29.44 (SD 17.54), Central 29.29 (SD 17.54), East 29.41 (SD 17.32), Northeast 30.11 (SD 17.26), West 30.21 (SD 17.26), and South 29.64 (SD 17.44), with a significant difference of ANOVA (F-value 13.74, $p < 0.001$).

Figure 6.2 compares the nutritional status of the children studied in the zonal division (simple line) to the WHO standard (dotted line). Despite the z-scores of the nutritional indicators in this zonal division having a normal distribution, they were on the negative side of the WHO standard Z-score curve, suggesting poor nutritional status. The tails were thick and the overall plots were almost asymmetrical. BAZ was almost evenly distributed across all zones, being much closer to the WHO, except for the West. There was a similarity across the zones in HAZ, where the tail density was more prominent and the distribution was platykurtic and nearly asymmetrical. The WHZ in the Central, North, Northeast, and South was found to be

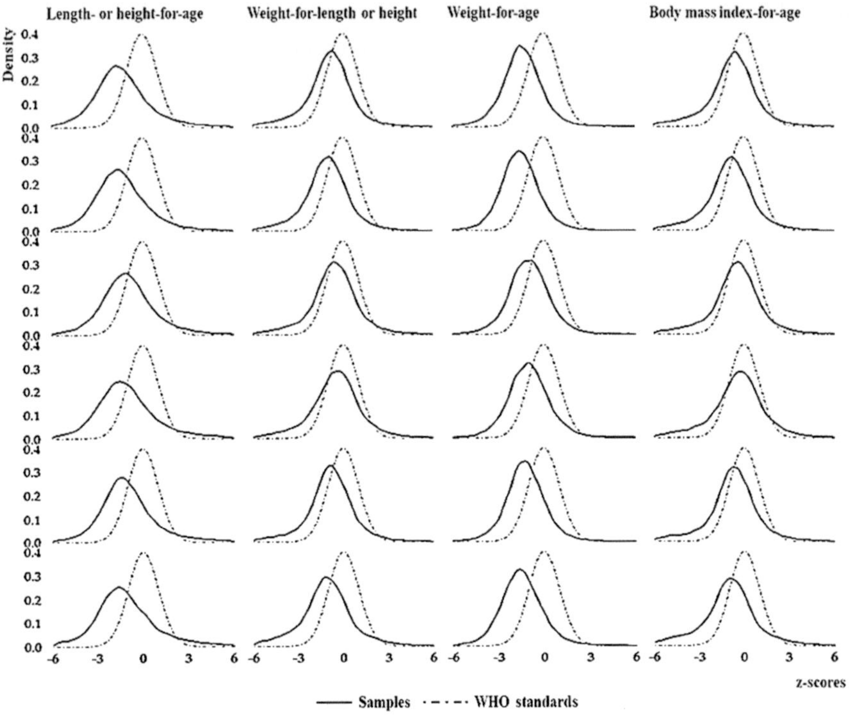

Fig. 6.2 Z-score distribution of nutritional indicators across the zone in India compared to WHO standards

symmetrical, with a reduction in tail density and plots were slightly closer to the WHO standard. In the North and Northeast, WAZ was asymmetrically distributed, while the tail density decreased. The West, Central, and East zones had very poor nutritional status in terms of HAZ, WHZ and WAZ, children's height and weight were below WHO requirements.

It was observed that there were significant differences in mean z-scores of each nutritional indicator, such as HAZ, WHZ, WAZ, and BAZ, among the zonal divisions, with the F-value of the ANOVA test being highly significant ($p < 0.001$) (Table 6.1).

The zonal distribution of undernutrition among under-five children in India is depicted in Fig. 6.3. The East (38.51) and Central (38.46) had the highest prevalence of stunting, while the North (29.56) and South (29.66) had the lowest. The highest prevalence of wasting was found in the West (25.40) and East (21.57), while the lowest was found in the North (14.74) and South (17.19). Underweight prevalence was highest in the West (37.26) and East (36.95), while it was lowest in the North (24.04) and South (27.22). The highest prevalence of thinness was found in the West (23.07) and East (19.34), while the lowest was found in the North (14.15) and South (15.77). Stunting and underweight were common and major issues in each zone, whereas thinness was less frequent in Indian children (Fig. 6.4). More

Table 6.1 Zonal differences in the mean Z-scores of nutritional indicators

Indicators	Central	East	North	Northeast	South	West	*F*-value	*p*-value
HAZ	−1.44 (1.79)	−1.44 (1.80)	−1.13 (1.76)	−1.26 (1.91)	−1.14 (1.75)	−1.29 (1.94)	225.61	<0.001
WHZ	−0.81 (1.45)	−0.98 (1.48)	−0.62 (1.49)	−0.74 (1.62)	−0.80 (1.47)	−1.07 (1.60)	339.21	<0.001
WAZ	−1.49 (1.30)	−1.60 (1.29)	−1.16 (1.33)	−1.35 (1.38)	−1.31 (1.30)	−1.59 (1.34)	581.09	<0.001
BAZ	−0.68 (1.50)	−0.84 (1.52)	−0.53 (1.52)	−0.62 (1.67)	−0.69 (1.51)	−0.94 (1.63)	261.86	<0.001

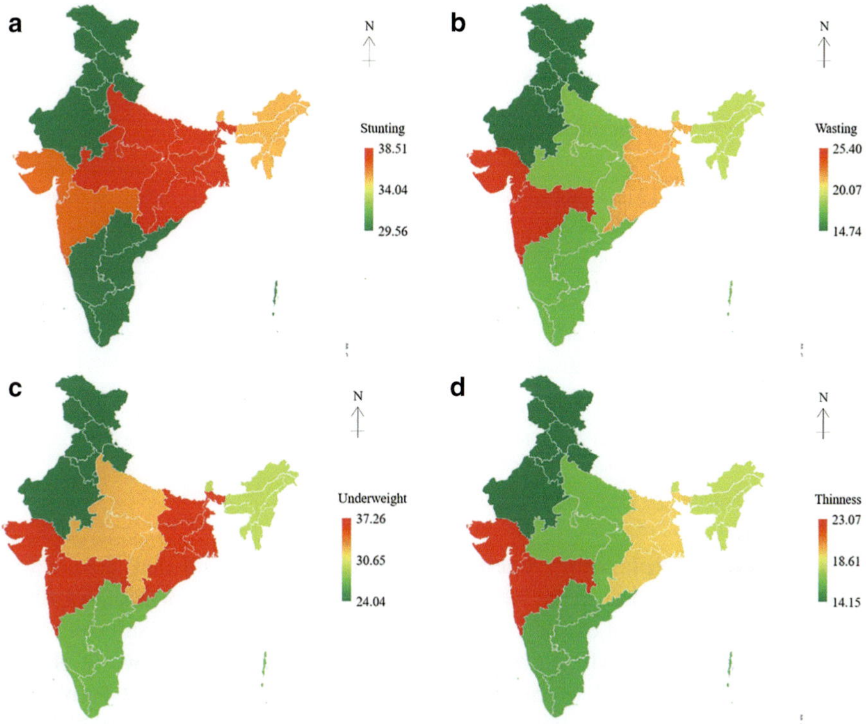

Fig. 6.3 Prevalence of undernutrition among under-five children in India across the geographical zones, (**a**) stunting, (**b**) wasting, (**c**) underweight, (**d**) thinness. Note: The figures were drawn by one of the authors. However, it came out to be like that of Kundu et al. (2024)

than one in every three children in the Central, East, Northeast, and West were suffering from stunting, accounting for 69.85 percent of the children. Similarly, in the East and West zones, more than one out of every three children was underweight. The Chi-square test revealed that the measures of variability of each indicator differed significantly between the zones, with *p* values of <0.001 for each indicator (Table 6.2).

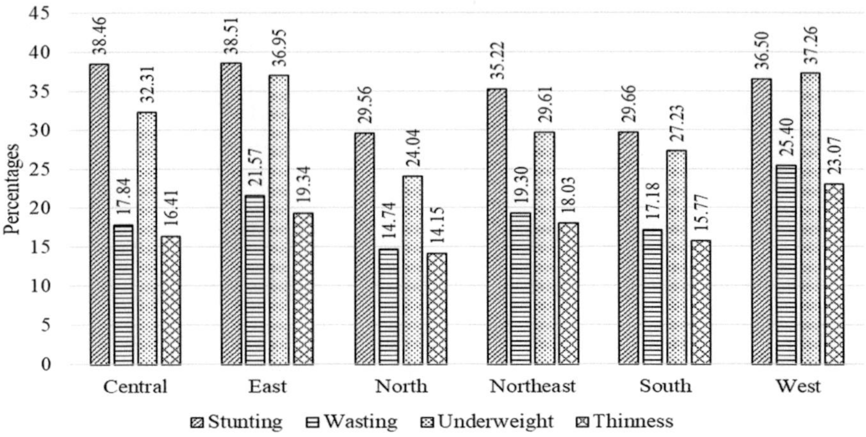

Fig. 6.4 Distribution of nutritional status across the zones

Table 6.2 Prevalence of undernutrition among under-five Indian children by different zones

Nutritional status	Central % (*n*)	East % (*n*)	North % (*n*)	Northeast % (*n*)	South % (*n*)	West % (*n*)	χ^2-value[a]	*p*-value
Stunting	38.46 (21,288)	38.51 (20,936)	29.56 (8106)	35.22 (2741)	29.66 (9951)	36.50 (9253)	1361.44	<0.001
Wasting	17.84 (9684)	21.57 (11,533)	14.74 (3976)	19.30 (1460)	17.18 (5632)	25.40 (6276)	1295.65	<0.001
Underweight	32.31 (18,250)	36.95 (20,502)	24.04 (6720)	29.61 (2368)	27.23 (9356)	37.26 (9683)	2146.90	<0.001
Thinness	16.41 (8935)	19.34 (10,382)	14.15 (3824)	18.03 (1367)	15.77 (5176)	23.07 (5701)	969.87	<0.001

[a]Pearson Chi-Square (χ^2) test within the zones

Distribution of Explanatory Factors by Zones It was found that anemia was more common in children in the West (73.51%), North (70.09%), and East (69.40%), with more than three out of every five children under the age of five suffering from anemia in these zones. The percentage gap between boys and girls was higher in North (5.26%), followed by South (4.10%) and East (3.93%). The number of orphans was varied by zone, with the Northeast having the most prevalence (1.16%). Up to two children were more common in each zone, with the highest prevalence in the South (85.03%). Maternal education varied significantly between zones, with the most non-educated (formal education) mothers in the East (29.39%) and the higher-educated mothers in the South (28.21%). Rural areas predominated in each zone, with the Northeast having the highest (85.29%). In each zone, majority of children belonged to the OBC community, except for the Northeast, where 39.42% of the children belonged to the ST community. The number of non-nuclear families was higher than the number of nuclear families in all zones except for Northeast. There was wide variation between zones in terms of wealth index, with poor households inhabiting in the Central (53.31%), East (70.79%), and Northeast (72.61%), while rich households spearheaded in the North (56.09%), West (49.32%), and South (52.22%) (Table 6.3).

Table 6.3 Explanatory factors and their distribution according to the zonal divisions

Explanatory	Central	East	North	Northeast	South	West	χ^2—across	p-value
Factors	% (n)	% (n)	% (n)	% (n)	% (n)	% (n)	Zones	
Anemia in children								
Anemic	68.66 (32,829)	69.40 (33,922)	70.09 (16,827)	64.26 (4521)	60.55 (18,300)	73.51 (17,058)	1243.36	<0.001
Non-anemic	31.34 (14,988)	30.60 (14,958)	29.91 (7180)	35.74 (2515)	39.45 (11,924)	26.49 (6147)		
Gender of children								
Boy	51.42 (31,141)	51.99 (30,134)	52.63 (15,647)	50.60 (4164)	52.05 (19,263)	51.91 (14,465)	18.01	0.003
Girl	48.58 (29,426)	48.01 (27,823)	47.37 (14,085)	49.40 (4066)	47.95 (17,749)	48.09 (13,402)		
Parents alive								
Alive	98.98 (59,929)	99.11 (57,415)	99.21 (29,493)	98.84 (8127)	98.99 (36,606)	99.17 (27,629)	22.18	<0.001
Not alive	1.02 (619)	0.89 (518)	0.79 (235)	1.16 (95)	1.01 (372)	0.83 (232)		
Birth order								
1st & 2nd	65.98 (39,314)	68.75 (39,182)	75.46 (22,061)	73.51 (5984)	85.03 (31,138)	78.47 (21,475)	5209.43	<0.001
3rd & more	34.02 (20,271)	31.25 (17,810)	24.54 (7175)	26.49 (2156)	14.97 (5483)	21.53 (5892)		
Mother's education								
Non-educated	26.08 (15,796)	29.39 (17,026)	20.95 (6229)	14.98 (1233)	7.53 (2788)	11.43 (3185)	16,621.22	<0.001
Primary	13.76 (8331)	13.90 (8052)	13.70 (4073)	16.52 (1360)	6.27 (2319)	10.37 (2889)		
Secondary	45.40 (27,498)	48.19 (27,921)	46.80 (13,915)	61.20 (5037)	57.99 (21,464)	61.35 (17,096)		

(continued)

Table 6.3 (continued)

Explanatory	Central	East	North	Northeast	South	West	χ^2—across	*p*-value
Higher	14.76 (8940)	8.53 (4942)	18.55 (5514)	7.30 (601)	28.21 (10,440)	16.86 (4698)		
Residence								
Rural	79.40 (48,090)	82.74 (47,956)	68.80 (20,455)	85.29 (7020)	61.07 (22,605)	59.56 (16,598)	10,265.85	<0.001
Urban	20.60 (12,476)	17.26 (10,001)	31.20 (9277)	14.71 (1211)	38.93 (14,407)	40.44 (11,269)		
Social category								
ST	9.23 (5519)	11.32 (5963)	8.46 (2436)	39.42 (2266)	6.53 (2353)	17.14 (4447)	15,896.76	<0.001
SC	25.38 (15,182)	27.92 (14,713)	29.35 (8455)	15.79 (908)	24.13 (8692)	16.31 (4232)		
OBC	50.02 (29,922)	41.47 (21,855)	34.24 (9862)	25.64 (1474)	58.90 (21,220)	36.30 (9419)		
General	15.37 (9193)	19.29 (10,168)	27.95 (8052)	19.15 (1101)	10.45 (3764)	30.25 (7850)		
Family type								
Nuclear	36.74 (22,251)	42.78 (24,792)	30.22 (8986)	50.19 (4131)	38.12 (14,108)	30.76 (8572)	2488.62	<0.001
Non-nuclear	63.26 (38,315)	57.22 (33,165)	69.78 (20,746)	49.81 (4099)	61.88 (22,904)	69.24 (19,295)		
Wealth index								
Poor	53.31 (32,290)	70.79 (41,028)	24.71 (7346)	72.61 (5976)	19.52 (7225)	28.38 (7909)	40583.62	<0.001
Middle	17.88 (10,830)	15.42 (8937)	19.20 (5709)	15.55 (1280)	28.26 (10,460)	22.30 (6215)		
Rich	28.80 (17,446)	13.79 (7992)	56.09 (16,677)	11.83 (974)	52.22 (19,327)	49.32 (13,743)		

6.5 Factors Affecting Undernutrition

Tables 6.4, 6.5, 6.6 and 6.7 shows the contribution of explanatory factors on child undernutrition in zonal divisions using binary logistic regression. Stunting, wasting, underweight, and thinness were used to characterize child undernutrition (coded as

Table 6.4 Model illustrates the role of explanatory factors on stunting among under-five children in Indian zones

	Central	East	North	Northeast	South	West
Explanatory factors	AOR (95% CI)	AOR (95% CI)	AOR (95% CI)	AOR (95% CI)	AOR (95% CI)	AOR (95% CI)
Anemia in children (Ref. Non-anemic)						
Anemic	1.32 (1.27, 1.38)***	1.25 (1.20, 1.30)***	1.29 (1.21, 1.37)***	1.31 (1.15, 1.49)***	1.44 (1.37, 1.52)***	1.38 (1.29, 1.48)***
Gender of children (Ref. Girl)						
Boy	1.09 (1.05, 1.13)***	1.02 (0.98, 1.06)	1.15 (1.08, 1.21)***	1.09 (0.96, 1.23)	1.04 (0.99, 1.09)	1.05 (0.99, 1.11)
Parents alive (Ref. Alive)						
Not alive	1.10 (0.92, 1.32)	0.88 (0.71, 1.09)	1.02 (0.74, 1.39)	1.15 (0.67, 1.98)	0.88 (0.68, 1.13)	1.05 (0.78, 1.40)
Birth order (Ref. 1st & 2nd)						
3rd & more	1.11 (1.06, 1.16)***	1.18 (1.12, 1.23)***	1.18 (1.10, 1.26)***	1.20 (1.03, 1.39)*	1.20 (1.12, 1.29)***	1.12 (1.04, 1.20)**
Mother's education (Ref. Higher)						
Non-educated	1.80 (1.68, 1.94)***	2.39 (2.17, 2.64)***	1.55 (1.38, 1.73)***	2.06 (1.47, 2.88)***	1.75 (1.56, 1.95)***	1.68 (1.48, 1.91)***
Primary	1.65 (1.52, 1.79)***	1.81 (1.64, 2.01)***	1.61 (1.44, 1.81)***	2.13 (1.53, 2.96)***	1.63 (1.46, 1.83)***	1.74 (1.54, 1.98)***
Secondary	1.33 (1.25, 1.42)***	1.48 (1.35, 1.62)***	1.43 (1.31, 1.57)***	1.55 (1.16, 2.07)**	1.30 (1.21, 1.38)***	1.42 (1.30, 1.56)***
Residence (Ref. Urban)						
Rural	1.01 (0.96, 1.07)	0.95 (0.90, 1.01)	1.11 (1.05, 1.17)***	1.04 (0.86, 1.27)	1.13 (1.07, 1.20)***	1.20 (1.14, 1.26)***
Social category (Ref. General)						
ST	1.12 (1.03, 1.22)**	1.13 (1.05, 1.22)**	1.16 (1.03, 1.31)*	1.13 (0.95, 1.35)	1.37 (1.20, 1.56)***	1.44 (1.31, 1.58)***
SC	1.37 (1.29, 1.47)***	1.17 (1.10, 1.24)***	1.25 (1.15, 1.35)***	1.05 (0.85, 1.29)	1.27 (1.15, 1.41)***	1.49 (1.36, 1.62)***
OBC	1.19 (1.13, 1.27)***	1.14 (1.07, 1.20)***	1.17 (1.08, 1.26)***	0.90 (0.74, 1.09)	1.15 (1.05, 1.27)**	1.31 (1.22, 1.41)***
Family type (Ref. Non-nuclear)						
Nuclear	1.06 (1.02, 1.11)**	1.01 (0.97, 1.06)	1.08 (1.01, 1.15)*	1.13 (1.00, 1.29)	0.92 (0.87, 0.97)**	0.95 (0.89, 1.01)
Wealth index (Ref. Rich)						
Poor	1.62 (1.53, 1.71)***	1.99 (1.84, 2.16)***	1.64 (1.51, 1.79)***	1.56 (1.22, 1.99)***	1.66 (1.54, 1.80)***	1.79 (1.64, 1.94)***
Middle	1.33 (1.25, 1.42)***	1.43 (1.31, 1.55)***	1.43 (1.32, 1.55)***	1.20 (0.92, 1.55)	1.31 (1.22, 1.39)***	1.42 (1.31, 1.54)***

Significant ***$p < 0.001$, **$p < 0.01$, *$p < 0.05$

Table 6.5 Model illustrates the role of explanatory factors on wasting among under-five children in Indian zones

	Central	East	North	Northeast	South	West
Explanatory factors	AOR (95% CI)	AOR (95% CI)	AOR (95% CI)	AOR (95% CI)	AOR (95% CI)	AOR (95% CI)
Anemia in children (Ref. Non-anemic)						
Anemic	1.08 (1.02, 1.14)**	1.27 (1.21, 1.34)***	1.10 (1.01, 1.20)*	1.10 (0.94, 1.29)	1.07 (1.00, 1.14)	1.12 (1.04, 1.21)**
Gender of children (Ref. Girl)						
Boy	1.11 (1.06, 1.17)***	1.09 (1.04, 1.14)***	1.16 (1.07, 1.25)***	1.17 (1.01, 1.36)*	1.15 (1.07, 1.22)***	1.13 (1.06, 1.20)***
Parents alive (Ref. Alive)						
Not alive	1.14 (0.91, 1.43)	1.03 (0.80, 1.31)	0.76 (0.48, 1.21)	0.95 (0.47, 1.91)	0.94 (0.68, 1.29)	0.88 (0.63, 1.24)
Birth order (Ref. 1st & 2nd)						
3rd & more	1.02 (0.96, 1.08)	1.10 (1.04, 1.16)**	1.02 (0.93, 1.12)	0.93 (0.76, 1.12)	0.94 (0.86, 1.03)	1.00 (0.92, 1.08)
Mother's education (Ref. Higher)						
Non-educated	1.22 (1.11, 1.34)***	1.04 (0.93, 1.16)	1.23 (1.06, 1.42)**	1.30 (0.87, 1.94)	1.40 (1.23, 1.61)***	0.89 (0.77, 1.02)
Primary	1.10 (0.99, 1.22)	0.92 (0.82, 1.04)	1.29 (1.11, 1.50)**	1.30 (0.88, 1.92)	1.10 (0.95, 1.27)	0.98 (0.86, 1.12)
Secondary	1.10 (1.01, 1.20)*	0.94 (0.85, 1.04)	1.22 (1.08, 1.37)**	0.99 (0.71, 1.40)	1.09 (1.00, 1.18)*	0.91 (0.83, 1.01)
Residence (Ref. Urban)						
Rural	0.91 (0.86, 0.96***	1.07 (1.01, 1.13)*	0.92 (0.84, 1.01)	1.15 (0.90, 1.47)	1.09 (1.02, 1.15)**	1.15 (1.07, 1.24)***
Social category (Ref. General)						
ST	1.43 (1.29, 1.59)***	1.27 (1.16, 1.40)***	1.38 (1.19, 1.61)***	0.70 (0.56, 0.87)**	1.38 (1.18, 1.62)***	1.61 (1.45, 1.78)***
SC	1.12 (1.02, 1.22)*	1.31 (1.22, 1.41)***	1.14 (1.02, 1.27)*	1.09 (0.86, 1.40)	1.16 (1.02, 1.32)*	0.98 (0.89, 1.09)
OBC	1.14 (1.05, 1.23)**	1.16 (1.08, 1.24)***	1.16 (1.05, 1.29)**	1.00 (0.80, 1.25)	1.08 (0.96, 1.21)	1.27 (1.17, 1.37)***
Family type (Ref. Non-nuclear)						
Nuclear	1.03 (0.98, 1.09)	1.04 (0.99, 1.09)	1.02 (0.94, 1.11)	0.97 (0.83, 1.14)	1.01 (0.95, 1.08)	1.29 (1.20, 1.38)***

(continued)

Table 6.5 (continued)

Explanatory factors	Central AOR (95% CI)	East AOR (95% CI)	North AOR (95% CI)	Northeast AOR (95% CI)	South AOR (95% CI)	West AOR (95% CI)
Wealth index (Ref. Rich)						
Poor	1.14 (1.06, 1.22)**	1.25 (1.14, 1.37)***	1.25 (1.11, 1.39)***	1.53 (1.12, 2.08)**	1.36 (1.24, 1.50)***	1.09 (1.00, 1.2)
Middle	1.01 (0.93, 1.10)	1.01 (0.91, 1.11)	1.18 (1.06, 1.31)**	1.19 (0.85, 1.65)	1.15 (1.06, 1.24)**	1.00 (0.91, 1.09)

Significant ***$p < 0.001$, **$p < 0.01$, *$p < 0.05$

Table 6.6 Model illustrates the role of explanatory factors on underweight among under-five children in Indian zones

Explanatory factors	Central AOR (95% CI)	East AOR (95% CI)	North AOR (95% CI)	Northeast AOR (95% CI)	South AOR (95% CI)	West AOR (95% CI)
Anemia in children (Ref. Non-anemic)						
Anemic	1.15 (1.10, 1.20)***	1.25 (1.20, 1.31)***	1.23 (1.15, 1.32)***	1.34 (1.16, 1.53)***	1.25 (1.18, 1.32)***	1.23 (1.15, 1.32)***
Gender of children (Ref. Girl)						
Boy	1.11 (1.06, 1.15)***	1.00 (0.96, 1.04)	1.14 (1.07, 1.22)***	1.22 (1.07, 1.39)**	1.09 (1.03, 1.15)**	1.14 (1.08, 1.21)***
Parents alive (Ref. Alive)						
Not alive	1.03 (0.85, 1.25)	1.21 (0.98, 1.49)	0.81 (0.57, 1.15)	0.88 (0.48, 1.60)	1.10 (0.86, 1.42)	1.06 (0.79, 1.41)
Birth order (Ref. 1st & 2nd)						
3rd & more	1.08 (1.04, 1.13)***	1.21 (1.16, 1.27)***	1.18 (1.10, 1.27)***	1.07 (0.92, 1.26)	1.21 (1.12, 1.30)***	1.16 (1.08, 1.24)***
Mother's education (Ref. Higher)						
Non-educated	1.64 (1.52, 1.77)***	1.96 (1.78, 2.16)***	1.75 (1.55, 1.99)***	2.44 (1.68, 3.55)***	1.90 (1.70, 2.13)***	1.43 (1.26, 1.63)***
Primary	1.42 (1.31, 1.54)***	1.45 (1.31, 1.61)***	1.94 (1.71, 2.20)***	2.23 (1.54, 3.22)***	1.67 (1.49, 1.88)***	1.48 (1.31, 1.67)***
Secondary	1.22 (1.14, 1.31)***	1.30 (1.19, 1.42)***	1.52 (1.37, 1.69)***	1.59 (1.14, 2.21)**	1.38 (1.29, 1.48)***	1.27 (1.16, 1.39)***
Residence (Ref. Urban)						
Rural	1.28 (1.22, 1.34)***	1.40 (1.34, 1.47)***	1.15 (1.08, 1.22)***	1.15 (0.93, 1.42)	1.01 (0.95, 1.07)	1.06 (0.99, 1.13)
Social category (Ref. General)						
ST	1.48 (1.36, 1.61)***	1.37 (1.27, 1.48)***	1.32 (1.17, 1.50)***	0.68 (0.57, 0.82)***	1.40 (1.22, 1.60)***	1.54 (1.41, 1.69)***
SC	1.33 (1.24, 1.43)***	1.35 (1.27, 1.44)***	1.22 (1.12, 1.33)***	0.95 (0.77, 1.18)	1.26 (1.13, 1.40)***	1.26 (1.16, 1.38)***
OBC	1.22 (1.15, 1.30)***	1.19 (1.12, 1.26)***	1.17 (1.07, 1.27)***	0.86 (0.71, 1.04)	1.13 (1.03, 1.24)*	1.37 (1.28, 1.47)***

(continued)

Table 6.6 (continued)

Explanatory factors	Central AOR (95% CI)	East AOR (95% CI)	North AOR (95% CI)	Northeast AOR (95% CI)	South AOR (95% CI)	West AOR (95% CI)
Family type (Ref. Non-nuclear)						
Nuclear	1.03 (0.99, 1.08)	1.05 (1.01, 1.09)*	1.11 (1.04, 1.19)**	1.06 (0.92, 1.21)	0.96 (0.90, 1.01)	1.15 (1.08, 1.22)***
Wealth index (Ref. Rich)						
Poor	1.58 (1.49, 1.67)***	1.97 (1.82, 2.13)***	1.50 (1.37, 1.64)***	1.94 (1.47, 2.56)***	1.94 (1.80, 2.10)***	1.66 (1.53, 1.80)***
Middle	1.26 (1.18, 1.34)***	1.36 (1.25, 1.48)***	1.36 (1.25, 1.48)***	1.43 (1.07, 1.92)*	1.35 (1.26, 1.44)***	1.25 (1.16, 1.35)***

Significant ***$p < 0.001$, **$p < 0.01$, *$p < 0.05$

Table 6.7 Model illustrates the role of explanatory factors on thinness among under-five children in Indian zones

Explanatory factors	Central AOR (95% CI)	East AOR (95% CI)	North AOR (95% CI)	Northeast AOR (95% CI)	South AOR (95% CI)	West AOR (95% CI)
Anemia in children (Ref. Non-anemic)						
Anemic	1.05 (0.99, 1.11)	1.23 (1.17, 1.30)***	1.05 (0.97, 1.15)	1.11 (0.94, 1.31)	1.05 (0.98, 1.12)	1.10 (1.02, 1.19)*
Sex child (Ref. Girl)						
Boy	1.04 (0.99, 1.09)	0.99 (0.95, 1.04)	1.09 (1.01, 1.18)*	1.09 (0.93, 1.28)	1.06 (0.99, 1.13)	1.03 (0.97, 1.11)
Parents alive (Ref. Alive)						
Not alive	1.13 (0.89, 1.45)	0.96 (0.73, 1.25)	0.80 (0.50, 1.28)	1.07 (0.53, 2.15)	0.94 (0.67, 1.31)	0.91 (0.64, 1.29)
Birth order (Ref. 1st & 2nd)						
3rd & more	1.04 (0.98, 1.11)	1.04 (0.98, 1.10)	0.99 (0.90, 1.09)	0.86 (0.70, 1.05)	0.93 (0.84, 1.02)	0.95 (0.87, 1.04)
Mother's education (Ref. Higher)						
Non-educated	1.15 (1.04, 1.27)**	0.98 (0.88, 1.10)	1.12 (0.96, 1.31)	1.16 (0.77, 1.73)	1.33 (1.15, 1.53)***	0.84 (0.72, 0.97)*
Primary	1.01 (0.91, 1.13)	0.88 (0.78, 0.99)*	1.14 (0.97, 1.33)	1.19 (0.80, 1.76)	1.00 (0.86, 1.17)	0.96 (0.83, 1.11)
Secondary	1.05 (0.97, 1.14)	0.91 (0.82, 1.00)	1.12 (1.00, 1.27)	0.95 (0.68, 1.34)	1.09 (1.00, 1.19)*	0.90 (0.82, 1.00)*
Residence (Ref. Urban)						
Rural	0.89 (0.85, 0.95)***	1.01 (0.96, 1.07)	0.93 (0.85, 1.03)	1.13 (0.88, 1.44)	1.04 (0.98, 1.01)	1.14 (1.05, 1.23)**

(continued)

Table 6.7 (continued)

	Central	East	North	Northeast	South	West
Explanatory factors	AOR (95% CI)	AOR (95% CI)	AOR (95% CI)	AOR (95% CI)	AOR (95% CI)	AOR (95% CI)
Social category (Ref. General)						
ST	1.44 (1.29, 1.61)***	1.20 (1.09, 1.32)***	1.24 (1.06, 1.46)**	0.72 (0.57, 0.90)**	1.36 (1.16, 1.61)***	1.51 (1.35, 1.68)***
SC	1.14 (1.04, 1.25)**	1.24 (1.15, 1.34)***	1.04 (0.93, 1.17)	1.07 (0.83, 1.37)	1.09 (0.96, 1.24)	0.94 (0.85, 1.05)
OBC	1.14 (1.05, 1.24)**	1.10 (1.02, 1.18)*	1.13 (1.02, 1.26)*	0.96 (0.76, 1.21)	1.02 (0.91, 1.15)	1.23 (1.13, 1.34)***
Family type (Ref. Non-nuclear)						
Nuclear	1.01 (0.96, 1.07)	1.03 (0.98, 1.08)	1.04 (0.95, 1.14)	0.96 (0.82, 1.14)	1.03 (0.96, 1.11)	1.27 (1.18, 1.37)***
Wealth index (Ref. Rich)						
Poor	1.05 (0.98, 1.14)	1.12 (1.02, 1.23)*	1.18 (1.05, 1.32)**	1.28 (0.94, 1.73)	1.22 (1.11, 1.36)***	1.02 (0.92, 1.13)
Middle	0.96 (0.88, 1.04)	0.95 (0.86, 1.05)	1.14 (1.02, 1.28)*	1.03 (0.74, 1.43)	1.03 (0.95, 1.12)	0.98 (0.90, 1.08)

Significant ***$p < 0.001$, **$p < 0.01$, *$p < 0.05$

1), with non-stunting, non-wasting, non-underweight, and non-thinness standing as a reference category (coded as 0) in the logistic regression. The Omnibus Chi-square for stunting, wasting, underweight, and thinness being 703.67, 119.83, 660.64, and 49.90 for North; 1848.77, 187.00, 1289.79, and 126.52 for Central; 2284.22, 43.76, 2223.91, and 164.35 for East; 166.35, 65.43, 198.54, and 38.97 for Northeast; 944.87, 272.97, 898.74, and 172.89 for West; and 1166.62, 176.81, 1212.64, and 93.24 for South, with a significant level of $p < 0.01$. The correct percentages of prediction of the model for stunting, wasting, underweight, and thinness in the North are 70.03%, 86.20%, 76.43%, and 87.30%; Central 61.05%, 83.13%, 67.20%, and 85.14%; East 61.39%, 78.89%, 62.67%, and 81.74%; Northeast 65.83%, 82.22%, 72.63%, and 83.62%; West 63.78%, 75.01%, 63.75%, and 78.01%; South 69.46%, 83.68%, 72.69%, and 85.43%, respectively. Both of these facts indicate that the models for each zonal division were well-fitted to the data. The models revealed the following information. The VIF demonstrated that there was no evidence of a multicollinearity problem among the predictor variables for all logistic models.

Stunting Child anemia was common in all zones, but the effect of anemia on stunting was the highest in the South, where it was 1.44 times more prevalent than the non-anemic child, followed by the West and Central, where it was 1.38 times and 1.32 times more prevalent, respectively. Boys were more likely to suffer from stunting, it was 1.15 and 1.09 times more prevalent in North and Central zones, respectively. Birth order was a common factor in each zone, stunting was 1.20 times more probable in the third or more birth order compared to the first and second child in both Northeast and South. Lower maternal education was found to be a common factor and being positively associated with stunting, with lower or non-educated mothers having a higher risk to have a stunting child than higher-educated mothers. Rural children were more likely to be stunted than urban children in the North, South, and West, while the prevalence in the West peaked at 1.20 times higher. Except for the Northeast, social category was shown to be a common factor in each zone. In the North, Central, East, and West, SC children were more likely to have stunting than general caste children, while ST children were more affected in the South. Children from nuclear families were 1.08 and 1.06 times more likely to be stunting in the north and Central zones, respectively, whereas 0.92 times less likely to have stunting in nuclear families of South. Stunting was shown to be more common in children belonging to poor and middle-wealth index households than in rich households.

Wasting Anemic children were more likely to be wasting than their non-anemic peers, except in the Northeast and South. Wasting was more common among boys in each zonal division, with rates of 1.17 times and 1.16 times higher in the Northeast and North, respectively. Wasting was 1.10 times more prevalent in the third or more birth order in the East compared to the first and second child. In the North, Central, and South, lower or non-educated mothers have a higher probability of having a wasting child than higher-educated mothers. In comparison to urban areas in the East, South, and West zone, children in rural areas were more likely to be wasting, while urban children in the Central zone were 22 percent more likely to be wasting. The ST children were more likely than general caste children to suffer from wasting, except in the Northeast. ST children in the North, Central, West, and South were more prone to wasting, while in East SC children were more sufferer. In the West, children from nuclear families were 1.29 times more likely to suffer from wasting. Children from the poor wealth index families were more likely to suffer from wasting, it was 1.53 and 1.21 times more common in the Northeast and South, respectively.

Underweight Underweight was more common in anemic children than in non-anemic counterparts. Boys were more likely to be underweight than girls in each zone except in the East. Underweight was more prevalent in the third or higher birth order compared to the first and second child, except for Northeast zone. Mother's education was a common factor in all zones; mothers who did not receive any formal education had a higher risk of their child being underweight, which was shown to be 2.44 times in Northeast, 1.96 times in East, and 1.90 times in South. In the Central, East, and North zones, children in rural areas were more likely to be underweight than those in urban areas. The ST children were more likely to be underweight than the general caste, but the situation was reversed in the Northeast, where they were 0.68 times less likely to be underweight. Underweight was more common in children from nuclear families in the North, East, and West. Children belonging to poor and middle-wealth index families were more likely to be underweight than those belonging to wealthy families in each zonal division. The wealth index had a greater impact in the East, with impoverished children being 1.97 times more likely to be underweight.

Thinness Anemic children were 1.23 and 1.10 times more likely to be thin than their non-anemic peers in the East and West zones, respectively. Boys in the North were 1.03 times more likely than girls to be thin. Children of non-educated mothers were more likely to be thin in the Central and South, whereas children of higher-educated mothers were thin in the East and West. Rural children were less likely to be thin than urban children in the Central, but more likely to be thin in the West. The ST children were more likely to be thin than general caste children in each zone, with the exception of the Northeast, where ST children were 0.72 times less likely to be thin. Among the West, being thin was 1.27 times more common in children of nuclear families. Children from low-income families were more likely to be thin; it was 1.18, 1.12, and 1.22 times more common in the North, East, and South, respectively.

6.6 Discussion

The purpose of this study was to determine the zonal prevalence of stunting, wasting, underweight, and thinness in under-five Indian children, as well as how child-related, maternal, and sociodemographic factors influenced undernutrition. The facts on nutritional status were synthesized in the following outcomes: First, there were zonal disparities in child's nutritional status, but stunting and underweight were the serious issues in each zone. Second, child malnutrition was associated with child-related, maternal, and sociodemographic characteristics, with some coexisting in all zones but others differing. There were considerable zonal variations in the prevalence of undernutrition, even when comparing the population curve to the WHO's reference curve in stunting, wasting, underweight, and thinness shows a propensity to vulnerability. The lowest z-score value of height-for-age (HAZ) was observed in the East and Central zones, weight-for-height (WHZ) in West, weight-for-age (WAZ) in East, and BMI-for-age (BAZ) in West. WHO notes that various forms of malnutrition have diverse outcomes, wasting can influence the immune system directly, stunting frequently results in delayed mental development, poor academic performance, and lower intellectual ability, and being underweight increases the risk of death (WHO 2010, 2019).

The child-related characteristics that had an impact on the nutritional indicators, were the child's anemia, gender, and birth order. Children with anemia tend to be stunted and underweight in all zones, but it can also cause wasting and thinness in specific zones. Undernutrition has been linked to gender disparities in children, boys were more prone than girls to experience undernutrition, and wasting was common in boys across the zones. Stunting was found to be frequently influenced by birth order, with third or subsequent children in each zone being more at chance than the first and second child. This suggests that families who follow the family planning norms and only have up to two kids, which will improve their child's nutritional condition since those kids were less prone to stunting. In India, orphans were not undernourished in any zone, indicating that if parents pass away before their children turn five, there was no scarcity of food, nourishment, or care, which was noteworthy for the nation. In maternal factors, children with less educated mothers were at a higher risk of undernutrition. Lower maternal education influences each type of child undernutrition, while it was a common cause of stunting and underweight in all zones. Similar findings that have been obtained from China, Indonesia, Nigeria, and Uganda have demonstrated the coexistence of lower mother education with child undernutrition (Beal et al. 2018; Nwosu and Ataguba 2020; Odei Obeng-Amoako et al. 2021; Zhang et al. 2018).

The prevalence of undernutrition varied by social category; Children from the ST community in the South were at risk of undernutrition, but the situation was quite the opposite in the Northeast, where the nutritional status of ST children was better than in any other zone in India. Children from SC communities and those from OBC communities in North, Central, East, and West have very poor nutritional conditions. The majority of undernourished children were found in rural areas in the East, North, South, and West than in urban areas. In the North, Central, East, and West, children from nuclear families were more prone to be undernourished. The Poor Wealth Index had a significant impact on child undernutrition, stunting, wasting, underweight, and thinness were more prevalent in children from poor families than in children from wealthier families. Ethiopia, Indonesia, Uganda, and Papua New Guinea have all seen a similar trend, indicating that the lack of maternal education and poor wealth index coexist with child undernutrition (Beal et al. 2018; Odei Obeng-Amoako et al. 2021; Pham et al. 2021; Yayo Negasi 2021).

6.7 Conclusion

This study was an attempt to find the zonal distribution of four undernutrition parameters of child health, namely, stunting, wasting, underweight and thinness, among children under the age of five in India. The study's six geographical zones are Central, East, North, Northeast, South, and West. Substantial zonal disparities were found in the prevalence of undernutrition. However, the zones in the middle belt, or the East, Central, and West were most affected. Some of these factors were found to have a significant effect on the health parameters of under-five children across all zones. These were anemia, higher birth order, lower education level of mothers and poor families for stunting, boys, and scheduled tribes for wasting, anemia, lower education level, scheduled tribes, poor families for underweight and scheduled tribes for thinness. Usually for children, BMI is not considered, and it is unlikely to give good results. It was also seen that the health status of children in Northeast zone had better health status than in most other zones. Thus, if Northeast zone and thinness were left out, then some more explanatory factors would become significant as determinants of the nutrition level.

The recommendation should be based on the explanatory variables for which there are scopes to change the status of the variables and thus our recommendation would be (a) to educate mothers, (b) not to have more than two children, if possible, and (c) to upgrade economic status. Above all, parents should be aware of how to take care of children so they may put that knowledge into practice in their own families.

6.8 Strength and Limitation of the Study

This study was based on the most recent DHS Survey of India, which was conducted between 2019 and 2021. It was feasible to offer a recent picture of the nutritional condition of children under the age of five in India by zonal division through this study. Also, this study was to determine the factors that contribute to child undernutrition. This enabled the development of zone-specific policies or the revision of existing policies to make them more advantageous and well-timed. In this study, the zone was given particular attention, due to factors like geographic location, language, culture, climate, ethnicity, and historical context that separate one zone from another. Apart from zonal division, if a similar study was conducted on each state of the country, then state-specific policies could have been developed. However, in order to understand the issue of child undernutrition holistically, much more research was required.

Acknowledgments The authors would like to acknowledge the IRB for approving the use of DHS data in this study.

Ethical Approval The Demographic and Health Surveys (DHS) provided the data utilized in this study. The survey methodology and participant confidentiality have been evaluated and approved by the ICF Institutional Review Board (IRB) and the host country's ethics committee of IIPS in India. The ICF IRB abides by the standards set out by the US Department of Health and Human Services for the confidentiality and protection of human subjects. Therefore, the use of the DHS data had already received ethical approval, and no more approval was needed.

Conflict of Interest The authors declared no potential conflicts of interest concerning the research, authorship, and/or publication of this article.

Funding This research received no specific grant from any funding agency, commercial entity, or not-for-profit organization.

References

Aboagye RG, Seidu AA, Ahinkorah BO, Arthur-Holmes F, Cadri A, Dadzie LK et al (2021) Dietary diversity and undernutrition in children aged 6-23 months in Sub-Saharan Africa. Nutrients 13:10. https://doi.org/10.3390/nu13103431

Beal T, Tumilowicz A, Sutrisna A, Izwardy D, Neufeld LM (2018) A review of child stunting determinants in Indonesia. Matern Child Nutr 14(4):e12617. https://doi.org/10.1111/mcn.12617

Berhe K, Weldegerima L, Gebrearegay F, Kahsay A, Tesfahunegn A, Rejeu M, Gebremariam B (2021) Effect of under-nutrition during pregnancy on low birth weight in Tigray regional state, Ethiopia; a prospective cohort study. BMC Nutr 7(1):72. https://doi.org/10.1186/s40795-021-00475-7

Bishwajit G, Ide S, Ghosh S (2014) Social determinants of infectious diseases in South Asia. Int Sch Res Notices 2014:135243. https://doi.org/10.1155/2014/135243

Blankenship JL, Gwavuya S, Palaniappan U, Alfred J, deBrum F, Erasmus W (2020) High double burden of child stunting and maternal overweight in the Republic of the Marshall Islands. Matern Child Nutr *16*(Suppl 2):e12832. https://doi.org/10.1111/mcn.12832

Cameron N (2007) Body mass index cut offs to define thinness in children and adolescents. BMJ 335(7612):166–167. https://doi.org/10.1136/bmj.39281.439178.80

Cheng J, Sun J, Yao K, Xu M, Cao Y (2022) A variable selection method based on mutual information and variance inflation factor. Spectrochim Acta A Mol Biomol Spectrosc 268:120652. https://doi.org/10.1016/j.saa.2021.120652

Geda NR, Feng CX, Henry CJ, Lepnurm R, Janzen B, Whiting SJ (2021) Multiple anthropometric and nutritional deficiencies in young children in Ethiopia: a multi-level analysis based on a nationally representative data. BMC Pediatr 21(1):11. https://doi.org/10.1186/s12887-020-02467-1

Ghosh S, Varerkar SA (2019) Undernutrition among tribal children in Palghar district, Maharashtra, India. PLoS One 14(2):e0212560. https://doi.org/10.1371/journal.pone.0212560

Griffiths P, Hindet A, Matthews Z (2001) Infant and child mortality in three culturally contrasting states of India. J Biosoc Sci 33(4):603–622. https://doi.org/10.1017/s0021932001006034

Hasan MM, Uddin J, Pulok MH, Zaman N, Hajizadeh M (2020) Socioeconomic inequalities in child malnutrition in Bangladesh: do they differ by region? Int J Environ Res Public Health 17:3. https://doi.org/10.3390/ijerph17031079

Islam MR, Moinuddin M, Ahmed A, Rahman SM (2021) Association of sickle cell disease with anthropometric indices among under-five children: evidence from 2018 Nigeria demographic and Health survey. BMC Med 19(1):5. https://doi.org/10.1186/s12916-020-01879-1

Jain I, Oberoi S, Jain A, Balgir RS, Sandhu MK, Lugani Y (2020) Factors affecting nutritional status of Anganwadi children: a cross-sectional study. J Family Med Prim Care 9(9):4613–4617. https://doi.org/10.4103/jfmpc.jfmpc_410_20

Kar A (2014) The Thar or the Great Indian Sand Desert. In World Geomorphological Landscapes. Berlin: Springer pp. 79–90. Available at https://doi.org/10.1007/978-94-017-8029-2_7

Kundu RN, Gautam RK, Chatterjee A, Bharati P, Liczbińska G, Malina RM (2024) Nutritional status of infants and young children in India across three decades: analysis of five national family health surveys. Eur J Clin Nutr 78(7):591–606. https://doi.org/10.1038/s41430-024-01427-7

Matariya ZR, Lodhiya KK, Mahajan RG (2016) Environmental correlates of undernutrition among children of 3-6 years of age, Rajkot, Gujarat, India. J Family Med Prim Care 5(4):834–839. https://doi.org/10.4103/2249-4863.201152

Meitei WB (2020) Nutritional status of under-five children in Northeast India: effect of household socioeconomic status. Indian J Public Health Res Dev 11(7):1003–1008. https://doi.org/10.37506/ijphrd.v11i7.10220

Mukhopadhyay R, Karisiddaiah SM (2014) The Indian Coastline: Processes and Landforms. In: Kale, V. (eds) Landscapes and Landforms of India. World Geomorphological Landscapes. Springer, Dordrecht. https://doi.org/10.1007/978-94-017-8029-2_8

Murarkar S, Gothankar J, Doke P, Pore P, Lalwani S, Dhumale G et al (2020) Prevalence and determinants of undernutrition among under-five children residing in urban slums and rural area, Maharashtra, India: a community-based cross-sectional study. BMC Public Health 20(1):1559. https://doi.org/10.1186/s12889-020-09642-0

Narayan J, John D, Ramadas N (2019) Malnutrition in India: status and government initiatives. J Public Health Policy 40(1):126–141. https://doi.org/10.1057/s41271-018-0149-5

NHM (2011) Janani Shishu Suraksha Karyakaram. National Health Mission. Retrieved from https://nhm.gov.in/index1.php?lang=1&level=3&sublinkid=842&lid=308

NHM (2013a) Rashtriya Bal Swasthya Karyakram. National Health Mission. Retrieved from https://nhm.gov.in/index1.php?lang=1&level=4&sublinkid=1190&lid=583

NHM (2013b) Reproductive, maternal, newborn, child and adolescent Health (RMNCH+A). National Health Mission. Retrieved from https://nhm.gov.in/index1.php?lang=1&level=1&sublinkid=794&lid=168
NHM (2014) India newborn action plan. National Health Mission. Retrieved from https://nhm.gov.in/index4.php?lang=1&level=0&linkid=153&lid=174
Nwosu CO, Ataguba JE (2020) Explaining changes in wealth inequalities in child health: the case of stunting and wasting in Nigeria. PLoS One 15(9):e0238191. https://doi.org/10.1371/journal.pone.0238191
Odei Obeng-Amoako GA, Karamagi CAS, Nangendo J, Okiring J, Kiirya Y, Aryeetey R et al (2021) Factors associated with concurrent wasting and stunting among children 6-59 months in Karamoja, Uganda. Matern Child Nutr 17(1):e13074. https://doi.org/10.1111/mcn.13074
Padmapriyadarsini C, Shobana M, Lakshmi M, Beena T, Swaminathan S (2016) Undernutrition & tuberculosis in India: situation analysis & the way forward. Indian J Med Res 144(1):11–20. https://doi.org/10.4103/0971-5916.193278
Pandit P, Galande S, Iris F (2021) Maternal malnutrition and anaemia in India: dysregulations leading to the 'thin-fat' phenotype in newborns. J Nutr Sci 10:e91. https://doi.org/10.1017/jns.2021.83
Pati S, Mahapatra S, Sinha R, Pati S, Samal SN (2018) Community management of acute malnutrition (CMAM) in Odisha, India: a multi-stakeholder perspective. Front Public Health 6:158. https://doi.org/10.3389/fpubh.2018.00158
Pham BN, Silas VD, Okely AD, Pomat W (2021) Measuring wasting and stunting prevalence among children under 5 years of age and associated risk factors in Papua New Guinea: new evidence from the comprehensive health and epidemiological surveillance system. Front Nutr 8:622660. https://doi.org/10.3389/fnut.2021.622660
Pike V, Bradley B, Rappaport AI, Zlotkin S, Perumal N (2021) A scoping review of research on policies to address child undernutrition in the Millennium Development Goals era. Public Health Nutr 24(13):4346–4357. https://doi.org/10.1017/S1368980021001890
Reddy D, Ma Y, Lakshminarayanan S, Sahu S, White LF, Reshma A et al (2021) Severe undernutrition in children affects tuberculin skin test performance in Southern India. PLoS One 16(7):e0250304. https://doi.org/10.1371/journal.pone.0250304
Roshania RP, Giri R, Cunningham SA, Young MF, Webb-Girard A, Das A et al (2022) Early life migration and undernutrition among circular migrant children: an observational study in the brick kilns of Bihar, India. J Glob Health 12:04008. https://doi.org/10.7189/jogh.12.04008
Singh KD, Alagarajan M, Ladusingh L (2015) What explains child malnutrition of indigenous people of Northeast India? PLoS One 10(6):e0130567. https://doi.org/10.1371/journal.pone.0130567
Soni A, Fahey N, Ash A, Bhutta Z, Li W, Simas TM et al (2022) Predictive algorithm to stratify newborns at-risk for child undernutrition in India: secondary analysis of the National Family Health Survey-4. J Glob Health 12:04040. https://doi.org/10.7189/jogh.12.04040
Stiller CK, Golembiewski SKE, Golembiewski M, Mondal S, Biesalski HK, Scherbaum V (2020) Prevalence of undernutrition and anemia among Santal Adivasi children, Birbhum District, West Bengal, India. Int J Environ Res Public Health 17:1. https://doi.org/10.3390/ijerph17010342
Tandoh MA, Appiah AO, Edusei AW (2021) Prevalence of anemia and undernutrition of adolescent females in selected schools in Ghana. Journal of Nutrition and Metabolism 1–5. Available at https://doi.org/10.1155/2021/6684839
Teferi H, Teshome T (2021) Magnitude and associated factors of undernutrition among children aged 6-59 months in Ethiopian orphanage Centres. Pediatric Health Med Ther 12:141–150. https://doi.org/10.2147/phmt.S289809
Tesema GA, Yeshaw Y, Worku MG, Tessema ZT, Teshale AB (2021) Pooled prevalence and associated factors of chronic undernutrition among under-five children in East Africa: a multilevel analysis. PLoS One 16(3):e0248637. https://doi.org/10.1371/journal.pone.0248637
Tesfaw LM, Fenta HM (2021) Multivariate logistic regression analysis on the association between anthropometric indicators of under-five children in Nigeria: NDHS 2018. BMC Pediatr 21(1):193. https://doi.org/10.1186/s12887-021-02657-5

UNICEF (Producer). (2021, April) UNICEF data: monitoring the situation of children and women: malnutrition. *UNICEF for every child.* Retrieved from https://data.unicef.org/topic/nutrition/malnutrition/

UNICEF/WHO/WBG (2017) Levels and trends in child malnutrition, UNICEF/WHO/World Bank Group joint malnutrition estimates: key findings of the *2017th edition.* World Health Organization, Washington, DC

UNICEF/WHO/WBG (2021) Levels and trends in child malnutrition: key findings of the 2021 edition of the joint child malnutrition estimates. World Health Organization, Geneva

Victora CG, Christian P, Vidaletti LP, Gatica-Domínguez G, Menon P, Black RE (2021) Revisiting maternal and child undernutrition in low-income and middle-income countries: variable progress towards an unfinished agenda. Lancet 397(10282):1388–1399. https://doi.org/10.1016/s0140-6736(21)00394-9

Wachs TD (2008) Multiple influences on children' nutritional deficiencies: a systems perspective. Physiol Behav 94(1):48–60. https://doi.org/10.1016/j.physbeh.2007.11.018

Wells JCK, Briend A, Boyd EM, Berkely JA, Hall A, Isanaka S, Webb P, Khara T, Dolan C (2019) Beyond wasted and stunted-a major shift to fight child undernutrition. Lancet Child Adolesc Health (11):831–834. https://doi.org/10.1016/S2352-4642(19)30244-5

WHO (2006) WHO Child Growth Standards: Length/height-for-age, weight-for-age, weight-for-length, weight-for-height and body mass index-for-age: methods and development. WHO Press, Geneva

WHO (2010) Nutrition landscape information system (NLIS) country profile indicators: interpretation guide. World Health Organization, Geneva

WHO (2014) Global nutrition targets 2025: Stunting policy brief. Retrieved from Geneva: https://apps.who.int/iris/bitstream/handle/10665/149019/WHO_N?sequence=1

WHO (Producer) (2017, 20 June 2022). The double burden of malnutrition: policy brief. WHO/NMH/NHD/17.3. Retrieved from https://www.who.int/publications/i/item/WHO-NMH-NHD-17.3

WHO (2019) Nutrition landscape information system (NLiS) country profile indicators: interpretation guide, 2nd edn. World Health Organization, Geneva

WHO (2021) Malnutrition. Retrieved from https://www.who.int/news-room/fact-sheets/detail/malnutrition

Yayo Negasi M (2021) Dynamics of inequality in child under-nutrition in Ethiopia. Int J Equity Health 20(1):182. https://doi.org/10.1186/s12939-021-01478-3

Yirga AA, Mwambi HG, Ayele DG, Melesse SF (2019) Factors affecting child malnutrition in Ethiopia. Afr Health Sci 19(2):1897–1909. https://doi.org/10.4314/ahs.v19i2.13

Zhang Y, Huang X, Yang Y, Liu X, Yang C, Wang A et al (2018) Double burden of malnutrition among children under 5 in poor areas of China. PLoS One 13(9):e0204142. https://doi.org/10.1371/journal.pone.0204142

Burden of Cesarian Delivery and its Impact on Preschool Children in Bangladesh: Survey in Rajshahi District

7

Md. Aslam Hossain, Md. Reazul Karim, and Md. Golam Hossain

7.1 Introduction

Cesarian section (C-section) is a life-saving surgery performed when the mother's or child's life is in danger (Zakerihamidi et al. 2015). Globally, C-section rates have risen dramatically from 12.1% in 2000 to 21.1% in 2015 (Boerma et al. 2018). Recent data (2010–2018) from 154 countries show that 21.1% of women worldwide gave birth by C-section, with rates ranging from 5% in Sub-Saharan Africa to 42.8% in Latin America and the Caribbean. Eastern and Southern Asia experienced the greatest increases (44.9 and 19.0 percentage points, respectively). Since 1990, C-sections have increased in all regions (Betran et al. 2021). In Bangladesh, C-sections rose from 3.5% in 2004 to 33% in 2018 (NIPORT and ICF 2020). Unnecessary C-sections have surged in Latin America (Magne et al. 2017), often without medical indications (Thomas et al. 2001). The World Health Organization (WHO) recommends C-sections only when medically necessary (WHO 2015).

In Bangladesh, several factors increase the risk of C-sections, including maternal education, wealth index, age, age at first birth, residence, parity, antenatal visits, husband's occupation, and private sector deliveries (Hasan et al. 2019; M. M. Rahman et al. 2018). Maternal anemia is also a risk factor (Adam et al. 2019). Short-term risks for C-sectioned mothers include infection, hemorrhage, visceral injury, and venous thromboembolism (NICE 2011). C-section babies have higher risks of asthma, food allergies, type 1 diabetes, obesity, anemia, Crohn's disease, and other conditions (Begum et al. 2017; Keag et al. 2018; Magne et al. 2017; Si et al. 2022). Autism spectrum disorders and ADHD are now also linked to C-sections (Zhang

M. A. Hossain (✉) · M. R. Karim · M. G. Hossain
Health Research Group, Department of Statistics, University of Rajshahi, Rajshahi, Bangladesh

M. Pal et al. (eds.), *Public Health and Nutrition*,
https://doi.org/10.1007/978-981-97-7890-4_7

et al. 2019). To achieve the Sustainable Development Goals (SDGs), addressing the global increase in C-sections is essential.

Several studies in Bangladesh have examined how socio-demographic, maternal, and child characteristics affect childhood diseases. For instance, Imran et al. investigated risk factors for early childhood acute respiratory infections, while Hasan et al. studied the link between C-sections and early childhood diseases (Hasan et al. 2020; Imran et al. 2019; Yusuf et al. 2019). As far as we know, no studies have been done in Bangladesh to look into how C-sections affect young children under the age of five. As a result, our primary goal was to investigate the prevalence of C-sections and their impact on preschool children in Bangladesh.

7.2 Methods

This cross-sectional study used both quantitative and qualitative methods in Rajshahi district, located in northwestern Bangladesh. The district covers 2425.37 square km with a population of 2,699,688, of which 17.33% are urban and 82.67% are rural (BSS 2011, adjusted on March 16, 2012). The main respondents were preschool children and their mothers living in the catchment area of community clinics in the district. Data was collected through a field survey conducted from October to December 2016, with interviews carried out by expert community health workers.

7.3 Sample Size Determination

A multistage sampling technique was utilized to select the samples for this study. The sample size was determined using the formula:

$$n = \frac{N}{1 + Nd^2}$$

where n is the sample size, N is the household size (in this study N = 271,302 N = 271,302 N = 271,302), and d is the margin of error (set at 0.05 for this study). With a 95% confidence level, this formula indicated that 399 respondents were needed for the study. However, to obtain more accurate results, data was collected from 540 respondents.

7.4 Sample Selection Procedure

In Rajshahi district, which has 233 community clinics across nine Upazilas (BBS 2011), samples were collected using a multistage sampling technique. First, two community clinics were randomly selected from each Upazila. Then, two villages were chosen from each clinic's catchment area. Finally, 15 households with children under five were randomly selected from each village, totaling 540 respondents. The mothers from these households were interviewed.

7.5 Outcome Variable

The outcome variable in this study was whether the delivery was via cesarian section or not. Participants were asked to indicate the type of delivery: (a) Yes, for cesarian delivery, or (b) No, for normal delivery.

7.6 Exposure Variables

The explanatory variables are listed below with their corresponding groups in parentheses.

7.6.1 Maternal Socio-Demographic Variables

Marginalized group (no, yes); drinking water facility (unhygienic, hygienic); toilet facility (unhygienic, hygienic); husband's occupation (farmer, labor, business, and service holder); husband's education level (illiterate, primary, high school, and higher education); maternal age (in years) (<20, 20–24, 25–29, ≥30), maternal BMI (underweight, normal, over weight); maternal occupation (housewife, others); and maternal education level (illiterate, primary, high school, and higher education) were considered as the maternal socio-demographic variables.

7.6.2 Maternal Reproductive and Pregnancy Variables

Maternal reproductive and pregnancy variables include the birth interval (in months) (<25, ≥25); severe headache with blurred vision problems (no, yes); edema problem (no, yes); anemic mother (no, yes); vaginal bleeding (no, yes); received antenatal care services (no, yes); iron-folic supplementary (no, yes); and taking extra rest (no, yes).

7.6.3 Child-Related Variables

Sex of the children (boy, girl); Mid-upper arm circumference of the children (severe acute malnutrition, moderate acute malnutrition, normal); stunting of the children (not stunted, stunted); wasting of the children (not wasting, wasting); initial breastfeeding (no, yes); jaundice complications after the birth (no, yes); pneumonia problem after the birth (no, yes); unable to suck problem after the birth (no, yes); exclusive breastfeeding within 0–6 months (no, yes); Zink treatment during diarrhea (no, yes); receive antibiotic during pneumonia (no, yes); and receive iron supplementation within 6–23 months (no, yes) were considered as the independent variables.

7.6.4 Mother's Anthropometric Measurement

The mother's weight and height were measured using a portable stadiometer and digital scales, respectively. Height was measured according to Martin and Saller's technique (Martin and Saller 1957): standing on the stadiometer without shoes, looking straight ahead, and keeping shoulders level. Weight was measured with the mother wearing light clothing. Both weight and height were recorded in kilograms (kg) and meters (m), respectively. Body Mass Index (BMI) was calculated using the standard formula:

$$\text{BMI} = \frac{\text{weight}(\text{kg})}{\text{height}(\text{m})^2}$$

7.6.5 Child's Anthropometric Measurement

Stunting A child is considered stunted if their height-for-age index falls below −2 standard deviations (SD) from the median of the standard growth curve. Severe stunting is diagnosed if it falls below −3 SD (WHO 2006).

Wasting This refers to a recent nutritional deficiency resulting from sudden food deprivation or poor nutrient absorption, leading to weight loss. Wasting is identified when weight-for-height is below −2 SD from the NCHS/WHO median value. Severe wasting is diagnosed if it falls below −3 SD (WHO 2006).

Moderate Acute Malnutrition (MAM) MAM is characterized by moderate wasting, defined as weight-for-height below −2 SD and greater than or equal to −3 SD for children under 5 years, or mid-upper arm circumference (MUAC) below 125 mm and greater than or equal to 115 mm for children aged 6-59 months (WHO 2006).

Severe Acute Malnutrition (SAM) SAM is diagnosed by severe wasting: WFH < −3 z-score for children under 5 years or MUAC <115 mm for children aged 6–59 months (WHO 2006).

7.7 Statistical Analysis

Descriptive statistics were used to summarize the study variables. The association between cesarian delivery and socio-demographic, reproductive, pregnancy, and child-related factors was analyzed using the χ^2 test. Binary logistic regression was employed to assess the overall impact of these factors on cesarian delivery, with standard error (SE) used to detect multicollinearity, confirming no issues (Chan 2004). Statistical significance was set at $p < 0.05$. The analysis was conducted using STATA software, version 14.2.

7.8 Results

7.8.1 Basic Characteristics

The descriptive statistics and chi-square distributions of cesarian deliveries in the Rajshahi district of Bangladesh are shown in Table 7.1. During the survey period, the prevalence of cesarian deliveries in Rajshahi district was around 34.4% (Fig. 7.1). Table 7.1 shows that cesarian delivery was significantly ($p = 0.001$) associated with the marginalized group of people in Rajshahi district, with about 96.0% chance of having a cesarian delivery for mothers who were not from the marginalized group. With cesarian delivery, the toilet facility was statistically significant ($p = 0.001$). The mothers who used the hygienic toilet had an 83.3% chance of having a cesarian delivery. In the study area, the husband's educational level and occupation were also significant factors in cesarian delivery. Mothers whose husband's education level was primary and whose husband was a farmer had a 38.0% chance of having a cesarian delivery. If the mother's own education level was in the secondary stage, however, they had a 51.0% chance of having a cesarian delivery. Cesarian delivery was found to be significantly ($p = 0.030$) related to birth interval, with 92.5% of mothers who had a 25-month or longer birth interval having a cesarian delivery. It is also observed that if the mothers have a severe headache with blurred vision problems, edema problems, and anemia problems during their pregnancy period, then there was 78.5%, 88.2%, and 95.7%, respectively, chance of being having a cesarian delivery for the mothers in the study area. Again the received ANC services of the mothers were also a significant ($p = 0.040$) predictor of the cesarian delivery for the mothers. There was 88.7% chance of having a cesarian delivery for the mothers who received ANC services. The percentage of cesarian delivery for the mothers is significantly high ($p \leq 0.001$) for the mothers who were taking extra rest during their pregnancy period (90.9%).

Table 7.2 indicates the most influential risk factors of cesarian delivery in Rajshahi district, Bangladesh. Marginalized group, toilet facility, maternal education level, edema problems, anemia problems, and taking extra rest were significantly associated with cesarian delivery for the mothers (Table 7.2). The mothers who have no anemia problems during their pregnancy period had 4.6 [AOR = 4.62, 95% CI = (1.10–19.39), $p = 0.036$] times higher chances of having a cesarian delivery than the mothers who have anemia problems during their pregnancy period. The probability of cesarian delivery among the mothers who were not taking extra rest was 3.1 [AOR = 3.06, 95% CI = (1.64-5.70), $p \leq 0.001$] times higher than the mothers who were taking extra rest. If the mothers came from marginalized group, then there are 2.6 [AOR = 2.63, 95% CI = (1.13-6.13), $p = 0.025$] times higher probability of having the cesarian delivery among the mothers than their counterparties. The

Table 7.1 Univariate and bivariate distributions of caesarian delivery in Rajshahi district according to the risk factors socio-economic, demographic, and pregnancy-related variable

Study variables	*N* (%)	Caesarian delivery		χ^2-values	*p*-values
		Yes, *N* (%)	No, *N* (%)		
Marginalized group				**20.03**	**<0.001**
No	468 (86.67)	178 (95.70)	290 (81.92)		
Yes	72 (13.33)	8 (4.30)	64 (18.08)		
Drinking water facility				**0.007**	**0.932**
Unimproved	56 (10.37)	19 (10.22)	37 (10.45)		
Improved	484 (89.63)	167 (89.78)	317 (89.55)		
Toilet facility				**27.62**	**<0.001**
Unhygienic	168 (31.11)	31 (16.67)	137 (38.70)		
Hygienic	372 (68.89)	155 (83.33)	217 (61.30)		
Husband's occupation				**13.33**	**0.004**
Farmer	225 (41.67)	71 (38.17)	154 (43.50)		
Labour	192 (35.56)	58 (31.18)	134 (37.85)		
Business	83 (15.37)	34 (18.28)	49 (13.84)		
Service holder	40 (7.41)	23 (12.37)	17 (4.80)		
Husband's education level				**31.62**	**<0.001**
Illiterate	102 (18.89)	18 (9.68)	84 (23.73)		
Primary	184 (34.07)	70 (37.63)	114 (32.20)		
High school	140 (25.93)	39 (20.97)	101 (28.53)		
Higher education	114 (21.11)	59 (31.72)	55 (15.54)		
Maternal age group				**7.21**	**0.066**
< 20 years	41 (7.59)	15 (8.06)	26 (7.34)		
20-24 years	173 (32.04)	52 (27.96)	121 (34.18)		
25-29 years	182 (33.70)	76 (40.86)	106 (29.94)		
> = 30 years	144 (26.67)	43 (23.12)	101 (28.53)		
Maternal BMI				**0.30**	**0.860**

(continued)

Table 7.1 (continued)

Study variables	*N* (%)	Caesarian delivery		χ^2-values	*p*-values
		Yes, *N* (%)	No, *N* (%)		
Underweight (<18.5 kg/m^2)	96 (17.78)	31 (16.67)	65 (18.36)		
Normal weight (18.5–24.99 kg/m^2)	341 (63.15)	118 (63.44)	223 (62.99)		
Overweight (> = 25 kg/m^2)	103 (19.07)	37 (19.89)	66 (18.64)		
Maternal occupation				**1.02**	**0.311**
Housewife	520 (96.30)	177 (95.16)	343 (96.89)		
Others	20 (3.70)	9 (4.84)	11 (3.11)		
Maternal education level				**31.94**	**<0.001**
Illiterate	76 (14.07)	9 (4.84)	67 (18.93)		
Primary	121 (22.41)	35 (18.82)	86 (24.29)		
High school	252 (46.67)	95 (51.08)	157 (44.35)		
Higher education	91 (16.85)	47 (25.27)	44 (12.43)		
Birth interval				**4.72**	**0.030**
<25 months	63 (11.67)	14 (7.53)	49 (13.84)		
≥25 months	477 (88.33)	172 (92.47)	305 (86.16)		
Severe headache with blurred vision problems				**4.008**	**0.045**
No	448 (82.96)	146 (78.49)	302 (85.31)		
Yes	92 (17.04)	40 (21.51)	52 (14.69)		
Edema problems				**6.48**	**0.011**
No	498 (92.22)	164 (88.17)	334 (94.35)		
Yes	42 (7.78)	22 (11.83)	20 (5.65)		
Anemic mother				**7.28**	**0.007**
No	529 (97.96)	178 (95.70)	351 (99.15)		
Yes	11 (2.04)	8 (4.30)	3 (0.85)		
Vaginal bleeding during pregnancy				**0.63**	**0.427**
No	524 (97.04)	179 (96.24)	345 (97.46)		
Yes	16 (2.96)	7 (3.76)	9 (2.54)		
Received ANC services				**4.24**	**0.040**
No	85 (15.74)	21 (11.29)	64 (18.08)		

(continued)

Table 7.1 (continued)

Study variables	N (%)	Caesarian delivery		χ^2-values	p-values
		Yes, N (%)	No, N (%)		
Yes	455 (84.26)	165 (88.71)	290 (81.92)		
Taking iron-folic supplementary				**0.19**	**0.657**
No	51 (9.44)	19 (10.22)	32 (9.04)		
Yes	489 (90.56)	167 (89.78)	322 (90.96)		
Taking extra rest				**16.54**	**<0.001**
No	100 (18.52)	17 (9.14)	83 (23.45)		
Yes	440 (81.48)	169 (90.86)	271 (76.55)		

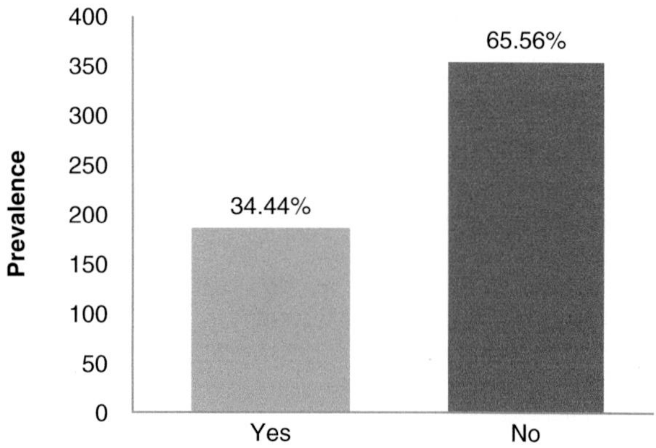

Fig. 7.1 Prevalence of caesarian delivery. Source: Hossain et al. (2023)

mothers who have no edema problems had 2.4 [AOR = 2.38, 95% CI = (1.14-4.93), $p = 0.020$] times higher chance of a cesarian delivery than the mothers who have edema problems during their pregnancy period. Again, the mothers who were using the unhygienic toilet had 2.1 [AOR = 2.12, 95% CI = (1.27–3.54), $p = 0.004$] times higher probability of a cesarian delivery than their counterparties. This study found mothers problem of severe headache with blurred vision was more prone to CS delivery [AOR = 1.69, 95% CI = (1.01–2.84), $p = <0.048$].

Table 7.3 describes the descriptive statistics and chi-square distributions of the risk factors which have health impact on the children due to cesarian delivery in Rajshahi district, Bangladesh. Mid-Upper Arm Circumference (MUAC) of the children was statistically significant ($p = 0.046$) with having the health impact on the children due to cesarian delivery. There was a 95.2% chance of having the health impact on the children due to cesarian deliver if the MUAC of the children was in normal (>12.5 cm) condition. Having the health impact on the children due to cesarian delivery was significantly ($p = <0.001$) related with initial breastfeeding where 88.7% chance of having the health impact on the children due to cesarian delivery for the mothers who were breastfeeding their children immediately after the birth.

Table 7.2 Multiple logistic regression analysis for finding the most influential risk factors of caesarian delivery in Rajshahi district

	Caesarian delivery					
	Unadjusted			Adjusted		
Study variables	UOR	(95% CI)	*p*-value	AOR	(95% CI)	*p*-value
Marginalized group						
No	Reference			Reference		
Yes	4.91	2.30–10.48	<0.001	2.63	1.13–6.13	0.025
Toilet facility						
Unhygienic	3.16	2.03–4.91	<0.001	2.12	1.27–3.54	0.004
Hygienic	Reference			Reference		
Husband's occupation						
Farmer	Reference			Reference		
Labour	1.06	0.70–1.61	0.767	1.31	0.82–2.08	0.262
Business	0.66	0.39–1.12	0.123	1.10	0.62–1.96	0.746
Service holder	0.34	0.17–0.67	0.002	0.88	0.38–2.09	0.772
Husband's education level						
Illiterate	Reference			Reference		
Primary	0.35	0.19–0.62	<0.001	0.58	0.29–1.16	0.126
High school	0.55	0.29–1.04	0.067	1.12	0.53–2.37	0.765
Higher education	0.19	0.11–0.37	<0.001	0.63	0.27–1.46	0.276
Maternal education level						
Illiterate	Reference			Reference		
Primary	0.33	0.15–0.73	0.007	0.54	0.22–1.34	0.185
High school	0.22	0.10–0.46	<0.001	0.42	0.17–1.01	0.051
College & Higher education	0.12	0.06–0.28	<0.001	0.31	0.11–0.83	0.020
Birth interval						
<25 months	Reference			Reference		
≥25 months	0.51	0.27–0.94	0.032	0.71	0.35–1.44	0.338
Severe headache with blurred vision problems						
No	1.59	1.01–2.51	0.046	1.69	1.01–2.84	0.048
Yes	Reference			Reference		
Edema problems						
No	2.24	1.18–4.22	0.013	2.38	1.14–4.93	0.020
Yes	Reference			Reference		
Anemic mother						
No	5.25	1.38–20.06	0.015	4.62	1.10–19.39	0.036
Yes	Reference			Reference		
Received ANC services						
No	1.73	1.02–2.94	0.041	0.89	0.48–1.64	0.709
Yes	Reference			Reference		
Taking extra rest						
No	3.04	1.75–5.31	<0.001	3.06	1.64–5.70	<0.001
Yes	Reference			Reference		

Table 7.3 Univariate and bivariate distributions of the characteristics which have health impact on the children due to caesarian delivery

Study variables	Total, *N* (%)	Caesarian delivery		χ^2-values	*p*-values
		Yes, *N* (%)	No, *N* (%)		
Child sex				**0.81**	**0.368**
Boy	273 (50.56)	99 (53.23)	174 (49.15)		
Girl	267 (49.44)	87 (46.77)	180 (50.85)		
Child MUAC				**6.17**	**0.046**
Severe Acute Malnutrition	12 (2.22)	1 (0.54)	11 (3.11)		
Moderate Acute Malnutrition	35 (6.48)	8 (4.30)	27 (7.63)		
Normal	493 (91.30)	177 (95.16)	316 (89.27)		
Initial breastfeeding				**19.57**	**<0.001**
No	29 (5.37)	21 (11.29)	8 (2.26)		
Yes	511 (94.63)	165 (88.71)	346 (97.74)		
Jaundice complications after the birth				**0.82**	**0.366**
No	493 (91.30)	167 (89.78)	326 (92.09)		
Yes	47 (8.70)	19 (10.22)	28 (7.91)		
Unable to suck problem after the birth				**0.87**	**0.351**
No	532 (98.52)	182 (97.85)	350 (98.87)		
Yes	8 (1.48)	4 (2.15)	4 (1.13)		
Exclusive breastfeeding (0–6 months)				**0.07**	**0.792**
No	31 (5.74)	10 (5.38)	21 (5.93)		
Yes	509 (94.26)	176 (94.62)	333 (94.07)		
Zink treatment during diarrhea				**6.82**	**0.009**
No	277 (51.30)	81 (43.55)	196 (55.37)		
Yes	263 (48.70)	105 (56.45)	158 (44.63)		
Receive antibiotic during pneumonia				**1.22**	**0.268**
No	365 (67.59)	120 (64.52)	245 (69.21)		
Yes	175 (32.41)	66 (35.48)	109 (30.79		
Receive iron supplementation (6-23 months)				**0.15**	**0.697**
No	401 (74.26)	140 (75.27)	261 (73.73)		
Yes	139 (25.74)	46 (24.73)	93 (26.27)		

Table 7.4 Multiple logistic regression analysis for finding the most influential factors that have health impact on the children due to caesarian delivery in Rajshahi district

	Caesarian delivery					
	Unadjusted			Adjusted		
Study variables	UOR	(95% CI)	*p*-value	AOR	(95% CI)	*p*-value
Child MUAC						
Severe Acute Malnutrition (<11.5 cm)	6.16	0.79-48.12	0.083	4.95	0.63-38.91	0.129
Moderate Acute Malnutrition (11.5–12.5 cm)	1.89	0.84-4.25	0.123	1.80	0.78-4.15	0.164
Normal (>12.5 cm)	Reference			Reference		
Initial breastfeeding						
No	5.50	2.39-12.69	<0.001	6.04	2.58-14.13	<0.001
Yes	Reference			Reference		
Zink treatment during diarrhea						
No	Reference			Reference		
Yes	1.61	1.12-2.29	0.009	1.67	1.15-2.42	0.006

Zink treatment during diarrhea was also a significant ($p = 0.009$) factor for having the health impact on the children due to cesarian delivery in the study area. Approximately 56.5% chance of having the health impact on the children due to cesarian delivery for the mothers who taken the Zink treatment during diarrhea.

Table 7.4 highlights the most influential factors which have health impact on the children due to cesarian delivery in Rajshahi district, Bangladesh. The initial breastfeeding and the Zink treatment during diarrhea were the significant risk factors which have health impact on the children due to cesarian delivery in the study area. There is a 6.1 [AOR = 6.04, 95% CI = (2.58–14.13), $p = <0.001$] times higher chance of having a health impact on the children due to cesarian delivery among the mothers who were not breastfeeding their children immediately after the birth than mothers who were breastfeeding their children immediately after the birth. If the mothers take the Zink treatment during diarrhea, then there is a 1.7 [AOR = 1.67, 95% CI = (1.15–2.42), $p = 0.006$] times higher chance of having the health impact on the children due to cesarian delivery among the mothers than their counterparties.

7.9 Discussion

The prevalence of cesarian delivery (C-section) in this study was 34.4%, which is higher than national survey reports. According to the Bangladesh Demographic and Health Survey (BDHS), C-section rates increased from 23% in 2014 to 33% in 2017 (NIPORT and ICF 2020). Another study reported an urban C-section prevalence of 36.9% among Bangladeshi mothers in 2021 (Ahmmed et al. 2021). In developed countries like those in Latin America, C-section rates are also high and continue to rise, reaching 40.5% (Betrán et al. 2007, 2016). The World Health Organization (WHO) guideline suggests that C-sections should ideally not exceed 10–15% of births and should only be performed when medically necessary (WHO 2015).

Our study found that mothers who had access to hygienic toilet facilities were more likely to undergo C-sections. This indicates that families with better economic status, often residing in urban areas, may opt for C-sections due to their ability to cover the associated costs (Chu et al. 2010). Similar findings from studies in Indonesia and Bangladesh have also linked higher wealth indices to increased C-section risks (Hasan et al. 2019; Wyatt et al. 2020). It is crucial to counsel pregnant mothers about the risks associated with unnecessary C-sections, which can lead to adverse health outcomes for both mothers and children.

C-section rates are significantly influenced by mothers' educational levels. In this study, higher-educated women were less likely to undergo C-section deliveries. Conversely, research from Northern Bangladesh suggested that higher educational attainment was associated with an increased likelihood of C-sections (Rahman et al. 2014). A meta-analysis from Iran also found a higher prevalence of C-sections among women with higher academic backgrounds (Rafiei et al. 2018). This discrepancy suggests the need for further evidence-based studies to clarify the relationship between C-section rates and maternal educational qualifications, potentially influenced by varying awareness of the long-term health implications for both mothers and children.

The present study also found that non-anemic mothers were less likely to have C-section than anemic mothers. However, this result was the opposite of a study conducted in Taiwan (Chu et al. 2020). We may suggest conducting advanced research to find out a plausible relationship between maternal anemia and mode of delivery in the Bangladeshi context.

This study revealed that women who did not receive antenatal care (ANC) visits were less inclined to opt for C-section deliveries. Conversely, research has shown that mothers who attended ANC visits during pregnancy were more likely to choose C-sections (Kamal et al. 2016). ANC visits are considered crucial for monitoring and ensuring a complication-free normal pregnancy. The observed difference in C-section preferences may stem from healthcare providers' influence during ANC visits, potentially motivating women toward surgical delivery.

Migraine is a common cause of headaches during pregnancy (Burch 2019), significantly affecting women of reproductive age (Robbins 2018). Our study identified severe headaches with blurred vision as a significant risk factor for C-section deliveries. Migraine often presents with severe headaches and blurred vision (Leonardi and Raggi 2013), and previous research has linked migraine to an increased likelihood of C-sections (Skajaa et al. 2019; Aarhus University 2019). Behavioral interventions and lifestyle adjustments are foundational in managing migraines during pregnancy, with neuromodulation and neurostimulation devices serving as additional treatment options (Parikh et al. 2020).

The swelling of the lower limbs is increased during pregnancy for enlarging uterus (Sikora-Szubert et al. 2012). Our study showed that edema problem during pregnancy is associated risk factor for cesarian delivery. Exercise is a safe, fruitful, and enjoyable complement for reduction of gestational-dependent edema (Hartmann and Huch 2005).

Our study revealed that mothers who don't take rest during pregnancy are associated with risk factor for cesarian delivery. More studies showed that women with poor sleep quality during pregnancy were at the high risk of cesarian delivery (Li et al. 2017; Teong et al. 2017).

Colostrum provides essential nutrients to newborn infants within one hour of birth, offering immunological and anti-inflammatory properties crucial for their health (Shrimpton 2017; Lawrence and Lawrence 2015). Breast milk further supports long-term benefits such as reducing obesity risk and enhancing psychosocial development (Patra et al. 2017). However, our study revealed that infants delivered via C-section face significant challenges in initiating breastfeeding, consistent with findings by Hobbs et al. (2016), which reported a 78% lower odds of early breastfeeding initiation compared to vaginal births (Exavery et al. 2015).

Furthermore, infants born through C-sections show distinct differences in gut microbiota development and are more likely to require zinc treatment during diarrhea, as observed in our study and supported by prior research on microbial diversity and immune-related disorders (Jakobsson et al. 2014; Palmer et al. 2007; Huurre et al. 2008; Sevelsted et al. 2015). These findings underscore potential long-term health implications associated with mode of delivery, reflecting the broader impact on neonatal health beyond the immediate postnatal period.

It is important to acknowledge limitations in our study, including focusing exclusively on live births in hospitals and clinics within Rajshahi district, Bangladesh, which may not fully represent all childbirth scenarios. Additionally, while we analyzed primary data, the study is constrained by inherent limitations of the dataset, such as incomplete medical records and the exclusion of certain influential factors documented in literature. Future studies should address these gaps to provide a comprehensive understanding of the complexities surrounding childbirth outcomes and their implications for maternal and infant health.

7.10 Conclusions

The rate of C-sections in Bangladesh remains higher than recommended by the WHO, leading to strain on the healthcare system due to unsafe practices and overuse. Factors such as belonging to marginalized groups, inadequate toilet facilities, low maternal education, severe headaches with blurred vision, edema, anemia, and prolonged rest during pregnancy were found to significantly predict C-sections in our study. Urgent measures are needed to implement strict guidelines and increase public awareness about the risks of unnecessary C-sections in Bangladesh. Counseling programs for women on delivery options should be prioritized to mitigate these effects. Our research highlights that C-sections adversely impact initial breastfeeding and increase the likelihood of zinc treatment during diarrhea for offspring. Addressing these issues is crucial for achieving Sustainable Development

Goals (SDGs) in the coming decade, making it imperative to focus globally on comprehensive strategies to manage C-section rates.

Ethical Approval This study was approved by the Ethical Review Committee of the Institute of Biological Sciences, University of Rajshahi, Bangladesh (Memo No 69/320/IAMEBBC/IBSC).

References

Aarhus University. (2019, June 26). Migraine increases the risk of complications during pregnancy and childbirth. Science Daily. Retrieved from www.sciencedaily.com/releases/2019/06/190626125111

Adam I, Kheiri S, Sharif ME, Ahmed ABA, Rayis DA (2019) Anaemia is associated with an increased risk for caesarean delivery. Int J Gynaecol Obstet 147(2):202–205. https://doi.org/10.1002/ijgo.12946

Ahmmed F, Manik MMR, Hossain MJ (2021) Caesarian section (CS) delivery in Bangladesh: a nationally representative cross-sectional study. PLoS One 16(7):e0254777. https://doi.org/10.1371/journal.pone.0254777

BBS (2011) Population and Housing Census 2011 Bangladesh Bureau of Statistics (BBS). Ministry of Planning, Government of the People's Republic of Bangladesh, Dhaka

Begum T, Rahman A, Nababan H, Hoque DME, Khan AF, Ali T, Anwar I (2017) Indications and determinants of caesarean section delivery: evidence from a population-based study in Matlab, Bangladesh. PLoS One 12(11):e0188074. https://doi.org/10.1371/journal.pone.0188074

Betrán AP, Merialdi M, Lauer JA, Bing-Shun W, Thomas J, Van Look P, Wagner M (2007) Rates of caesarean section: analysis of global, regional and national estimates. Paediatr Perinat Epidemiol 21(2):98–113. https://doi.org/10.1111/j.1365-3016.2007.00786

Betrán AP, Ye J, Moller AB, Zhang J, Gülmezoglu AM, Torloni MR (2016) The increasing trend in caesarean section rates: global, regional and national estimates: 1990–2014. PLoS One 11(2):e0148343. https://doi.org/10.1371/journal.pone.0148343

Betran AP, Ye J, Moller AB, Souza JP, Zhang J (2021) Trends and projections of caesarean section rates: global and regional estimates. BMJ Glob Health 6:6. https://doi.org/10.1136/bmjgh-2021-005671

Boerma T, Ronsmans C, Melesse DY, Barros AJD, Barros FC, Juan L et al (2018) Global epidemiology of use of and disparities in caesarean sections. Lancet 392(10155):1341–1348. https://doi.org/10.1016/s0140-6736(18)31928-7

Burch R (2019) Headache in pregnancy and the puerperium. Neurol Clin 37(1):31–51. https://doi.org/10.1016/j.ncl.2018.09.004

Chan YH (2004) Biostatistics 202: logistic regression analysis. Singapore Med J 45(4):149–153

Chu KH, Tai CJ, Hsu CS, Yeh MC, Chien LY (2010) Women's preference for cesarean delivery and differences between Taiwanese women undergoing different modes of delivery. BMC Health Serv Res 10:138. https://doi.org/10.1186/1472-6963-10-138

Chu FC, Shaw SW, Lo LM, Hsieh TT, Hung TH (2020) Association between maternal anemia at admission for delivery and adverse perinatal outcomes. J Chin Med Assoc 83(4):402–407. https://doi.org/10.1097/jcma.0000000000000215

Exavery A, Kanté AM, Hingora A, Phillips JF (2015) Determinants of early initiation of breastfeeding in rural Tanzania. Int Breastfeed J 10:27. https://doi.org/10.1186/s13006-015-0052-7

Hartmann S, Huch R (2005) Response of pregnancy leg edema to a single immersion exercise session. Acta Obstet Gynecol Scand 84(12):1150–1153. https://doi.org/10.1111/j.0001-6349.2005.00829

Hasan F, Alam MM, Hossain MG (2019) Associated factors and their individual contributions to caesarean delivery among married women in Bangladesh: analysis of Bangladesh demographic and health survey data. BMC Pregnancy Childbirth 19(1):433. https://doi.org/10.1186/s12884-019-2588-9

Hasan MN, Chowdhury MAB, Jahan J, Jahan S, Ahmed NU, Uddin MJ (2020) Cesarean delivery and early childhood diseases in Bangladesh: an analysis of demographic and health survey (BDHS) and multiple indicator cluster survey (MICS). PLoS One 15(12):e0242864. https://doi.org/10.1371/journal.pone.0242864

Hobbs AJ, Mannion CA, McDonald SW, Brockway M, Tough SC (2016) The impact of caesarean section on breastfeeding initiation, duration and difficulties in the first four months postpartum. BMC Pregnancy Childbirth 16:90. https://doi.org/10.1186/s12884-016-0876-1

Hossain MA, Karim MR, Mamun ASMA, Islam MS, Hossain MG (2023) Logistic regression analysis of mode of delivery influencing nutritional status among under-five children in Bangladesh: survey in rural area of Rajshahi District. Int J Stat Sci 23(2):107–116

Huurre A, Kalliomäki M, Rautava S, Rinne M, Salminen S, Isolauri E (2008) Mode of delivery—effects on gut microbiota and humoral immunity. Neonatology 93(4):236–240. https://doi.org/10.1159/000111102

Imran MIK, Inshafi MUA, Sheikh R, Chowdhury MAB, Uddin MJ (2019) Risk factors for acute respiratory infection in children younger than five years in Bangladesh. Public Health 173:112–119. https://doi.org/10.1016/j.puhe.2019.05.011

Jakobsson HE, Abrahamsson TR, Jenmalm MC, Harris K, Quince C, Jernberg C et al (2014) Decreased gut microbiota diversity, delayed Bacteroidetes colonisation and reduced Th1 responses in infants delivered by caesarean section. Gut 63(4):559–566. https://doi.org/10.1136/gutjnl-2012-303249

Kamal N, Curtis S, Hasan MS, Jamil K (2016) Trends in equity in use of maternal health services in urban and rural Bangladesh. Int J Equity Health 15:27. https://doi.org/10.1186/s12939-016-0311-2

Keag OE, Norman JE, Stock SJ (2018) Long-term risks and benefits associated with cesarean delivery for mother, baby, and subsequent pregnancies: systematic review and meta-analysis. PLoS Med 15(1):e1002494. https://doi.org/10.1371/journal.pmed.1002494

Lawrence RA, Lawrence RM (2015) Breastfeeding: a guide for the medical profession. Elsevier Health Sciences

Leonardi M, Raggi A (2013) Burden of migraine: international perspectives. Neurol Sci 34(Suppl 1):S117–S118. https://doi.org/10.1007/s10072-013-1387-8

Li R, Zhang J, Zhou R, Liu J, Dai Z, Liu D et al (2017) Sleep disturbances during pregnancy are associated with cesarean delivery and preterm birth. J Matern Fetal Neonatal Med 30(6):733–738. https://doi.org/10.1080/14767058.2016.1183637

Magne F, Puchi Silva A, Carvajal B, Gotteland M (2017) The elevated rate of cesarean section and its contribution to non-communicable chronic diseases in Latin America: the growing involvement of the microbiota. Front Pediatr 5:192. https://doi.org/10.3389/fped.2017.00192

Martin R, Saller K (1957) Lehrbuch der anthropologie. Gustav Fischer Verlag, Stuttgart

NICE (Producer). (2011, January 2018). Caesarean section: Clinical guideline. Caesarean section. Retrieved from https://www.nice.org.uk/guidance/CG132

NIPORT, ICF (2020) Bangladesh Demographic and Health Survey 2017–18. Retrieved from Dhaka, Bangladesh: https://www.dhsprogram.com/pubs/pdf/FR344/FR344.pdf

Palmer C, Bik EM, DiGiulio DB, Relman DA, Brown PO (2007) Development of the human infant intestinal microbiota. PLoS Biol 5(7):e177. https://doi.org/10.1371/journal.pbio.0050177

Parikh SK, Delbono MV, Silberstein SD (2020) Managing migraine in pregnancy and breastfeeding. Prog Brain Res 255:275–309. https://doi.org/10.1016/bs.pbr.2020.07.011

Patra K, Hamilton M, Johnson TJ, Greene M, Dabrowski E, Meier PP, Patel AL (2017) NICU human milk dose and 20-month neurodevelopmental outcome in very low birth weight infants. Neonatology 112(4):330–336. https://doi.org/10.1159/000475834

Rafiei M, Saei Ghare M, Akbari M, Kiani F, Sayehmiri F, Sayehmiri K, Vafaee R (2018) Prevalence, causes, and complications of cesarean delivery in Iran: a systematic review and meta-analysis. Int J Reprod Biomed 16(4):221–234

Rahman M, Ahmad Shariff A, Shafie A, Saaid R, Md Tahir R (2014) Determinants of caesarean risk factor in northern region of Bangladesh: a multivariate analysis. Iran J Public Health 43(1):16–27

Rahman MM, Haider MR, Moinuddin M, Rahman AE, Ahmed S, Khan MM (2018) Determinants of caesarean section in Bangladesh: cross-sectional analysis of Bangladesh demographic and health survey 2014 data. PLoS One 13(9):e0202879. https://doi.org/10.1371/journal.pone.0202879

Robbins MS (2018) Headache in pregnancy. Continuum (Minneap Minn) 24(4, Headache):1092–1107. https://doi.org/10.1212/con.0000000000000642

Sevelsted A, Stokholm J, Bønnelykke K, Bisgaard H (2015) Cesarean section and chronic immune disorders. Pediatrics 135(1):e92–e98. https://doi.org/10.1542/peds.2014-0596

Shrimpton R (2017) Early initiation of breastfeeding. e-Library of Evidence for Nutrition Actions (eLENA). Retrieved from https://www.who.int/tools/elena/commentary/earlybreastfeeding

Si KY, Li HT, Zhou YB, Li ZW, Zhang L, Zhang YL et al (2022) Cesarean delivery on maternal request and common child health outcomes: a prospective cohort study in China. J Glob Health 12:11001. https://doi.org/10.7189/jogh.12.11001

Sikora-Szubert A, Kowalska-Koprek U, Karowicz-Bilińska A (2012) The analysis of selected biochemical parameters concentration in pregnant women with idiopathic edema of the lower limbs—preliminary report. Ginekol Pol 83(9):660–664

Skajaa N, Szépligeti SK, Xue F, Sørensen HT, Ehrenstein V, Eisele O, Adelborg K (2019) Pregnancy, birth, neonatal, and postnatal neurological outcomes after pregnancy with migraine. Headache 59(6):869–879. https://doi.org/10.1111/head.13536

Teong ACA, Diong AX, Omar SZ, Tan PC (2017) The impact of self-reported sleep on caesarean delivery in women undergoing induction of labour: a prospective study. Sci Rep 7(1):12339. https://doi.org/10.1038/s41598-017-12410-7

Thomas, J., Paranjothy, S., Obstetricians, R. C. o., & Unit, G. C. E. S. (2001). National Sentinel Caesarean Section Audit Report. Retrieved from London: https://orca.cardiff.ac.uk/id/eprint/93112/1/nscs_audit.pdf

WHO (2006) WHO child growth standards : length/height-for-age, weight-for-age, weightfor-length, weight -for-height and body mass index-for-age : methods and development. World Health Organization, Geneva

WHO (2015) WHO statement on caesarean section rates. Reprod Health Matters 23(45):149–150. https://doi.org/10.1016/j.rhm.2015.07.007

Wyatt S, Silitonga P, Febriani E, Long Q (2020) Factors associated with rising Csection rate in Indonesia: findings from the Indonesian demographic and health surveys from 1998—2017. Authorea. doi:https://doi.org/10.22541/au.160071103.39107601

Yusuf A, Mamun A, Kamruzzaman M, Saw A, Abo El-Fetoh NM, Lestrel PE, Hossain MG (2019) Factors influencing childhood anaemia in Bangladesh: a two level logistic regression analysis. BMC Pediatr 19(1):213. https://doi.org/10.1186/s12887-019-1581-9

Zakerihamidi M, Latifnejad Roudsari R, Merghati Khoei E (2015) Vaginal delivery vs. cesarean section: a focused ethnographic study of Women's perceptions in the north of Iran. Int J Community Based Nurs Midwifery 3(1):39–50

Zhang T, Sidorchuk A, Sevilla-Cermeño L, Vilaplana-Pérez A, Chang Z, Larsson H et al (2019) Association of cesarean delivery with risk of neurodevelopmental and psychiatric disorders in the offspring: a systematic review and meta-analysis. JAMA Netw Open 2(8):e1910236. https://doi.org/10.1001/jamanetworkopen.2019.10236

Maternal and Child Nutritional Status in South and Southeast Asia: A Comparative Analysis Across Bangladesh, Cambodia, India, Maldives, Nepal, Pakistan, and Timor-Leste

8

Ramendra Nath Kundu, Arna Chatterjee, Zannatun Nyma, Manoranjan Pal, Susmita Bharati, Md. Golam Hossain, and Premananda Bharati

Abbreviations

ANOVA	Analysis of variance
BAZ	BMI for age Z-score
BDHS	Bangladesh Demographic and Health Survey
BMI	Body Mass Index
CDHS	Cambodia Demographic and Health Survey
CI	Confidence Interval
DHS	Demographic and Health Surveys

R. N. Kundu
Former UGC Sr. Research Fellow, Department of Anthropology, West Bengal State University, Barasat, West Bengal, India

A. Chatterjee
Junior Research Fellow, Anthropological Survey of India, SRC, Mysuru, India

Z. Nyma
Shiga University of Medical Science, Setatsukinowacho, Shiga, Japan

M. Pal
Economic Research Unit, Indian Statistical Institute (ISI), Kolkata, West Bengal, India

S. Bharati
Sociological Research Unit, Indian Statistical Institute, Kolkata, West Bengal, India

M. G. Hossain
Department of Statistics, University of Rajshahi, Rajshahi, Bangladesh

P. Bharati (✉)
Biological Anthropology Unit, Indian Statistical Institute (ISI), Kolkata, West Bengal, India

M. Pal et al. (eds.), *Public Health and Nutrition*,
https://doi.org/10.1007/978-981-97-7890-4_8

HAZ	Height/length for age Z-score
LMICs	Low- and Middle-Income Countries
MDHS	Maldives Demographic and Health Survey
NDHS	Nepal Demographic and Health Survey
NFHS	National Family Health Survey
PDHS	Pakistan Demographic and Health Survey
S-SE	South and Southeast
TLDHS	Timor-Leste Demographic and Health Survey
UNICEF	United Nations Children's Fund; Maternal, Newborn, Child and Adolescent Health
WAZ	Weight for age Z-score
WHO	World Health Organization
WHZ	Weight for height/length Z-score

8.1 Introduction

Annually, undernutrition accounts for at least half of all the deaths in children under five globally (Kundu et al. 2024; UNICEF/WHO/WBG 2023). An estimated 6.3 million liveborn children worldwide died before the age of 5 years in 2013 (UNICEF/WHO/WBG/UN 2013). The World Health Organization (WHO) reports that globally in 2016, 155 million children under five were stunted, 52 million were wasted, and 99 million were underweight (Black et al. 2013; WHO 2017). According to WHO (2006), a z-score less than -2SD is considered as stunting, wasting, underweight or thinness, respectively, for height-for-age, weight-for-height, weight-for-age, and BMI-for-age. In 2020, 149.2 million under-five children were reported as stunted and 45.4 million as wasted globally, whereas Asian countries accounted for 79 million being stunted and 31.9 million being wasted (UNICEF/WHO/WBG 2021).

Undernutrition is a widespread problem in low- and middle-income countries (LMICs), especially in South Asia, Southeast Asia, and Africa (Arora 2009; Marotz 2012). The prevalence of stunting is very high (≥40%) in many countries of Sub-Saharan Africa, South Central Asia, and Southeast Asia (de Onis and Blössner 2003). India, Pakistan, and Bangladesh have particularly high rates of undernutrition in the South Asian regions (Headey et al. 2016). Pakistan is ranked 22nd in the world for under-five child mortality, and undernutrition is considered the main reason for this mortality (Bhutta et al. 2013; UNICEF 2016b). According to the Pakistan Demographic and Health Survey (2017–18), 37.6% of under-five children were stunted and 23.1% were underweight (NIPS and ICF 2019).

Numerous studies have shown that the first 23 months of a child's life are of utmost importance for their physical and cognitive growth (UNICEF 2016a). During this time, children experience rapid development, both physically and cognitively, which lays the foundation for their overall health and well-being. Undernutrition has a significant impact on the cognitive and physical development of children, leading to an increased risk of infections and longer recovery times, and ultimately contributing to morbidity and mortality (Pelletier and Frongillo 2003; Pelletier et al. 1995). Multiple interlinked factors cause undernutrition, which has short and long-term detrimental health effects on children (Bomela 2009; WHO 2013).

Maternal nutritional status during gestation is directly linked to the appropriate growth of the fetus and infant (Hasan et al. 2019; Mohamed et al. 2022). Maternal insufficient gestational weight gain and undernutrition are responsible for poor fetal growth and low birth weight, whereas maternal excessive pregnancy weight gain and obesity are linked with excessive fetal growth, childhood obesity, and even late antepartum death (Kaar et al. 2014; King 2003; Lawlor et al. 2012; Ruager-Martin et al. 2010; Triunfo and Lanzone 2015). Low body mass index (BMI), indicative of maternal undernutrition, contributes to fetal growth restriction, which increases the risk of neonatal deaths and increases the risk of stunting, especially for children ≥2 years of age (Black et al. 2013). In Pakistan, a mother's low BMI, short stature, and low education level can significantly contribute to her child's underweight status (Khan et al. 2019). Similar findings were observed in Nepal, where a mother's BMI was found to be an important determinant of childhood stunting (Tiwari et al. 2014). It is not just a mother's weight, height, and BMI that play a role, but also her age (Nankinga et al. 2019; Nigatu et al. 2018). Children born to younger mothers (aged 15–24 years) are more likely to be stunted (Nankinga et al. 2019).

There have been some notable gaps in the research on the relationship between maternal and child nutrition in South and Southeast Asia, specifically in using national-level data to compare multiple countries. Previous studies examining the factors affecting child nutritional status have been limited to certain regions or counties (Khan et al. 2019; Nigatu et al. 2018; Tiwari et al. 2014). A comparative study is necessary to address these gaps and gain a more comprehensive understanding of the issue. The aim of this study is to explore the effect of maternal demographic, anthropometric, and nutritional characteristics on under-five child nutrition in seven South and Southeast Asian countries, using nationally representative data.

8.2 Methods

8.2.1 Data Source

The latest Demographic and Health Surveys (DHS) Program conducted in South and Southeast (S-SE) Asian countries provided unit-level data. This program primarily focuses on children and mothers' health, mortality, and sociodemographic characteristics. For this study, a total of seven countries in S-SE Asia were selected, and a systematic household survey was conducted by the DHS in the last 10 years, adhering to the standard guidelines. The countries selected for this study were Bangladesh (BDHS, 2017–2018), Cambodia (CDHS, 2021–2022), India (NFHS, 2019–2021), Maldives (MDHS, 2016–2017), Nepal (NDHS 2023), Pakistan (PDHS, 2017–2018), and Timor-Leste (TLDHS 2018) (GDS, MoF, and ICF 2018; IIPS and ICF 2021;

MOH and ICF 2018; MoHP, NERA, and ICF 2022; NIPORT and ICF 2020; NIPS and ICF 2019; NIS, MoH, and ICF 2023). The surveys provided nationally representative data on mothers and their children, which was used for the analysis. A total of 2,73,337 reproductive-age women and their 2,63,068 alive children were primarily selected for the study. Excluding 46,023 mother-child pairs as invalid samples, 2,17,045 mother-child pairs were finally selected for this study. Invalid samples included crucial data beyond reasonable limits or missing values. Figure 8.1 demonstrates the data inclusion and exclusion criteria in the flow chart.

8.2.2 Study Variables

Demographic Variables The study considered age and gender as demographic variables. Specifically, the age range of the mothers who were included in the study was between 15 and 49 years, which is referred to as reproductive age. The study considered both boys and girls up to the age of 59 months.

Anthropometric Variables During the household survey, anthropometric measurements were taken in accordance with the DHS guidelines that follow standard protocols. Anthropometric variables such as body height (in cm) and weight (in kg) were considered for both mothers and their children. The body length of children under 24 months of age was measured while they were lying down (recumbent) on the board, whereas the height of children aged 24 months and above was measured while they were standing. The mother's height, on the other hand, was measured while she was standing. A portable anthropometer and weighing machine were used to measure the body height and weight, respectively. The anthropometric measurements were taken with utmost care and precision to ensure accurate and reliable results.

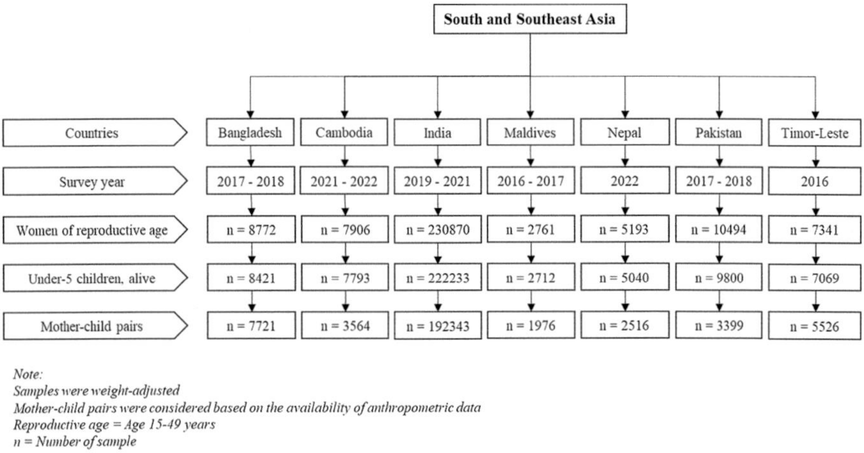

Fig. 8.1 Data selection procedure for this study

Nutritional Variables We assessed the nutritional status of the mothers by calculating their body mass index (BMI). For the children, we utilized height/length for age Z-score (HAZ), weight for age Z-score (WAZ), weight for height/length Z-score (WHZ), and BMI for age Z-score (BAZ) measurements, as recommended by the World Health Organization.

8.2.3 Statistical Analysis

This study used various statistical techniques to investigate the relationship between maternal factors and child nutritional conditions in different countries. Descriptive analysis was used to determine the mean and standard deviation (SD) of the mean for quantitative variables. The ANOVA test was employed to see the variation of mean demographic, anthropometric, and nutritional indicators across different countries. Stepwise multiple linear regression was used to identify which maternal factors contribute significantly to child nutritional conditions. We examined the statistical significance using p-value with ≤ 0.05 considered as significant. The Statistical Package for the Social Sciences (SPSS, version 25.0) was used for statistical analysis.

8.3 Results

Table 8.1 presents a comprehensive statistical summary of the characteristics of mothers in S-SE countries. The table shows the mean and standard deviation (SD) for each variable and sees whether the mean values differ significantly among the countries (ANOVA, $p < 0.001$). The mean age of the mother in Bangladesh (25.65 years) was much less than that of Maldives (30.47 years). On the other hand, Maldives mothers had higher mean weight and BMI (weight: 60.19 kg, BMI: 25.90 kg/m^2), while Pakistan had a higher mean height (154.57 cm).

Table 8.2 provides an overview of basic demographic and anthropometric measurements, which include the age, weight, and height/length of children from different S-SE Asian countries. The mean age of the children varied significantly (ANOVA, $p < 0.001$) across countries but was mostly around 28 to 31 months. The mean weight and height/length exhibited significant differences (ANOVA, $p < 0.001$) across the countries. The children's weight ranged from 10 to 12 kg, while their height/length varied from 82 to 87 cm.

Table 8.3 presents a descriptive overview of four key nutritional measures for children in S-SE Asia, including HAZ, WAZ, WHZ, and BAZ. The data clearly illustrate considerable differences in each nutritional measure across the countries (ANOVA, $p < 0.001$). For overall children, the mean HAZ and WAZ were the highest in the Maldives and the lowest in Timor-Leste, while the highest WHZ and BAZ are found in Pakistan and the lowest in Timor-Leste.

Table 8.4 presents the Pearson correlation coefficients between various maternal variables (Age, Weight, Height, BMI) and child variables (Weight, Height, HAZ,

Table 8.1 Descriptive analysis of mother's demographic and anthropometric variables

S-SE Asian countries	N	Mother's age (years)	Mother's weight (kg)	Mother's height (cm)	Mother's BMI (kg/m^2)
		Mean (SD)	Mean (SD)	Mean (SD)	Mean (SD)
Bangladesh	7721	25.65 (5.62)	51.85 (10.01)	151.02 (5.39)	22.69 (3.98)
Cambodia	3564	30.32 (6.14)	55.32 (9.54)	154.04 (5.19)	23.28 (3.64)
India	192,343	26.96 (4.82)	50.57 (10.28)	151.76 (5.94)	21.92 (4.06)
Maldives	1976	30.47 (5.27)	60.19 (11.88)	152.38 (5.43)	25.90 (4.86)
Nepal	2516	26.59 (5.30)	52.03 (10.01)	152.06 (5.36)	22.48 (4.01)
Pakistan	3399	28.95 (5.84)	58.87 (13.05)	154.57 (5.77)	24.61 (5.11)
Timor-Leste	5526	30.42 (6.55)	49.00 (8.50)	151.57 (5.28)	21.31 (3.42)
ANOVA: F [*p*-value]		1037.12 [$p < 0.001$]	799.65 [$p < 0.001$]	241.58 [$p < 0.001$]	676.38 [$p < 0.001$]

S-SE South and Southeast; *SD* standard deviation

Table 8.2 Descriptive analysis of child's demographic and anthropometric variables

S-SE Asian countries	N	Age (month)	Weight (kg)	Height/length (cm)
		Mean (SD)	Mean (SD)	Mean (SD)
Overall children				
Bangladesh	7721	28.58 (17.47)	10.81 (3.35)	83.20 (14.28)
Cambodia	3564	29.25 (17.22)	11.27 (3.36)	84.95 (13.73)
India	192,343	30.07 (17.20)	10.82 (3.27)	84.31 (13.80)
Maldives	1976	30.86 (17.10)	11.82 (3.66)	86.98 (14.47)
Nepal	2516	29.87 (16.89)	11.16 (3.16)	84.81 (13.31)
Pakistan	3399	28.87 (17.28)	10.93 (3.36)	82.64 (13.56)
Timor-Leste	5526	30.20 (16.89)	10.49 (2.98)	83.60 (13.12)
ANOVA: F [*p*-value]		13.87 [$p < 0.001$]	55.67 [$p < 0.001$]	32.95 [$p < 0.001$]
Boys				
Bangladesh	4024	28.50 (17.37)	11.06 (3.34)	83.82 (14.12)
Cambodia	1801	29.05 (17.55)	11.40 (3.33)	85.12 (13.70)
India	99,237	30.21 (17.19)	11.08 (3.25)	84.98 (13.66)
Maldives	1003	31.75 (17.14)	12.22 (3.67)	88.36 (14.14)
Nepal	1306	29.32 (17.01)	11.39 (3.17)	85.09 (13.27)
Pakistan	1731	28.71 (17.11)	11.16 (3.28)	83.17 (13.19)
Timor-Leste	2752	30.57 (16.75)	10.71 (2.92)	84.19 (12.91)
ANOVA: F [*p*-value]		11.86 [$p < 0.001$]	31.39 [$p < 0.001$]	21.4 [$p < 0.001$]
Girls				
Bangladesh	3697	28.67 (17.58)	10.54 (3.35)	82.53 (14.42)
Cambodia	1763	29.46 (16.89)	11.14 (3.38)	84.79 (13.76)
India	93,106	29.92 (17.22)	10.55 (3.27)	83.61 (13.92)
Maldives	973	29.95 (17.01)	11.40 (3.61)	85.56 (14.67)
Nepal	1210	30.47 (16.75)	10.92 (3.13)	84.50 (13.34)
Pakistan	1668	29.04 (17.47)	10.69 (3.43)	82.10 (13.92)
Timor-Leste	2774	29.84 (17.03)	10.27 (3.02)	83.01 (13.30)
ANOVA: F [*p*-value]		4.19 [$p < 0.001$]	26.55 [$p < 0.001$]	13.92 [$p < 0.001$]

S-SE South and Southeast, *SD* standard deviation

Table 8.3 Descriptive analysis of child's nutritional indicators based on WHO recommendations

S-SE Asian countries	*N*	HAZ Mean (SD)	WAZ Mean (SD)	WHZ Mean (SD)	BAZ Mean (SD)
Overall children					
Bangladesh	7721	−1.38 (1.28)	−1.15 (1.10)	−0.52 (1.13)	−0.42 (1.13)
Cambodia	3564	−1.05 (1.34)	−0.93 (1.13)	−0.49 (1.29)	−0.40 (1.30)
India	192,343	−1.40 (1.68)	−1.41 (1.21)	−0.85 (1.44)	−0.74 (1.48)
Maldives	1976	−0.87 (1.21)	−0.81 (1.17)	−0.47 (1.29)	−0.42 (1.29)
Nepal	2516	−1.25 (1.16)	−1.10 (1.06)	−0.55 (1.05)	−0.46 (1.02)
Pakistan	3399	−1.56 (1.57)	−1.12 (1.21)	−0.29 (1.16)	−0.16 (1.20)
Timor−Leste	5526	−1.66 (1.93)	−1.63 (1.28)	−0.98 (1.58)	−0.82 (1.63)
ANOVA: *F* [*p*-value]		90.67 [$p < 0.001$]	308.06 [$p < 0.001$]	228.97 [$p < 0.001$]	207.18 [$p < 0.001$]
Boys					
Bangladesh	4024	−1.38 (1.29)	−1.15 (1.11)	−0.54 (1.17)	−0.42 (1.17)
Cambodia	1801	−1.12 (1.36)	−0.98 (1.17)	−0.52 (1.34)	−0.41 (1.34)
India	99,237	−1.44 (1.68)	−1.42 (1.20)	−0.88 (1.46)	−0.74 (1.50)
Maldives	1003	−0.87 (1.24)	−0.83 (1.22)	−0.52 (1.34)	−0.45 (1.34)
Nepal	1306	−1.20 (1.17)	−1.02 (1.07)	−0.50 (1.09)	−0.40 (1.05)
Pakistan	1731	−1.59 (1.60)	−1.12 (1.23)	−0.30 (1.16)	−0.13 (1.21)
Timor−Leste	2752	−1.79 (1.92)	−1.72 (1.25)	−1.04 (1.59)	−0.83 (1.64)
ANOVA: *F* [*p*-value]		60.03 [$p < 0.001$]	179.49 [$p < 0.001$]	125.51 [$p < 0.001$]	109.44 [$p < 0.001$]
Girls					
Bangladesh	3697	−1.38 (1.27)	−1.16 (1.09)	−0.51 (1.09)	−0.43 (1.09)
Cambodia	1763	−0.98 (1.31)	−0.88 (1.09)	−0.46 (1.24)	−0.39 (1.25)
India	93,106	−1.36 (1.69)	−1.39 (1.21)	−0.83 (1.42)	−0.74 (1.46)
Maldives	973	−0.88 (1.18)	−0.80 (1.12)	−0.42 (1.23)	−0.38 (1.23)
Nepal	1210	−1.30 (1.15)	−1.17 (1.05)	−0.60 (1.00)	−0.52 (0.98)
Pakistan	1668	−1.53 (1.54)	−1.12 (1.19)	−0.29 (1.15)	−0.19 (1.18)
Timor−Leste	2774	−1.52 (1.93)	−1.55 (1.31)	−0.93 (1.57)	−0.81 (1.61)
ANOVA: *F* [*p*-value]		36.36 [$p < 0.001$]	135.02 [$p < 0.001$]	104.97 [$p < 0.001$]	98.82 [$p < 0.001$]

S-SE South and Southeast, *SD* standard deviation, *HAZ* height/length for age Z-score; *WAZ* weight for age Z-score, *WHZ* weight for height/length Z-score, *BAZ* BMI for age Z-score

WAZ, WHZ, BAZ) across several S-SE Asian countries. The correlations are shown for overall children, boys, and girls separately. It is clear from the tables that Weight, Height, HAZ, WAZ, WHZ, and BAZ were significantly positively correlated with Age, Weight, Height, and BMI of mothers with very few exceptions.

Tables 8.5, 8.6, 8.7, 8.8, 8.9 and 8.10 present the results of stepwise multiple linear regression analyses of children weight, height, HAZ, WAZ, WHZ, and BAZ on mother's weight, height, age, and BMI for each country separately for boys, girls, and all children. The picture that emerged from these tables was uniform. All the coefficients were found to be positive except for a very few cases. This means that maternal factors significantly influenced child's status of health regardless of

Table 8.4 Exploring the correlation of variables between mothers and their children in South and Southeast Asian Countries

S-SE Asian countries		Overall children						Boys						Girls					
		Weight	Height	HAZ	WAZ	WHZ	BAZ	Weight	Height	HAZ	WAZ	WHZ	BAZ	Weight	Height	HAZ	WAZ	WHZ	BAZ
Bangladesh	Age	0.189**	0.210**	0.011	−0.022	−0.045**	−0.034**	0.206**	0.230**	0.028	−0.014	−0.048**	−0.039*	0.170**	0.188**	−0.008	−0.031	−0.041*	−0.028
	Weight	0.219**	0.170**	0.246**	0.273**	0.146**	0.125**	0.228**	0.174**	0.268**	0.290**	0.151**	0.125**	0.211**	0.165**	0.220**	0.254**	0.139**	0.124**
	Height	0.101**	0.081**	0.291**	0.248**	0.060**	0.037**	0.107**	0.082**	0.297**	0.253**	0.070**	0.041**	0.098**	0.080**	0.285**	0.242**	0.048**	0.032
	BMI	0.199**	0.154**	0.151**	0.199**	0.135**	0.121**	0.207**	0.159**	0.176**	0.216**	0.136**	0.120**	0.190**	0.148**	0.124**	0.179**	0.133**	0.123**
Cambodia	Age	0.170**	0.197**	−0.004	−0.044**	−0.056**	−0.049**	0.166**	0.210**	−0.02	−0.073**	−0.073**	−0.074**	0.175**	0.183**	0.013	−0.013	−0.036	−0.022
	Weight	0.123**	0.072**	0.146**	0.212**	0.148**	0.132**	0.142**	0.086**	0.119**	0.205**	0.164**	0.150**	0.104**	0.057*	0.177**	0.221**	0.128**	0.112**
	Height	0.084**	0.042*	0.193**	0.221**	0.113**	0.092**	0.074**	0.03	0.196**	0.224**	0.116**	0.098**	0.096**	0.055*	0.189**	0.216**	0.109**	0.085**
	BMI	0.103**	0.065**	0.077**	0.139**	0.115**	0.107**	0.127**	0.085**	0.047*	0.129**	0.131**	0.123**	0.078**	0.043	0.110**	0.150**	0.096**	0.089**
India	Age	0.237**	0.245**	−0.003	0.010**	0.010**	0.018**	0.238**	0.244**	0.004	0.022**	0.016**	0.025**	0.237**	0.246**	−0.011**	−0.002	0.003	0.010**
	Weight	0.188**	0.128**	0.184**	0.271**	0.147**	0.124**	0.192**	0.134**	0.188**	0.272**	0.147**	0.121**	0.185**	0.122**	0.179**	0.271**	0.147**	0.128**
	Height	0.118**	0.098**	0.206**	0.213**	0.054**	0.029**	0.121**	0.099**	0.211**	0.219**	0.061**	0.032**	0.115**	0.097**	0.201**	0.207**	0.046**	0.027**
	BMI	0.156**	0.099**	0.115**	0.207**	0.138**	0.124**	0.160**	0.105**	0.118**	0.205**	0.135**	0.119**	0.154**	0.094**	0.111**	0.209**	0.142**	0.129**
Maldives	Age	0.187**	0.194**	0.032	0.041	0.017	0.029	0.167**	0.172**	0.027	0.032	0.019	0.021	0.212**	0.221**	0.039	0.053	0.015	0.039
	Weight	0.087**	0.032	0.155**	0.194**	0.141**	0.120**	0.077*	0.008	0.118**	0.203**	0.187**	0.167**	0.098**	0.057	0.198**	0.183**	0.088**	0.066*
	Height	0.073**	0.063**	0.248**	0.177**	0.033	0.02	0.102**	0.086**	0.255**	0.193**	0.055	0.039	0.036	0.035	0.240**	0.159**	0.008	−0.002
	BMI	0.064**	0.011	0.071**	0.137**	0.136**	0.118**	0.041	−0.026	0.028	0.141**	0.178**	0.162**	0.090**	0.049	0.118**	0.133**	0.089**	0.069*
Nepal	Age	0.220**	0.224**	0.015	0.004	−0.01	<0.001	0.201**	0.208**	0.011	0.002	−0.008	<0.001	0.236**	0.242**	0.013	−0.002	−0.018	−0.008
	Weight	0.157**	0.075**	0.296**	0.356**	0.254**	0.222**	0.118**	0.029	0.288**	0.362**	0.273**	0.242**	0.197**	0.122**	0.304**	0.347**	0.232**	0.199**
	Height	0.096**	0.078**	0.317**	0.238**	0.052**	0.019	0.066*	0.045	0.300**	0.226**	0.060*	0.025	0.126**	0.111**	0.335**	0.250**	0.041	0.011
	BMI	0.133**	0.051**	0.193**	0.287**	0.252**	0.230**	0.103**	0.016	0.192**	0.299**	0.267**	0.247**	0.163**	0.088**	0.193**	0.274**	0.234**	0.209**
Pakistan	Age	0.231**	0.247**	−0.002	0.008	0.005	0.021	0.196**	0.208**	0.013	0.027	0.025	0.033	0.267**	0.285**	−0.017	−0.011	−0.014	0.01
	Weight	0.207**	0.158**	0.231**	0.292**	0.172**	0.141**	0.184**	0.146**	0.227**	0.251**	0.133**	0.092**	0.233**	0.171**	0.234**	0.336**	0.213**	0.193**
	Height	0.121**	0.104**	0.257**	0.248**	0.071**	0.042*	0.124**	0.104**	0.285**	0.279**	0.086**	0.054*	0.122**	0.107**	0.224**	0.213**	0.054*	0.03
	BMI	0.177**	0.130**	0.156**	0.224**	0.158**	0.135**	0.150**	0.117**	0.140**	0.169**	0.113**	0.080**	0.204**	0.144**	0.172**	0.282**	0.204**	0.193**
Timor–Leste	Age	0.191**	0.213**	−0.014	−0.040**	−0.041**	−0.031*	0.199**	0.215**	0.014	−0.006	−0.034	−0.022	0.189**	0.214**	−0.045*	−0.076**	−0.050**	−0.040*
	Weight	0.151**	0.102**	0.057**	0.149**	0.109**	0.106**	0.175**	0.112**	0.051**	0.170**	0.138**	0.138**	0.128**	0.092**	0.066**	0.131**	0.081**	0.075**
	Height	0.099**	0.096**	0.141**	0.129**	0.003	−0.012	0.123**	0.131**	0.137**	0.111**	−0.016	−0.028	0.074**	0.060**	0.147**	0.148**	0.025	0.005
	BMI	0.119**	0.068**	0.001	0.105**	0.116**	0.119**	0.130**	0.062**	−0.008	0.130**	0.153**	0.158**	0.108**	0.074**	0.01	0.082**	0.079**	0.080**

HAZ height/length for age Z-score, *WAZ* weight for age Z-score, *WHZ* weight for height/length Z-score, *BAZ* BMI for age Z-score
Significant $^{**}p < 0.01$, $^{*}p < 0.05$

Table 8.5 Stepwise-multiple linear regression analysis of child's weight (kg) on maternal variables

		B	*p*-value	B	*p*-value	*B*	*p*-value
S-SE Asian countries	Maternal factors	Male		Female		Overall	
Bangladesh	Mother's weight (kg)	0.058	$p < 0.001$	0.090	$p < 0.001$	0.058	$p < 0.001$
	Mother's age (year)	0.104	$p < 0.001$	0.079	$p < 0.001$	0.092	$p < 0.001$
	Mother's height (cm)	0.032	0.002	−0.074	0.036	0.026	$p < 0.001$
	R-Square	0.079		0.062		0.070	
Cambodia	Mother's weight (kg)	0.040	$p < 0.001$	–	–	−0.198	0.032
	Mother's age (year)	0.080	$p < 0.001$	0.104	$p < 0.001$	0.088	$p < 0.001$
	Mother's height (cm)	–	–	0.076	$p < 0.001$	0.207	0.002
	Mother's BMI (kg/m^2)	–	–	–	–	0.529	0.016
	R-Square	0.038		0.043		0.042	
India	Mother's weight (kg)	0.040	$p < 0.001$	0.040	$p < 0.001$	−0.001	0.870
	Mother's age (year)	0.143	$p < 0.001$	0.146	$p < 0.001$	0.144	$p < 0.001$
	Mother's height (cm)	0.033	$p < 0.001$	0.029	$p < 0.001$	0.059	$p < 0.001$
	Mother's BMI (kg/m^2)	–	–	–	–	0.096	$p < 0.001$
	R-Square	0.075		0.076		0.075	
Maldives	Mother's weight (kg)	–	–	0.022	0.029	–	–
	Mother's age (year)	0.114	$p < 0.001$	0.158	$p < 0.001$	0.137	$p < 0.001$
	Mother's height (cm)	0.068	0.001	0.044	0.045	0.065	$p < 0.001$
	R-Square	0.035		0.059		0.043	
Nepal	Mother's weight (kg)	0.032	$p < 0.001$	0.039	$p < 0.001$	0.033	$p < 0.001$
	Mother's age (year)	0.110	$p < 0.001$	0.125	$p < 0.001$	0.120	$p < 0.001$
	Mother's height (cm)	–	–	0.040	0.021	0.032	0.008
	R-Square	0.050		0.081		0.066	
Pakistan	Mother's weight (kg)	0.083	$p < 0.001$	0.048	$p < 0.001$	0.043	$p < 0.001$
	Mother's age (year)	0.096	$p < 0.001$	0.130	$p < 0.001$	0.113	$p < 0.001$
	Mother's height (cm)	–	–	0.046	0.002	0.036	$p < 0.001$

(continued)

Table 8.5 (continued)

		B	*p*-value	B	*p*-value	*B*	*p*-value
S-SE Asian countries	Maternal factors	Male		Female		Overall	
	Mother's BMI (kg/m^2)	–0.107	0.015	–	–	–	–
	R-Square	0.065		0.112		0.086	
Timor-Leste	Mother's weight (kg)	0.094	$p < 0.001$	0.026	$p < 0.001$	0.034	$p < 0.001$
	Mother's age (year)	0.080	$p < 0.001$	0.091	$p < 0.001$	0.085	$p < 0.001$
	Mother's height (cm)	–	–	0.039	0.001	0.035	$p < 0.001$
	Mother's BMI (kg/m^2)	–0.125	0.001	–	–	–	–
	R-Square	0.050		0.051		0.049	

S-SE South and Southeast, *B* unstandardized coefficients

Table 8.6 Stepwise-multiple linear regression analysis of child's height (cm) on maternal variables

S-SE Asian countries	Predicted maternal factors	*B*	*p*-value	*B*	*p*-value	*B*	*p*-value
		Boys		Girls		Overall	
Bangladesh	Mother's age (year)	0.524	$p < 0.001$	0.447	$p < 0.001$	0.488	$p < 0.001$
	Mother's weight (kg)	0.169	$p < 0.001$	0.165	$p < 0.001$	0.167	$p < 0.001$
	Mother's height (cm)	0.139	0.002	0.127	0.007	0.131	$p < 0.001$
	R-Square	0.071		0.055		0.063	
Cambodia	Mother's age (year)	0.447	$p < 0.001$	0.444	$p < 0.001$	0.459	$p < 0.001$
	Mother's weight (kg)	0.097	0.003	–	–	–	–
	Mother's height (cm)	–	–	0.181	0.004	0.155	$p < 0.001$
	R-Square	0.047		0.040		0.043	
India	Mother's age (year)	0.662	$p < 0.001$	0.683	$p < 0.001$	0.673	$p < 0.001$
	Mother's weight (kg)	−0.134	0.015	−0.178	0.001	−0.156	$p < 0.001$
	Mother's height (cm)	0.297	$p < 0.001$	0.322	$p < 0.001$	0.311	$p < 0.001$
	Mother's BMI (kg/m^2)	0.515	$p < 0.001$	0.596	$p < 0.001$	0.556	$p < 0.001$
	R-Square	0.067		0.068		0.067	
Maldives	Mother's age (year)	0.503	$p < 0.001$	0.626	$p < 0.001$	0.536	$p < 0.001$
	Mother's height (cm)	0.309	$p < 0.001$	0.199	0.032	0.261	$p < 0.001$
	Mother's BMI (kg/m^2)	−0.244	0.010	–	–	–	–
	R-Square	0.044		0.042		0.038	
Nepal	Mother's age (year)	0.520	$p < 0.001$	0.644	$p < 0.001$	0.580	$p < 0.001$
	Mother's height (cm)			0.256	$p < 0.001$	0.195	$p < 0.001$
	R-Square	0.045		0.072		0.058	
Pakistan	Mother's age (year)	0.419	$p < 0.001$	0.572	$p < 0.001$	0.497	$p < 0.001$
	Mother's weight (kg)	0.308	$p < 0.001$	0.129	$p < 0.001$	0.129	$p < 0.001$
	Mother's height (cm)	–	–	0.199	0.001	0.155	$p < 0.001$
	Mother's BMI (kg/m^2)	−0.436	0.015	–	–	–	–
	R-Square	0.061		0.096		0.076	
Timor-Leste	Mother's age (year)	0.426	$p < 0.001$	0.468	$p < 0.001$	0.438	$p < 0.001$
	Mother's height (cm)	0.283	$p < 0.001$	0.183	$p < 0.001$	0.240	$p < 0.001$
	Mother's BMI (kg/m^2)	–	–	–	–	0.107	0.043
	R-Square	0.052		0.050		0.051	

S-SE South and Southeast, *B* unstandardized coefficients

Table 8.7 Stepwise-multiple linear regression analysis of child's HAZ on maternal variables

		B	*p*-value	B	*p*-value	*B*	Sig.
S-SE Asian countries	Predicted maternal factors	Boys		Girls			*p*-value
Bangladesh	Mother's height (cm)	0.071	$p < 0.001$	0.055	$p < 0.001$	0.068	$p < 0.001$
	Mother's weight (kg)	–	–	0.016	$p < 0.001$	–	–
	Mother's BMI (kg/m^2)	0.053	$p < 0.001$	–	–	0.045	$p < 0.001$
	R-Square	0.111		0.091		0.101	
Cambodia	Mother's height (cm)	0.055	$p < 0.001$	0.034	$p < 0.001$	0.042	$p < 0.001$
	Mother's weight (kg)	–	–	0.017	$p < 0.001$	0.012	$p < 0.001$
	R-Square	0.040		0.044		0.041	
India	Mother's height (cm)	0.058	$p < 0.001$	0.069	$p < 0.001$	0.066	$p < 0.001$
	Mother's BMI (kg/m^2)	0.048	$p < 0.001$	0.093	$p < 0.001$	0.081	$p < 0.001$
	Mother's weight (kg)	–	–	−0.020	0.005	−0.014	0.004
	Mother's age (year)	−0.008	$p < 0.001$	−0.013	$p < 0.001$	−0.011	$p < 0.001$
	R-Square	0.048		0.045		0.047	
Maldives	Mother's height (cm)	0.057	$p < 0.001$	0.063	$p < 0.001$	0.060	$p < 0.001$
	Mother's BMI (kg/m^2)	–	–	0.031	$p < 0.001$	0.018	0.001
	Mother's age (year)	–	–	0.018	0.016	0.014	0.006
	R-Square	0.065		0.085		0.073	
Nepal	Mother's height (cm)	0.051	$p < 0.001$	0.053	$p < 0.001$	0.052	$p < 0.001$
	Mother's weight (kg)	0.025	$p < 0.001$	0.024	$p < 0.001$	0.025	$p < 0.001$
	R-Square	0.129		0.148		0.138	
Pakistan	Mother's height (cm)	0.062	$p < 0.001$	0.137	$p < 0.001$	0.069	$p < 0.001$
	Mother's BMI (kg/m^2)			0.295	0.003	0.052	$p < 0.001$
	Mother's weight (kg)	0.019	$p < 0.001$	−0.099	0.015	–	–
	Mother's age (year)			−0.013	0.041	−0.009	0.039
	R-Square	0.097		0.085		0.089	
Timor-Leste	Mother's height (cm)	0.047	$p < 0.001$	0.053	$p < 0.001$	0.049	$p < 0.001$
	R-Square	0.014		0.017		0.015	

S-SE South and Southeast, *B* unstandardized coefficients, Sig. = *p*-value

Table 8.8 Stepwise- multiple linear regression analysis of child's WAZ on maternal variables

		B	*p*-value	*B*	*p*-value	*B*	*p*-value
S-SE Asian countries	Predicted maternal factors	Boys		Girls		Overall	
Bangladesh	Mother's weight (kg)	0.026	$p < 0.001$	0.022	$p < 0.001$	0.024	$p < 0.001$
	Mother's height (cm)	0.033	$p < 0.001$	0.030	$p < 0.001$	0.031	$p < 0.001$
	Mother's age (year)	−0.008	0.013	−0.012	$p < 0.001$	−0.010	$p < 0.001$
	R-Square	0.102		0.087		0.095	
Cambodia	Mother's weight (kg)	0.018	$p < 0.001$	–	–	0.020	$p < 0.001$
	Mother's height (cm)	0.034	$p < 0.001$	0.047	$p < 0.001$	0.034	$p < 0.001$
	Mother's age (year)	−0.018	$p < 0.001$	−0.009	0.044	−0.013	$p < 0.001$
	Mother's BMI (kg/m^2)	–	–	0.050	$p < 0.001$	–	–
	R-Square	0.067		0.072		0.069	
India	Mother's weight (kg)	0.027	$p < 0.001$	0.028	$p < 0.001$	0.007	0.048
	Mother's height (cm)	0.025	$p < 0.001$	0.022	$p < 0.001$	0.037	$p < 0.001$
	Mother's age (year)	−0.006	$p < 0.001$	−0.012	<0.001	−0.009	$p < 0.001$
	Mother's BMI (kg/m^2)	–	–	–	–	0.047	$p < 0.001$
	R-Square	0.073		0.073		0.073	
Maldives	Mother's weight (kg)	0.015	$p < 0.001$	0.052	$p < 0.001$	0.015	$p < 0.001$
	Mother's height (cm)	0.025	0.001	–	–	0.026	$p < 0.001$
	Mother's age (year)	–	–	0.015	0.032	–	–
	Mother's BMI (kg/m^2)	–	–	−0.087	$p < 0.001$	–	–
	R-Square	0.043		0.054		0.046	
Nepal	Mother's weight (kg)	0.036	$p < 0.001$	0.069	$p < 0.001$	0.069	$p < 0.001$
	Mother's height (cm)	0.023	$p < 0.001$	–	–	–	–
	Mother's age (year)	–	–	−0.014	0.011	−0.011	0.006
	Mother's BMI (kg/m^2)	–	–	−0.082	$p < 0.001$	−0.077	$p < 0.001$
	R-Square	0.147		0.143		0.145	
Pakistan	Mother's weight (kg)	–	–	−0.080	0.011	0.024	$p < 0.001$

(continued)

Table 8.8 (continued)

		B	*p*-value	*B*	*p*-value	*B*	*p*-value
S-SE Asian countries	Predicted maternal factors	Boys		Girls		Overall	
	Mother's height (cm)	0.058	$p < 0.001$	0.115	$p < 0.001$	0.037	$p < 0.001$
	Mother's age (year)	–	–	−0.010	0.038	–	–
	Mother's BMI (kg/m^2)	0.044	$p < 0.001$	0.265	<0.001	–	–
	R-Square	0.100		0.149		0.117	
Timor-Leste	Mother's weight (kg)	0.025	<0.001	−0.098	0.021	0.019	$p < 0.001$
	Mother's height (cm)			0.097	$p < 0.001$	0.016	$p < 0.001$
	Mother's age (year)			−0.020	$p < 0.001$	−0.012	$p < 0.001$
	Mother's BMI (kg/m^2)			0.262	0.008		
	R-Square	0.019		0.030		0.021	

S-SE South and Southeast, *B* unstandardized coefficients

Table 8.9 Stepwise- multiple linear regression analysis of child's WHZ on maternal variables

S-SE Asian countries	Predicted maternal factors	*B* Boys	*p*-value	*B* Girls	*p*-value	*B* Overall	*p*-value
Bangladesh	Mother's weight (kg)	0.019	$p < 0.001$	0.017	$p < 0.001$	0.018	$p < 0.001$
	Mother's age (year)	−0.015	$p < 0.001$	−0.013	$p < 0.001$	−0.014	$p < 0.001$
	R-Square	0.027		0.023		0.025	
Cambodia	Mother's weight (kg)	0.025	$p < 0.001$	0.015	$p < 0.001$	0.019	$p < 0.001$
	Mother's age (year)	−0.022	$p < 0.001$	−0.011	0.030	−0.016	$p < 0.001$
	Mother's height (cm)			0.016	0.011	0.013	0.004
	R-Square	0.037		0.023		0.031	
India	Mother's weight (kg)	0.021	$p < 0.001$	0.013	$p < 0.001$	0.017	$p < 0.001$
	Mother's age (year)	−0.004	$p < 0.001$	−0.007	$p < 0.001$	−0.005	$p < 0.001$
	Mother's BMI (kg/m^2)			0.020	$p < 0.001$	0.011	$p < 0.001$
	R-Square	0.019		0.020		0.020	
Maldives	Mother's weight (kg)	0.019	$p < 0.001$			0.015	$p < 0.001$
	Mother's BMI (kg/m^2)			0.023	0.005		
	R-Square	0.028		0.008		0.018	
Nepal	Mother's weight (kg)	0.030	$p < 0.001$			0.030	$p < 0.001$
	Mother's age (year)			−0.014	0.011	−0.012	0.002
	Mother's BMI (kg/m^2)			0.065	$p < 0.001$	−0.011	0.008
	R-Square	0.074		0.063		0.072	
Pakistan	Mother's weight (kg)	0.011	$p < 0.001$	0.018	$p < 0.001$	0.015	$p < 0.001$
	R-Square	0.015		0.041		0.026	
Timor-Leste	Mother's age (year)	−0.013	0.006	−0.014	0.003	−0.014	$p < 0.001$
	Mother's BMI (kg/m^2)	0.074	$p < 0.001$	0.039	$p < 0.001$	0.056	$p < 0.001$
	R-Square	0.023		0.008		0.014	

S-SE South and Southeast, *B* unstandardized coefficients

Table 8.10 Stepwise-multiple linear regression analysis of child's BAZ on maternal variables

		B	*p*-value	*B*	*p*-value	*B*	*p*-value
S-SE Asian countries	Predicted maternal factors	Boys		Girls		Overall	
Bangladesh	Mother's weight (kg)	0.015	$p < 0.001$	0.015	$p < 0.001$	0.017	$p < 0.001$
	Mother's age (year)	−0.011	0.001	−0.009	0.004	−0.011	$p < 0.001$
	Mother's height (cm)					−0.006	0.024
	R-Square	0.017		0.018		0.018	
Cambodia	Mother's weight (kg)	0.022	$p < 0.001$	0.015	$p < 0.001$	0.019	$p < 0.001$
	Mother's age (year)	−0.023	$p < 0.001$			−0.017	$p < 0.001$
	R-Square	0.030		0.012		0.022	
India	Mother's weight (kg)	0.010	$p < 0.001$	0.007	$p < 0.001$	0.008	$p < 0.001$
	Mother's age (year)			−0.005	$p < 0.001$	−0.002	0.001
	Mother's BMI (kg/m^2)	0.019	$p < 0.001$	0.031	$p < 0.001$	0.025	$p < 0.001$
	R-Square	0.013		0.015		0.014	
Maldives	Mother's weight (kg)	0.018	$p < 0.001$				
	Mother's BMI (kg/m^2)			0.018	0.028	0.031	$p < 0.001$
	R-Square	0.025		0.005		0.013	
Nepal	Mother's age (year)					−0.008	0.027
	Mother's BMI (kg/m^2)	0.065	$p < 0.001$	0.053	$p < 0.001$	0.062	$p < 0.001$
	R-Square	0.061		0.047		0.056	
Pakistan	Mother's weight (kg)	0.008	$p < 0.001$			0.013	$p < 0.001$
	Mother's BMI (kg/m^2)			0.043	<0.001		
	R-Square	0.008		0.035		0.019	
Timor-Leste	Mother's age (year)			−0.015	0.002	−0.012	0.001
	Mother's BMI (kg/m^2)	0.079	$p < 0.001$			0.061	$p < 0.001$
	Mother's height (cm)	−0.014	0.022	0.038	$p < 0.001$		
	R-Square	0.026		0.008		0.015	

S-SE South and Southeast, *B* unstandardized coefficients

their sex. The table also includes the R-Square value for each country's model, providing an insight into how much of the variance in child's weight was explained by these maternal variables combined.

A heatmap featured in Fig. 8.2 presents a summary of how various maternal factors impact child growth and nutrition across S-SE Asian countries. The heatmap

S & SE Asian countries	Mother's age (year)			Mother's weight (kg)			Mother's height (cm)			Mother's BMI (kg/m²)			R-Square		
	Boys	Girls	All	Boys	Girls	All	Boys	Girls	All	Boys	Girls	All	Boys	Girls	All
Dependent Variable: Child's weight (kg)															
Bangladesh	0.104	0.079	0.092	0.058	0.090	0.058	0.032	—	0.026	—	-0.074	—	0.079	0.062	0.070
Cambodia	0.080	0.104	0.088	0.040	—	-0.198	—	0.076	0.207	—	—	0.529	0.038	0.043	0.042
India	0.143	0.146	0.144	0.040	0.040	-0.001	0.033	0.029	0.059	—	—	0.096	0.075	0.076	0.075
Maldives	0.114	0.158	0.137	—	0.022	—	0.068	0.044	0.065	—	—	—	0.035	0.059	0.043
Nepal	0.110	0.125	0.120	0.032	0.039	0.033	—	0.040	0.032	—	—	—	0.050	0.081	0.066
Pakistan	0.096	0.130	0.113	0.083	0.048	0.043	—	0.046	0.036	-0.107	—	—	0.065	0.112	0.086
Timor-Leste	0.080	0.091	0.085	0.094	0.026	0.034	—	0.039	0.035	-0.125	—	—	0.050	0.051	0.049
Dependent Variable: Child's height (cm)															
Bangladesh	0.524	0.447	0.488	0.169	0.165	0.167	0.139	0.127	0.131	—	—	—	0.071	0.055	0.063
Cambodia	0.447	0.444	0.459	0.097	—	—	—	0.181	0.155	—	—	—	0.047	0.040	0.043
India	0.662	0.683	0.673	-0.134	-0.178	-0.156	0.297	0.322	0.311	0.515	0.596	0.556	0.067	0.068	0.067
Maldives	0.503	0.626	0.536	—	—	—	0.309	0.199	0.261	-0.244	—	—	0.044	0.042	0.038
Nepal	0.520	0.644	0.580	—	—	—	—	0.256	0.195	—	—	—	0.045	0.072	0.058
Pakistan	0.419	0.572	0.497	0.308	0.129	0.129	—	0.199	0.155	-0.436	—	—	0.061	0.096	0.076
Timor-Leste	0.426	0.468	0.438	—	—	—	0.283	0.183	0.240	—	—	0.107	0.052	0.050	0.051
Dependent Variable: Child's HAZ															
Bangladesh	—	—	—	—	0.016	—	0.071	0.055	0.068	0.053	—	0.045	0.111	0.091	0.101
Cambodia	—	—	—	—	0.017	0.012	0.055	0.034	0.042	—	—	—	0.040	0.044	0.041
India	-0.008	-0.013	-0.011	—	-0.020	-0.014	0.058	0.069	0.066	0.048	0.093	0.081	0.048	0.045	0.047
Maldives	—	0.018	0.014	—	—	—	0.057	0.063	0.060	—	0.031	0.018	0.065	0.085	0.073
Nepal	—	—	—	0.025	0.024	0.025	0.051	0.053	0.052	—	—	—	0.129	0.148	0.138
Pakistan	—	-0.013	-0.009	0.019	-0.099	—	0.062	0.137	0.069	—	0.295	0.052	0.097	0.085	0.089
Timor-Leste	—	—	—	—	—	—	0.047	0.053	0.049	—	—	—	0.014	0.017	0.015
Dependent Variable: Child's WAZ															
Bangladesh	-0.008	-0.012	-0.010	0.026	0.022	0.024	0.033	0.030	0.031	—	—	—	0.102	0.087	0.095
Cambodia	-0.018	-0.009	-0.013	0.018	—	0.020	0.034	0.047	0.034	—	0.050	—	0.067	0.072	0.069
India	-0.006	-0.012	-0.009	0.027	0.028	0.007	0.025	0.022	0.037	—	—	0.047	0.073	0.073	0.073
Maldives	—	0.015	—	0.015	0.052	0.015	0.025	—	0.026	—	-0.087	—	0.043	0.054	0.046
Nepal	—	-0.014	-0.011	0.036	0.069	0.069	0.023	—	—	—	-0.082	-0.077	0.147	0.143	0.145
Pakistan	—	-0.010	—	—	-0.080	0.024	0.058	0.115	0.037	0.044	0.265	—	0.100	0.149	0.117
Timor-Leste	—	-0.020	-0.012	0.025	-0.098	0.019	—	0.097	0.016	—	0.262	—	0.019	0.030	0.021
Dependent Variable: Child's WHZ															
Bangladesh	-0.015	-0.013	-0.014	0.019	0.017	0.018	—	—	—	—	—	—	0.027	0.023	0.025
Cambodia	-0.022	-0.011	-0.016	0.025	0.015	0.019	—	0.016	0.013	—	—	—	0.037	0.023	0.031
India	-0.004	-0.007	-0.005	0.021	0.013	0.017	—	—	—	—	0.020	0.011	0.019	0.020	0.020
Maldives	—	—	—	0.019	—	0.015	—	—	—	—	0.023	—	0.028	0.008	0.018
Nepal	—	-0.014	-0.012	0.030	—	0.030	—	—	-0.011	—	0.065	—	0.074	0.063	0.072
Pakistan	—	—	—	0.011	0.018	0.015	—	—	—	—	—	—	0.015	0.041	0.026
Timor-Leste	-0.013	-0.014	-0.014	—	—	—	—	—	—	0.074	0.039	0.056	0.023	0.008	0.014
Dependent Variable: Child's BAZ															
Bangladesh	-0.011	-0.009	-0.011	0.015	0.015	0.017	—	—	-0.006	—	—	—	0.017	0.018	0.018
Cambodia	-0.023	—	-0.017	0.022	0.015	0.019	—	—	—	—	—	—	0.030	0.012	0.022
India	—	-0.005	-0.002	0.010	0.007	0.008	—	—	—	0.019	0.031	0.025	0.013	0.015	0.014
Maldives	—	—	—	0.018	—	—	—	—	—	—	0.018	0.031	0.025	0.005	0.013
Nepal	—	—	-0.008	—	—	—	—	—	—	0.065	0.053	0.062	0.061	0.047	0.056
Pakistan	—	—	—	0.008	—	0.013	—	—	—	—	0.043	—	0.008	0.035	0.019
Timor-Leste	—	-0.015	-0.012	—	—	—	-0.014	—	—	0.079	0.038	0.061	0.026	0.008	0.015

B-values: Lowest … Highest

R-square: <0.050 … 0.050–0.100 … >0.100

Fig. 8.2 Summary model with heatmap for the effect of maternal factors on child outcomes

consists of multiple columns representing different maternal factors, like age, weight, height, and BMI, and each row represents country-wise child outcome metrics, such as child weight, height, HAZ, WAZ, WHZ, and BAZ. Different colors are used to indicate the strength and direction of the connection between maternal factors and child outcomes. This helps in identifying the maternal factors that consistently exhibit positive or negative impacts on child developmental outcomes.

The slope coefficients indicate child's weight and height and are positively related to maternal age for both boys and girls in most countries. Since this is not a time series data, these relations are to be interpreted very cautiously. For example, as the mother's age increased, the child's weight and height are expected to increase as well. This means that between two families, the child in the family with higher age of mother had an expected weight and height higher than the child in a family with lower age mother. The HAZ is predominantly linked to the mother's height, whereas WAZ is associated with the mother's weight, height, and BMI. As a result, if the mother had a higher weight, height, or BMI (country-specific), then the child had a higher expected WAZ score. Both WHZ and BAZ were positively related to the mother's weight and BMI. This means that if the mother had a higher weight and/or BMI, then the child had a higher expected value of WHZ and BAZ score.

8.4 Discussion

The primary goal of this study is to delve into the complex interplay between maternal and child nutritional status in South and Southeast Asian countries, notably Bangladesh, Cambodia, India, Maldives, Nepal, Pakistan, and Timor-Leste. These nations are grappling with a substantial burden of undernourished children, accounting for nearly half of the global total (UNICEF/WHO/WBG 2021). The findings in the study provide a comprehensive understanding of how maternal health influences child development in these settings. It underscores a significant association between maternal attributes, such as age, height, weight, and BMI, and various child development markers, including height, weight, HAZ, WAZ, WHZ, and BAZ. This nuanced comprehension, derived from the study, can play a pivotal role in the formulation and execution of effective maternal and child health programs in the region.

The study encompasses reproductive-age women aged between 15 and 49, reflecting the diverse maternal characteristics across the countries. The average distribution reveals that Bangladesh, Nepal, and India have younger mothers compared to other countries. In Maldives, mothers exhibit the highest body weight, with their BMI falling under the overweight category. On the other hand, Timor-Leste mothers have the lowest weight and BMI. This rich diversity in maternal characteristics underscores the complexity of the issue and its potential impact on their child's development.

Anthropometric measures differ across the countries among the children. The highest height and weight for boys and girls are found in Maldives and Cambodia. The lowest child weight is found in Timor-Leste, and the lowest height is found in Pakistan. In terms of nutritional scores such as HAZ, WAZ, WHZ, and BAZ,

Timor-Leste ranks the lowest for both boys and girls. Conversely, the Maldives have the highest HAZ and WAZ scores, while Pakistan has the highest WHZ and BAZ scores for both boys and girls.

The study reveals that maternal weight, height, and BMI are significant predictors of nutritional indicators in children. These findings support existing literature, suggesting that a mother's physical health can serve as a proxy for the intrauterine environment and children's early life nutritional status in Brazil, Guatemala, Philippines, South Africa, Ethiopia, and Sub-Saharan African countries (Addo et al. 2013; Farah et al. 2019; Karlsson and Dribe 2022). Notably, maternal height emerged as a particularly strong predictor across all countries analyzed, suggesting a possible genetic connection that may be further impacted by environmental factors such as access to healthcare (Addo et al. 2013).

Policy Implications These findings have profound policy implications, emphasizing the need for comprehensive maternal health programs that focus on the improvement of mother's health before conception. Initiatives aimed at improving maternal nutrition, healthcare access, and education can yield favorable outcomes for the child. Additionally, it is crucial to implement targeted measures to address the adverse health effects of early pregnancy on children.

Strength and Limitations The current study provides valuable insights into the link between maternal traits and child outcomes. However, it also points out the need for additional research to better understand the mechanisms behind this link. Conducting longitudinal studies can help us gain a more comprehensive understanding of causal relationships. Interventional studies can provide a means of testing specific strategies to improve maternal and child health outcomes. In addition, expanding the scope of research to include genetic and epigenetic data can help us identify the biological underpinnings of the observed correlations and guide more effective interventions.

8.5 Conclusion

This study reaffirms the critical role of maternal health in shaping child health and developmental outcomes in South and Southeast Asian contexts. It provides a strong empirical basis for enhancing maternal health services as a strategic approach to improving public health outcomes across generations, emphasizing the interconnected nature of maternal and child health. This study suggests that a child's height and weight can be influenced by the age of their mother. This, in turn, can be affected by factors such as demographic trends or the mother's nutritional status during her growth period. Moreover, a mother's own height, weight, and BMI can also play a role in determining their child's nutritional outcomes. In S-SE Asian children, HAZ and WAZ are mainly associated with maternal height and weight, respectively; WHZ is associated with maternal height and weight; and BAZ is associated with maternal BMI and weight. Based on the nutrition scores of children in S-SE Asian countries, Timor-Leste emerged as the most vulnerable country regarding childhood malnutrition. This highlights the urgent need for effective interventions to improve maternal and child health in this region.

The research findings highlight the importance of prioritizing maternal healthcare services to ensure better health outcomes for mothers and their children. Policymakers and healthcare providers should recognize the significance of maternal healthcare services and focus on improving maternal health to ensure that mothers and their children receive the best possible care.

8.6 Declarations

This study uses data that is nationally representative and obtained from the Demographic and Health Surveys (DHS) Program, which is publicly available. The study design and participant confidentiality were reviewed and approved by the ICF Institutional Review Board (IRB). The data used for this study were already ethically approved, so no additional ethical approval was necessary.

Acknowledgement The authors would like to acknowledge Demographic and Health Surveys (DHS) for providing data.

Availability of Data and Materials The datasets are available at https://dhsprogram.com/Data/.

Competing Interests The authors declare that they have no competing interests.

Funding This study had no grant, technical or corporate support.

Authors' Contributions RNK, PB, and MGH conceived the presented idea. RNK, and AC designed methodology. RNK involved in data curation. RNK and MP performed analysis. RNK, ZN, MP, and AC statistical data interpretation. RNK, AC, and ZN drafted the manuscript. MP, SB, MGH, and PB verified the analytical methods. MP and PB critically revised the manuscript. RNK and SB finalized the manuscript. PB supervised the study. All the authors read and approved the manuscript.

References

Addo OY, Stein AD, Fall CH, Gigante DP, Guntupalli AM, Horta BL et al (2013) Maternal height and child growth patterns. J Pediatr 163(2):549–554. https://doi.org/10.1016/j.jpeds.2013.02.002

Arora C (2009) Child Nutrition. ABD Publishers, Jaipur

Bhutta ZA, Hafeez A, Rizvi A, Ali N, Khan A, Ahmad F et al (2013) Reproductive, maternal, newborn, and child health in Pakistan: challenges and opportunities. Lancet 381(9884):2207–2218. https://doi.org/10.1016/s0140-6736(12)61999-0

Black RE, Victora CG, Walker SP, Bhutta ZA, Christian P, de Onis M et al (2013) Maternal and child undernutrition and overweight in low-income and middle-income countries. Lancet 382(9890):427–451. https://doi.org/10.1016/s0140-6736(13)60937-x

Bomela NJ (2009) Social, economic, health and environmental determinants of child nutritional status in three Central Asian Republics. Public Health Nutr 12(10):1871–1877. https://doi.org/10.1017/s1368980009004790

de Onis M, Blössner M (2003) The World Health Organization Global Database on Child Growth and Malnutrition: methodology and applications. Int J Epidemiol 32(4):518–526. https://doi.org/10.1093/ije/dyg099

Farah AM, Endris BS, Gebreyesus SH (2019) Maternal undernutrition as proxy indicators of their offspring's undernutrition: evidence from 2011 Ethiopia demographic and health survey. BMC Nutr 5:17. https://doi.org/10.1186/s40795-019-0281-z

GDS, MoF, ICF (2018) Timor-Leste Demographic and Health Survey 2016. Retrieved from Dili, Timor-Leste and Rockville, Maryland, USA. http://dhsprogram.com/pubs/pdf/FR329/FR329.pdf

Hasan SMT, Khan MA, Ahmed T (2019) Inadequate maternal weight gain in the third trimester increases the risk of intrauterine growth restriction in rural Bangladesh. PLoS One 14(2):e0212116. https://doi.org/10.1371/journal.pone.0212116

Headey D, Hoddinott J, Park S (2016) Drivers of nutritional change in four South Asian countries: a dynamic observational analysis. Matern Child Nutr 12(Suppl 1):210–218. https://doi.org/10.1111/mcn.12274

IIPS, ICF (2021) National Family Health Survey (NFHS-5), 2019–21: India. Retrieved from Mumbai: https://dhsprogram.com/publications/publication-OF43-Other-Fact-Sheets.cfm

Kaar JL, Crume T, Brinton JT, Bischoff KJ, McDuffie R, Dabelea D (2014) Maternal obesity, gestational weight gain, and offspring adiposity: the exploring perinatal outcomes among children study. J Pediatr 165(3):509–515. https://doi.org/10.1016/j.jpeds.2014.05.050

Karlsson O, Dribe M (2022) Maternal height and child health and schooling in sub-Saharan Africa: Decomposition and heterogeneity. Soc Sci Med 315:115480. https://doi.org/10.1016/j.socscimed.2022.115480

Khan S, Zaheer S, Safdar NF (2019) Determinants of stunting, underweight and wasting among children < 5 years of age: evidence from 2012-2013 Pakistan demographic and health survey. BMC Public Health 19(1):358. https://doi.org/10.1186/s12889-019-6688-2

King JC (2003) The risk of maternal nutritional depletion and poor outcomes increases in early or closely spaced pregnancies. J Nutr 133(5 Suppl 2):1732s–1736s. https://doi.org/10.1093/jn/133.5.1732S

Kundu RN, Hossain MG, Haque MA, Mahumud RA, Pal M, Bharati P (2024) Burden of undernutrition among under-five Bengali children and its determinants: Findings from Demographic and Health Surveys of Bangladesh and India. PLoS One 19(4):e0301808. https://doi.org/10.1371/journal.pone.0301808

Lawlor DA, Relton C, Sattar N, Nelson SM (2012) Maternal adiposity—a determinant of perinatal and offspring outcomes? Nat Rev Endocrinol 8(11):679–688. https://doi.org/10.1038/nrendo.2012.176

Marotz LR (2012) Health, safety, and nutrition for the young child, 8th edn. Wadsworth Cengage Learning, Belmont

MOH, ICF (2018) Maldives demographic and health survey 2016–17. Malé, Maldives, and Rockville, Maryland, USA. Retrieved from http://dhsprogram.com/pubs/pdf/FR349/FR349.pdf

Mohamed HJJ, Loy SL, Mitra AK, Kaur S, Teoh AN, Rahman SHA, Amarra MS (2022) Maternal diet, nutritional status and infant birth weight in Malaysia: a scoping review. BMC Pregnancy Childbirth 22(1):294. https://doi.org/10.1186/s12884-022-04616-z

MoHP, NERA, ICF (2023) Nepal Demographic and Health Survey 2022 (NDHS, 2023). Kathmandu, Nepal. Retrieved from https://www.dhsprogram.com/pubs/pdf/FR379/FR379.pdf

Nankinga O, Kwagala B, Walakira EJ (2019) Maternal employment and child nutritional status in Uganda. PLoS One 14(12):e0226720. https://doi.org/10.1371/journal.pone.0226720

Nigatu G, Assefa Woreta S, Akalu TY, Yenit MK (2018) Prevalence and associated factors of underweight among children 6-59 months of age in Takusa district, Northwest Ethiopia. Int J Equity Health 17(1):106. https://doi.org/10.1186/s12939-018-0816-y

NIPORT, ICF (2020) Bangladesh Demographic and Health Survey 2017–18 (BDHS, 2017–2018). Dhaka, Bangladesh, and Rockville, Maryland, USA. Retrieved from https://www.dhsprogram.com/pubs/pdf/FR344/FR344.pdf

NIPS, ICF (2019) Pakistan Demographic and Health Survey 2017–18 (PDHS, 2017–2018). Islamabad, Pakistan, and Rockville, Maryland, USA. Retrieved from http://dhsprogram.com/pubs/pdf/FR354/FR354.pdf
NIS, MoH, ICF (2023) Cambodia Demographic and Health Survey 2021–22 Final Report (CDHS, 2021–2022). Phnom Penh, Cambodia, and Rockville, Maryland, USA. Retrieved from https://dhsprogram.com/publications/publication-FR377-DHS-Final-Reports.cfm
Pelletier DL, Frongillo EA (2003) Changes in child survival are strongly associated with changes in malnutrition in developing countries. J Nutr 133(1):107–119. https://doi.org/10.1093/jn/133.1.107
Pelletier DL, Frongillo EA Jr, Schroeder DG, Habicht JP (1995) The effects of malnutrition on child mortality in developing countries. Bull World Health Organ 73(4):443–448
Ruager-Martin R, Hyde MJ, Modi N (2010) Maternal obesity and infant outcomes. Early Hum Dev 86(11):715–722. https://doi.org/10.1016/j.earlhumdev.2010.08.007
Tiwari R, Ausman LM, Agho KE (2014) Determinants of stunting and severe stunting among under-fives: evidence from the 2011 Nepal Demographic and Health Survey. BMC Pediatr 14:239. https://doi.org/10.1186/1471-2431-14-239
TLDHS (2018) Timor-Leste Demographic and Health Survey 2016. GDS, MoF, ICF. Retrieved from Dili, Timor-Leste and Rockville, Maryland, USA: http://dhsprogram.com/pubs/pdf/FR329/FR329.pdf
Triunfo S, Lanzone A (2015) Impact of maternal under nutrition on obstetric outcomes. J Endocrinol Investig 38(1):31–38. https://doi.org/10.1007/s40618-014-0168-4
UNICEF (2016a) From the first hour of life: Making the case for improved infant and young child feeding everywhere. Retrieved from New York: https://www.unicef.org/media/49801/file/From-the-first-hour-of-life-ENG.pdf
UNICEF (2016b) The State of the World's Children 2016: A fair chance for every child. Retrieved from New York: https://www.unicef.org/media/50076/file/UNICEF_SOWC_2016-ENG.pdf
UNICEF/WHO/WBG (2021) Levels and trends in child malnutrition: key findings of the 2021 edition of the joint child malnutrition estimates. World Health Organization, Geneva
UNICEF/WHO/WBG (2023) Levels and trends in child malnutrition: UNICEF/WHO/World Bank Group Joint Child Malnutrition Estimates: key findings of the 2023 edition. UNICEF and WHO, New York
UNICEF/WHO/WBG/UN (2013) Levels & trends in child mortality: report 2013. Retrieved from Washington DC: https://childmortality.org/wp-content/uploads/2018/12/UN-IGME-Child-Mortality-Report-2013.pdf
WHO (2006) WHO Child Growth Standards: length/height-for-age, weight-for-age, weight-for-length, weight-for-height and body mass index-for-age: methods and development. WHO Press, Geneva
WHO (2013) Guideline: updates on the management of severe acute malnutrition in infants and children. Retrieved from Geneva: https://www.who.int/publications/i/item/9789241506328
WHO (2017) The double burden of malnutrition. Policy brief. World Health Organization, Geneva

Part II

Health Care

Empowerment of Mothers and its Impact on the Health of Children: A Comparative Analysis of North-Eastern Region and the Rest of India

9

Manoranjan Pal and Utpal Kumar De

9.1 Introduction

It is widely accepted that mothers play a crucial role in nurturing a child. It is also taken for granted that mothers raise children better, especially in the early childhood days, than their male counterparts (Rohner 2016; Veneziano 2003; Gežová 2015; Pal et al. 2021). However, in this society mothers face several constraints and subjugation that prohibits them in exercising their roles effectively. A famous "object-relations theory" states that the behavior of people to others in their adult lives is shaped by family experiences during infancy and naturally mothers play an important role in it (Zgourides 2000). Therefore, mothers can play their important roles in shaping the future of their children only if they are truly empowered. On the other hand, Finley et al. (2008) found that mothers were rated as heavily involved in nearly all domains. Mothers have generally been found to be more involved than fathers in most studies in the literature (e.g., Craig 2006; Pal et al. 2021).

Using data from the Netherlands, West Germany, and the USA, Korupp et al. (2002) drew general conclusions that trends in educational reproduction did not change by adding the mother's influence on that of the fathers. But the children's educational attainment is substantively influenced by the mother's educational and occupational status (Bharati et al. 2012). Behrman and Rosenzweig (2002), however, saw that if one controls women's earnings, child-rearing ability endowments, and schooling of their husbands, then it may have a marginal adverse impact on the health of children.

There are many evidences showing that the mother's education and other empowerment characteristics are much important for child's health status and educational

M. Pal (✉)
Economic Research Unit, Indian Statistical Institute (ISI), Kolkata, West Bengal, India

U. K. De
Department of Economics, North-Eastern Hill University, Shillong, Meghalaya, India

M. Pal et al. (eds.), *Public Health and Nutrition*,
https://doi.org/10.1007/978-981-97-7890-4_9

attainment (Jerrim and Micklewright 2011). Furthermore, mother's education and earning capability influence her decision-making ability as well as her status and overall empowerment. Because mothers' status and position in the society determine their decision-making ability regarding child's education, healthcare, nutritional intake, etc., which ultimately determine the health condition, mental growth, and overall progress of the children.

The two national-level studies in 1992/93 and 1998/99 found that the rate of undernutrition among preschool children fell by 11% during this period (Gragnolati et al. 2005). Over the past three decades, the proportion of household expenditure on food items has decreased, partly due to the decrease in the relative prices of food grains and the increase in the access to subsidized food grains (Ramchandran 2007); and possibly due to the unequal intrahousehold food distribution within the family, which has an adverse effect on preschool children (NNMB 2006). It has also been argued that some socio-economic factors, such as gender, place of residence, parents' (particularly the mother's) educational status, religion, and caste, have a significant impact on the rate of undernutrition among children (Gragnolati et al. 2005, 20–22). Among these factors, mother's educational background, job profile, earning capacity, age, and the society or religion in which she belongs decide directly or indirectly the status of her empowerment. Therefore, indirectly these factors through mother's empowerment affect the health status of children from the beginning of their lives.

The objective of this study is to understand how empowerment level gauged by those aforesaid factors affects not only the health status of the mothers but also the health of children in North-East India vis a vis the rest of India.

9.2 Statement of the Problem

Analysis of possible regional and socioeconomic factors thought to influence child nutrition outcomes did not reveal any substantive causal relations or even strong patterns either in the cross-section or in the change (Alderman et al. 2007; Braveman and Gottlieb 2014; Compte et al. 2021). The rate of malnutrition was lower among children of educated mothers. With respect to the mother's occupation, the reduction was the greatest among nonworking mothers and the lowest among mothers with professional, technical, and clerical jobs. This is because higher-income mothers with professional, technical, or clerical jobs had already impacted the prevalence of child malnutrition. Moreover, mothers who work outside the home may have less time for child feeding and healthcare, with possible adverse nutritional outcomes (Radhakrishna and Ravi 2004). This implication has been reflected among the children of agricultural and low-paid manual workers in our study. Thus, Radhakrishna and Ravi (2004) suggest that the cause of the high-measured prevalence of childhood undernutrition in India may lie less in the way we treat our children and more in the way we treat our women.

North-East India despite being in a disadvantageous location and conceivably backward in terms of several opportunities as compared to the other regions of the country has been observed to acquiring more literacy, being advanced in taking maternal care, taking immunization of mothers during pregnancy and children, breastfeeding of baby and other healthcare measures in respect of mother and children. Hence, a study of North-East India in comparison to other parts of India in respect of women empowerment indicators vis-a-vis the health status of children under-five would provide an insight to this aspect and to taking some important policy measures.

9.3 Data and Methodology

We have obtained the relevant data from NFHS Round 5. Data on Child's (0–5 years) weight at birth, age, sex, height, status of BCG, DPT, Polio, Measles other vaccinations, hemoglobin, and mothers' level of education, mothers' age, various other healthcare measures have been used. Data on mothers' decision power on various issues, ability to think that beating of female members is not justified, wealth index, level of education, frequency of reading newspaper, frequency of seeing TV, and even mothers' health status constitute the level of empowerment of mothers. Some of these parameters like decision making power directly measure the empowerment and some parameters have affect the empowerment.

Statistical Analysis Bivariate frequency tables were computed, and Chi-square tests were performed to see if the relevant variables were dependent. Our main concern was to find out the frequency and/or percentage of children of certain child health parameters such as number and percentages of children with status of anemia, vaccination, Nutritional status through weight-for-age and height-for-age z-values, etc., corresponding to each combination of North-East and the rest of India. This gives us a valuable insight into the differences of these values of all the respective variables between North-East and other parts of India.

Again, we have run the logistic regression using unit-level data with the occurrence of status of each of some health variables of children like anemia, HAZ, WAZ, WHZ, etc. on various independent variables. The model for logistic regression is.

$$y = a + \sum bx + e,$$

where y is the log odd of the respective dependent variable, x represents vector of explanatory variables related to mother's socio-economic characteristics and various empowerment indicators. The explanatory variables can be described as—Place of Residence = Res (=0 if rural, =1 if urban), Sex of Household head = Sex (=0 for male, =1 for female), Wealth Index = WI (first three of five categories of NFHS is clubbed as poor (=0), and the rest is clubbed as rich (=1)), Household size = HH size (0 for <4, and 1 for 4 and above household size), Religion (=1 if the household is Hindu or Muslim and 0 for the rest), ST (=1 if the household is ST, 0 otherwise), BMI group (0 = underweight, 1 is normal and above), Newspaper (=1 if mother reads newspaper, 0 otherwise), TV (=1 if mother watches television, 0 otherwise),

Literate (=1 If mother is literate, 0 otherwise), Anemia (=1 if Anemic, 0 otherwise), Health Insurance (=1 if the mother has health insurance and 0 otherwise), Tetanus injection is taken during pregnancy—- Tet._Inj._Pregnancy (=1 if yes, 0 otherwise), Breast Feeding Month (=1 if breast feeding is done for more than 6 months, 0 otherwise), Antenatal Visit (=1 if yes, 0 otherwise), Place of Delivery (=1 if done in hospital, nursing home, etc., 0 otherwise), Taking part in decision making = Who Decides (on any matter regarding child welfare——treatment, immunization, education, etc. = 1 if done by mother alone or jointly with other member/s of the family, 0 if mother is not involved at all), Beating of wife is justified = Beating justified (=1 if mother supports it, 0 otherwise), Age of mother (1 for age equal to 35 years or more, 0 otherwise).

9.4 Results

A comparison of distribution of sample households in respect of some general characteristics like place of residence, sex of household head, wealth index, household size, and social and religious distribution is presented in Table 9.1. It is observed that sample households are mostly rural, which is 84.5% in case of North-East India, while it is 77.4% in case of the rest of India. About 18% of the households in North-East India are female headed, while it is 14.5% in case of the rest of India. In the overall sample, as the cut-off point suggests, the percentage of poor households is less than the non-poor households in the rest of India, while in the North-East the number of poor households is more than double of the non-poor households. Similarly, the percentage of households having size of 4 and more is over 91% and 84%, respectively, at the rest of India and North-East India. Percentage of Hindu and Muslim together is 95 in the rest of India, while it is below half (48.1%) in North-East India. While proportion of scheduled tribe is only 8.3% in the rest of India, it is about two-thirds (64.5%) in North-East India.

Overall, it can be said that proportion of rural, female headed, poor and non-Hindu-Muslim, and ST households are significantly more in North-East India than those in rest of India. Only the proportion of household size being 4 and above is more in the mainland India than that of North-East India.

If we look at the mother's health and socio-economic characteristics, we can say that in mainland India, other than North-East, about one-fifth are underweight, while in North-East it is only 11 percent (Table 9.2). Also, 59.7% of mothers are anemic in the rest of India whereas 52.4% of mothers in North-East India are anemic. In respect of these two parameters, mothers of North-East India have relatively better health conditions. This is even though incidence of poverty is more pronounced in North-East India and more households are female headed and hailed from ST communities.

Despite being in disadvantageous conditions the better health conditions reflected in less incidence of Anemia and underweight among the mothers in North-East India can be associated with the fact that mothers in North-East India are more literate (about 79 percent) than that of the rest of India (72.6%) (Table 9.3). However,

Table 9.1 General status of sample households

	Place of residence			
	Rest of India		**North-East**	
Place	*Sample size*	*Percentage*	*Sample size*	*Percentage*
Rural	115,657	77.4	23,211	84.5
Urban	33,726	22.6	4249	15.5
Total	149,383	100.0	27,460	100.0
	Sex of household head			
	Rest of India		**North-East**	
Sex	*Sample size*	*Percentage*	*Sample size*	*Percentage*
Male	127,683	85.5	22,536	82.1
Female	21,698	14.5	4924	17.9
Total	149,381	100.0	27,460	100.0
	Wealth index			
	Rest of India		**North-East**	
Status of Wealth	*Sample size*	*Percentage*	*Sample size*	*Percentage*
Poor	66,874	44.8	18,474	67.3
Not poor	82,509	55.2	8986	32.7
Total	149,383	100.0	27,460	100.0
	Household size			
	Rest of India		**North-East**	
Household Size	*Sample size*	*Percentage*	*Sample size*	*Percentage*
1–3	13,168	8.8	4254	15.5
4 or more	136,215	91.2	23,206	84.5
Total	149,383	100.0	27,460	100.0
	Religious distribution			
	Rest of India		**North-East**	
Religion	*Sample size*	*Percentage*	*Sample size*	*Percentage*
Others	7407	5.0	14,258	51.9
Hindu or Muslim	141,976	95.0	13,202	48.1
Total	149,383	100.0	27,460	100.0
	Distribution between scheduled tribes and others			
	Rest of India		**North-East**	
Category	*Sample size*	*Percentage*	*Sample size*	*Percentage*
Others	131,938	91.7	8227	35.5
Scheduled tribes	12,001	8.3	14,919	64.5
Total	143,939	100.0	23,146	100.0

relatively more mothers (about 29%) in the rest of India read newspaper regularly and that figure in North-East India is less than about 25%. Over 69% of mothers in other parts of India watch TV regularly, which is about 65% in North-East India. Even though mothers' literacy is more in North-East India percentage of mothers' reading newspaper, watching television is less in North-East India than in the other parts of India. Also, health insurance coverage in North-East India is less than that of other parts of India. Similarly, higher literacy rate in North-East India can be attributed to higher percentage of insurance of pregnant mothers than that of other

Table 9.2 Distribution of mothers in terms of BMI and anemia categories

	BMI Group (Mother)			
	Rest of India		**North-East**	
Status of BMI	**Sample size**	**Percentage**	**Sample size**	**Percentage**
Underweight	27,868	19.2	3083	11.3
Not underweight	117,039	80.8	24,104	88.7
Total	144,907	100.0	27,187	100.0
	Anemia			
	Rest of India		**North-East**	
Status of Anemia	**Sample size**	**Percentage**	**Sample size**	**Percentage**
Not anemic	57,743	40.3	12,810	47.6
Anemic	85,618	59.7	14,102	52.4
Total	143,361	100.0	26,912	100.0

Table 9.3 Literacy rate and habit of reading newspaper, watching television

	Literate			
	Rest of India		**North-East**	
	Sample size	***Percentage***	***Sample size***	***Percentage***
Illiterate	40,977	27.4	5796	21.1
Not illiterate	108,406	72.6	21,664	78.9
Total	149,383	100.0	27,460	100.0
	Reading newspaper			
	Rest of India		**North-East**	
	Sample size	***Percentage***	***Sample size***	***Percentage***
Does not read	106,154	71.1	20,639	75.2
Reads	43,229	28.9	6821	24.8
Total	149,383	100.0	27,460	100.0
	Watching TV			
	Rest of India		**North-East**	
	Sample size	***Percentage***	***Sample size***	***Percentage***
Does not see	46,024	30.8	9692	35.3
Sees	103,359	69.2	17,768	64.7
Total	149,383	100.0	27,460	100.0

parts of India (Table 9.5). Whereas higher percentage of reading newspaper or watching television are found to apparently have no influence on the health status in case of other parts of India than that in North-East India, as clear from the results. Now-a-days awareness appears to be more pronounced due to social media contacts, and various healthcare campaigns by government and different NGOs.

Percentage of mothers availing health insurance (39.2) is much higher than that of mainland India (25.3). This along with the mothers' health condition by aforesaid two criteria reveals better healthcare awareness of mothers in North-East India, which matches with a relatively higher literacy rate. It is further clear that this has been due to the higher literacy rate and awareness of the mothers in North-East

Table 9.5 Differences in extent of measures to protect mother and child

	Health insurance			
	Rest of India		**North-East**	
	Sample size	**Percentage**	**Sample size**	**Percentage**
Does not have health insurance	111,592	74.7	16,697	60.8
Has health insurance	37,791	25.3	10,763	39.2
Total	149,383	100.0	27,460	100.0
	Whether tetanus injection taken during pregnancy			
	Rest of India		**North-East**	
	Sample size	**Percentage**	**Sample size**	**Percentage**
No	6996	4.7	2701	9.9
Yes	141,637	95.3	24,461	90.1
Total	148,633	100.0	27,162	100.0
	Antenatal Visit			
	Rest of India		**North-East**	
	Sample size	**Percentage**	**Sample size**	**Percentage**
No	8250	5.6	3212	12.1
Yes	139,568	94.4	23,316	87.9
Total	147,818	100.0	26,528	100.0
	Place of Delivery			
	Rest of India		**North-East**	
	Sample size	**Percentage**	**Sample size**	**Percentage**
Home	14,756	9.9	6463	23.5
Hospital, etc.	134,627	90.1	20,997	76.5
Total	149,383	100.0	27,460	100.0
	Breastfeeding (Number of Months)			
	Rest of India		**North-East**	
	Sample size	**Percentage**	**Sample size**	**Percentage**
0–6	35,004	24.8	4954	19.9
7 or more	106,215	75.2	19,912	80.1
Total	141,219	100.0	24,866	100.0

India in comparison to other parts of India. The Pearson Chi^2 values are found to be significant on both occasions of BMI and Anemia (Table 9.4).

However, a lower percentage of mothers in North-East India (90.1%) have had tetanus injections during pregnancy when compared to other parts of India (95.3%) (see Table 9.5). Similar is the case for antenatal visit of mothers, and delivery of baby in hospital where percentage is much higher in the rest of India than that of North-East India. On the other hand, for longer period of breast feeding of baby (7 months and above), percentage of mothers in North-East India is significantly more (80.1) than that of rest of India (75.2). On the contrary to health indicators, all these facts reveal that mothers in rest of India utilize more precautionary measures through tetanus injection, antenatal visit, and using hospital for birth of baby in comparison to that of North-East India (Table 9.5). It may be because the mothers of North-East India are already healthy and have more physical fitness and more

Table 9.4 Relation between literacy rate and health characteristics

Mother BMI Group * Mother Literacy Crosstabulation						**Pearson Chi²**
			Illiterate	Not illiterate	Total	
Mother BMI group	Underweight	Number (%)	10,488 (23.0)	20,463 (16.2)	30,951 (18)	1064.17 (0.000)
	Not underweight	Number (%)	35,077 (77.0)	106,066 (83.8)	141,143 (82)	
Total		Number (%)	45,565 (100)	126,529 (100)	172,094 (100)	
Mother Anemia Group * Mother Literacy Crosstabulation						**Pearson Chi²**
			Illiterate	Not illiterate	Total	
Mother Anemia Group	Anemic	Number (%)	16,513 (36.7)	54,040 (43.1)	70,553 (41.4)	571.76 (0.000)
	Not Anemic	Number (%)	28,513 (63.3)	71,207 (56.9)	99,720 (58.6)	
Total		Number (%)	45,026 (100)	125,247 (100)	170,273 (100)	
Mother Health Insurance Group * Mother Literacy Crosstabulation						**Pearson Chi²**
			Illiterate	Not illiterate	Total	
Mother's Health Insurance	No	Number (%)	34,857 (74.5)	93,432 (71.8)	128,289 (72.5)	125.14 (0.000)
	Yes	Number (%)	11,916 (25.5)	36,638 (28.2)	48,554 (27.5)	
Total		Number (%)	46,773 (100)	130,070 (100)	176,843 (100)	

Note: *p*-values of Pearson Chi² test is given in parenthesis. *p*-value = 0.000 means that the actual *p*-value is less than 0.001

immunity or resistance power against most of the unbecoming health hazards faced by the mothers.

Table 9.6 reveals that decision on 4 or more categories is taken either by mother or jointly in relatively more proportion in North-East India than that of other parts of India. In a few cases the proportion of mother to take decision is comparatively lower in North-east India than that of other parts of India. In matters of justification of beating wife by husband majority disagrees. However, the proportion is more in North-East India. Furthermore, the proportion of mother aged above 35 years is significantly higher in North-East India (18%) in comparison to the other parts of India (9.5%). All these facts (literacy, independence, and disregarding husbands' subjugation, taking part in decision making) state that mothers in North-East India are more empowered and studies also show that women in North-East India are economically more empowered (De and Ghosh 2011; Ghosh and De 2007).

The higher empowerment status of mothers in North-East India is expected to have a significant bearing on the health, education, and other aspects of the children. In order to check that we compared the incidence of birthweight, post-natal checkup,

Table 9.6 Empowerment of mother and health of child

Who decides on all matters in family (mother or jointly 1, Else 0)				
	Rest of India		**North-East**	
	Sample size	**Percentage**	**Sample size**	**Percentage**
0–3 Cases	134,872	90.3	24,333	88.6
4–5 Cases	14,511	9.7	3127	11.4
Total	149,383	100.0	27,460	100.0
	Thinks beating wife is justified			
	Rest of India		**North-East**	
	Sample size	**Percentage**	**Sample size**	**Percentage**
Others Think not Justified	141,422	94.7	26,258	95.6
At Least in One Criterion	7961	5.3	1202	4.4
Total	149,383	100.0	27,460	100.0
	Mothers' Age			
	Rest of India		**North-East**	
	Sample size	**Percentage**	**Sample size**	**Percentage**
Age below 35	135,155	90.5	22,512	82.0
Age 35 or more	14,228	9.5	4948	18.0
Total	149,383	100.0	27,460	100.0
	Birth weight of baby			
	Rest of India		**North-East**	
	Sample size	**Percentage**	**Sample size**	**Percentage**
Underweight	24,491	17.7	2762	11.7
Normal	113,566	82.3	20,777	88.3
Total	138,057	100.0	23,539	100.0
	Baby post-natal check-up			
	Rest of India		**North-East**	
	Sample size	**Percentage**	**Sample size**	**Percentage**
No	78,126	52.3	19,987	72.9
Yes	71,202	47.7	7442	27.1
Total	149,328	100.0	27,429	100.0
	Anemia of children			
	Rest of India		**North-East**	
	Sample size	**Percentage**	**Sample size**	**Percentage**
Anemic	81,105	70.7	13,232	58.5
Not anemic	33,606	29.3	9370	41.5
Total	114,711	100.0	22,602	100.0

and anemic conditions of children in North-East India with that of other parts of India. The comparative picture displayed in Table 9.6 further reveals that percentage of underweight children is only 11.7% while that in other parts of India it is 17.7% (Table 9.6). Like less antenatal visit in case of mothers in North-East India (Table 9.5), percentage of baby going through post-natal checkup is also relatively less in North-East India (27.1%), which is significantly more (47.7%) in other parts of India (Table 9.6). In North-East India, 58.5% of the children are anemic and the percentage in other parts of India is 70.7%. On these above three criteria, we can easily state that the children in North-East India are relatively healthier and require less post-natal visit to doctors. The fewer post-natal visits may also be due to the relatively poor healthcare infrastructure and lower accessibility to a large section of population (De and Lyngdoh 2020).

By using the standard healthcare measure of WHO in terms of height for age, weight for age, weight for height, and BMI of under-five children we can also make a further comparison between the health status of children in North-East India and other parts of India (Table 9.7). In North-East India, significantly a lower percentage of under-five children are found to be stunted (as per height for age), underweight (as per weight for age), and wasted (as per weight for height) as compared to that of

Table 9.7 Comparison of health status of children in North-East and other parts of India by using the WHO criteria and vaccination status

	Child HAZ			
	Rest of India		**North-East**	
	Sample size	***Percentage***	***Sample size***	***Percentage***
Stunted	45,141	**33.8**	8321	**32.8**
Normal	88,258	66.2	17,080	67.2
Total	133,399	100.0	25,401	100.0
	Child WAZ			
	Rest of India		**North-East**	
	Sample size	***Percentage***	***Sample size***	***Percentage***
Underweight	42,596	**31.1**	6028	**23.1**
Normal	94,166	68.9	20,030	76.9
Total	136,762	100.0	26,058	100.0
	Child WHZ			
	Rest of India		**North-East**	
	Sample size	***Percentage***	***Sample size***	***Percentage***
Wasted	26,254	**20.1**	4102	**16.6**
Normal	104,095	79.9	20,678	83.4
Total	130,349	100.0	24,780	100.0
	Child BMI			
	Rest of India		**North-East**	
	Sample size	***Percentage***	***Sample size***	***Percentage***
Underweight	24,550	**18.8**	3941	**15.9**
Normal	106,266	81.2	20,904	84.1
Total	130,816	100.0	24,845	100.0
	Vaccination			
	Rest of India		**North-East**	
	Sample size	**Percentage**	**Sample size**	**Percentage**
0–7	79,857	53.5	17,910	65.2
8–10	69,526	46.5	9550	34.8
Total	149,383	100.0	27,460	100.0

Stunting, wasting, underweight, and thinness cut offs are defined as height-for-age, weight-for-height, weight-for-age, and BMI-for-age *z*-scores less than or equal to the corresponding-2 times standard deviation of the WHO Child growth standards medians WHO (2006).

rest of mainland India. In terms of body-mass index (BMI) also, a lower percentage of children (15.9%) of North-East India are found to be underweight than that of the rest of India (18.8%). However, if we look at the vaccination of children, a lower percentage (34.8%) in North-East India has completed 8 and above vaccinations as compared to that of rest of India (46.5%). About two-thirds of children have completed maximum of seven vaccinations or less in North-East India. By all the standard four criteria, status of health of children in North-East India is much better than those in other parts of India. Because of better health conditions immunity of children in North-East India appears to be more and their parents, especially mothers give less preference toward some costly vaccinations compared to free basic vaccinations.

9.5 Results of Logistic Regressions

The logistic regression of birthweight of children suggests birthweight of children is significantly and positively influenced by wealth index, because the chance of higher birthweight is more for wealthy households. However, there are variations as the coefficient of wealth index in the rest of India (0.158) is much less than that of North-East (NE) India (0.245) (Table 9.8). Similar is the case of literacy having a positive significant effect on birthweight for both NE and Rest of India children. Coefficient of religion is positive in case other parts of India while it is negative in case of North-East India, both being significant. Moreover, ST child has more chance of higher birthweight in NE whereas it is not significant in the Rest of India. NE India is dominated by non-Hindu, non-Muslim religions, and most of them are ST. They seem to have some privilege over other communities. Like before, mother's BMI, habit of watching TV, reading newspaper, education, and health insurance have significant impact on the birthweight, while mother's anemia has significant negative impacts. It is expected because anemic mothers are coded as 1. The measures like breastfeeding for longer period, tetanus during pregnancy, antenatal care, and age is significant in both regions. Coefficients of the other empowerment indicators like participation in decision making are significant positive and wife beating is significant negative meaning that empowerment of women acts indirectly to improve birthweight as they can take firm decision on any matter and go for healthcare of themselves as well as take care of babies. In North-East India, women are already more empowered and there is little variation in choosing hospital for delivery or taking part in decision making. Therefore, the coefficients of those variables are insignificant in case of North-East India.

Table 9.9 displays the logistic regression result of post-natal check-up of child on various socio-economic characteristics. The result reveals significant negative impacts of place of delivery in hospital and wealth index, in general as well as of family size in the rest of India with mothers' BMI group, ST in the North-East. Literacy of mothers has significant positive impact on preference for post-natal check-up of child along with the habits of reading newspaper and watching television. Also, breastfeeding, antenatal check-up of mother, taking tetanus injection,

Table 9.8 Logistic regression of child birthweight on socio-economic characteristics of mothers

	Rest of India					North-East				
Explanatory variables	Coef.	*p*-value	AOR	Lower limit	Upper limit	Coef.	*p*-value	AOR	Lower limit	Upper limit
Res	−0.061	0.003	0.941	0.905	0.979	−0.010	0.897	0.990	0.851	1.151
Sex	−0.008	0.700	0.992	0.950	1.035	−0.179	0.005	0.836	0.737	0.948
WI	0.158	0.000	1.171	1.128	1.215	0.245	0.000	1.277	1.126	1.449
HH size	0.126	0.000	1.134	1.076	1.194	0.059	0.399	1.061	0.925	1.216
Religion	0.078	0.031	1.081	1.007	1.159	−0.369	0.000	0.692	0.596	0.803
ST	0.006	0.835	1.006	0.953	1.061	0.438	0.000	1.549	1.339	1.791
BMI Group	0.249	0.000	1.283	1.237	1.331	0.390	0.000	1.476	1.285	1.697
Newspaper	0.078	0.000	1.081	1.041	1.122	0.038	0.562	1.039	0.914	1.181
TV	0.074	0.000	1.077	1.038	1.118	0.143	0.015	1.154	1.028	1.295
Literate	0.077	0.000	1.080	1.039	1.123	0.189	0.006	1.208	1.057	1.380
Anemia	−0.030	0.056	0.970	0.941	1.001	−0.195	0.000	0.823	0.741	0.914
Health insurance	0.087	0.000	1.090	1.053	1.129	−0.048	0.358	0.953	0.860	1.056
Tet. Inj._pregnancy	0.146	0.000	1.157	1.075	1.246	0.098	0.351	1.103	0.897	1.357
Breastfeeding month	0.234	0.000	1.264	1.222	1.307	0.247	0.000	1.280	1.137	1.441
Antenatal visit	0.191	0.000	1.211	1.129	1.299	0.393	0.000	1.481	1.234	1.777
Place of delivery	0.171	0.000	1.187	1.117	1.261	−0.046	0.572	0.955	0.816	1.119
Who decides	0.110	0.000	1.117	1.056	1.181	0.100	0.251	1.106	0.931	1.313
Beating justified	−0.086	0.018	0.917	0.854	0.985	0.065	0.651	1.067	0.806	1.412
Age_35	0.060	0.030	1.062	1.006	1.122	0.133	0.072	1.142	0.988	1.319
Constant	0.291	0.000	1.338			0.875	0.000	2.400		

Birthweight: 0 for underweight and 1 for normal
AOR adjusted odds ratio

Table 9.9 Logistic regression of post-natal check-up of child on socio-economic characteristics of mothers

	Rest of India					North-East				
Explanatory variables	Coef.	*p*-value	AOR	Lower limit	Upper limit	Coef.	*p*-value	AOR	Lower limit	Upper limit
Res	−0.155	0.000	0.857	0.832	0.882	−0.475	0.000	0.622	0.561	0.690
Sex	0.010	0.528	1.010	0.979	1.043	0.313	0.000	1.367	1.261	1.481
WI	−0.017	0.220	0.983	0.956	1.010	−0.102	0.013	0.903	0.833	0.979
HH size	−0.092	0.000	0.912	0.877	0.950	0.039	0.411	1.039	0.948	1.140
Religion	0.199	0.000	1.220	1.157	1.287	0.348	0.000	1.416	1.281	1.565
ST	0.277	0.000	1.319	1.266	1.374	−0.254	0.000	0.775	0.702	0.856
BMI group	0.036	0.012	1.037	1.008	1.067	−0.098	0.060	0.906	0.818	1.004
Newspaper	0.084	0.000	1.087	1.058	1.118	0.362	0.000	1.436	1.326	1.555
TV	0.236	0.000	1.266	1.231	1.302	0.100	0.012	1.105	1.023	1.193
Literate	0.115	0.000	1.122	1.089	1.155	0.117	0.013	1.124	1.025	1.232
Anemia	−0.003	0.782	0.997	0.974	1.020	0.120	0.000	1.127	1.054	1.205
Health insurance	0.107	0.000	1.113	1.085	1.142	0.370	0.000	1.447	1.353	1.547
Tet_Inj_pregnancy	0.344	0.000	1.411	1.333	1.493	0.437	0.000	1.547	1.342	1.784
Breast feeding month	0.081	0.000	1.084	1.057	1.112	0.133	0.002	1.142	1.051	1.240
Antenatal visit	1.118	0.000	3.058	2.884	3.243	0.634	0.000	1.886	1.655	2.148
Place of delivery	−0.365	0.000	0.694	0.668	0.722	−0.559	0.000	0.572	0.526	0.622
Who decides	0.077	0.000	1.080	1.037	1.124	0.028	0.604	1.029	0.924	1.146
Beating justified	−0.016	0.553	0.984	0.933	1.038	0.090	0.306	1.094	0.921	1.298
Age_35	0.046	0.020	1.047	1.007	1.089	0.006	0.891	1.006	0.923	1.097

Post-Natal Check-up = 1 if yes, and 0 otherwise
AOR adjusted odds ratio

health insurance, and decision making by women as well as their age have significant positive impacts on the post-natal check-up of child.

Almost, similar impacts of variables are found in the case of a child to be anemic (Table 9.10). Only household size of 4 or more, religion Hindu/Muslim and mother's anemia, 7 months or more breastfeeding have inverse impact on a child to be non-anemic. It means the chance of anemia rises with the rise in those variables. Household income and mother's education enhance the chance of a child to be non-anemic in both North-East and other regions of India and the impacts are more pronounced in other parts of India. Other empowerment-related variables are not however significant.

Similar impacts are found in case of those socio-economic variables on the children healthcare indices as measured by height for age (whether normal or stunted), weight for age (whether normal or underweight), weight for height (normal or wasted), and the results of logistic regressions are presented in Tables 9.11. In addition to those, place of delivery in hospital or formal health center increases the chance of completing eight vaccinations of child (Table 9.12), which is otherwise not significant on previous four cases.

Table 9.10 Logistic regression of child is non-anemic on socio-economic characteristics of mothers

	Rest of India					North-East				
Explanatory variables	Coef.	*p*-value	AOR	Lower limit	Upper limit	Coef.	*p*-value	AOR	Lower limit	Upper limit
Res	0.050	0.005	1.051	1.015	1.088	0.109	0.024	1.115	1.014	1.226
Sex	0.052	0.009	1.053	1.013	1.095	−0.073	0.084	0.929	0.855	1.010
WI	0.109	0.000	1.115	1.078	1.154	0.097	0.016	1.102	1.019	1.192
HH size	−0.043	0.080	0.958	0.912	1.005	−0.107	0.018	0.899	0.822	0.982
Religion	−0.004	0.914	0.996	0.934	1.063	−0.490	0.000	0.613	0.555	0.676
ST	−0.219	0.000	0.803	0.761	0.848	0.015	0.772	1.015	0.919	1.120
BMI group	0.231	0.000	1.260	1.215	1.307	0.228	0.000	1.256	1.126	1.401
Newspaper	0.066	0.000	1.068	1.034	1.104	0.143	0.000	1.153	1.065	1.249
TV	0.086	0.000	1.089	1.052	1.128	0.131	0.001	1.140	1.056	1.230
Literate	0.175	0.000	1.192	1.149	1.237	0.118	0.009	1.126	1.030	1.230
Anemia	−0.520	0.000	0.594	0.578	0.611	−0.562	0.000	0.570	0.534	0.608
Health insurance	0.067	0.000	1.069	1.036	1.102	0.055	0.108	1.057	0.988	1.131
Tet_Inj_pregnancy	0.006	0.855	1.006	0.939	1.079	−0.057	0.360	0.945	0.837	1.067
Breast feeding month	−0.102	0.000	0.903	0.866	0.942	−0.194	0.001	0.824	0.733	0.925
Antenatal visit	0.067	0.044	1.069	1.002	1.142	−0.084	0.135	0.919	0.823	1.027
Place of delivery	−0.060	0.016	0.942	0.897	0.989	−0.066	0.122	0.937	0.862	1.018
Who decides	0.039	0.125	1.039	0.989	1.092	0.007	0.893	1.007	0.906	1.120
Beating justified	−0.011	0.747	0.989	0.926	1.057	0.001	0.987	1.001	0.844	1.188
Age_35	0.263	0.000	1.300	1.243	1.360	0.253	0.000	1.288	1.187	1.397

Child is Non-Anemic = 1 if yes, and 0 otherwise
AOR adjusted odds ratio

Table 9.11 Logistic regression of child HAZ, child WAZ and child WHZ on socio-economic characteristics of mothers

	Child_HAZ				Child_WAZ				Child_WHZ			
Explanatory variables	Rest of India		North-East		Rest of India		North-East		Rest of India		North-East	
	B	Sig.	*B*	Sig.	*B*	Sig.	*B*	Sig.	*B*	Sig.	*B*	Sig.
Res	0.037	0.027	0.026	0.606	−0.020	0.250	0.075	0.196	−0.052	0.008	0.054	0.401
Sex	−0.019	0.287	−0.180	0.000	0.021	0.236	0.038	0.415	0.050	0.018	0.210	0.000
WI	0.361	0.000	0.394	0.000	0.424	0.000	0.392	0.000	0.228	0.000	0.211	0.000
HH size	−0.077	0.001	−0.040	0.381	−0.053	0.021	0.020	0.691	−0.054	0.045	−0.024	0.686
Religion	−0.137	0.000	−0.015	0.764	−0.157	0.000	−0.228	0.000	−0.173	0.000	−0.224	0.000
ST	0.044	0.050	−0.114	0.021	−0.112	0.000	0.167	0.002	−0.141	0.000	0.052	0.404
BMI group	0.272	0.000	0.256	0.000	0.460	0.000	0.463	0.000	0.315	0.000	0.284	0.000
Newspaper	0.094	0.000	0.029	0.486	0.102	0.000	0.087	0.066	−0.007	0.723	0.174	0.001
TV	0.096	0.000	0.102	0.006	0.093	0.000	0.168	0.000	0.044	0.016	−0.017	0.715
Literate	0.235	0.000	0.106	0.014	0.239	0.000	0.197	0.000	0.120	0.000	0.121	0.025
Anemia	−0.067	0.000	−0.112	0.001	−0.076	0.000	−0.096	0.010	−0.021	0.156	0.033	0.435
Health insurance	0.018	0.200	−0.147	0.000	0.001	0.949	−0.190	0.000	0.050	0.003	−0.122	0.005
Tet_Inj_Pregnancy	0.043	0.165	0.109	0.068	0.034	0.266	−0.034	0.624	0.026	0.468	−0.020	0.801
Breast feeding month	−0.442	0.000	−0.390	0.000	−0.174	0.000	−0.197	0.000	0.215	0.000	0.073	0.170
Antenatal visit	−0.016	0.578	0.011	0.844	0.038	0.186	0.033	0.595	0.027	0.418	0.035	0.628
Place of delivery	0.164	0.000	0.090	0.028	0.132	0.000	0.044	0.350	0.021	0.399	−0.007	0.898
Who decides	0.013	0.579	−0.018	0.729	0.024	0.306	−0.032	0.590	0.023	0.386	−0.071	0.294
Beating justified	−0.079	0.008	0.028	0.747	−0.044	0.144	0.099	0.317	0.031	0.387	0.066	0.551
Age_35	0.037	0.091	−0.012	0.774	−0.003	0.899	−0.017	0.727	0.036	0.166	0.105	0.061

HAZ, WAZ WHZ = 1 for normal, 0 otherwise

Table 9.12 Logistic regression of child vaccination on socio-economic characteristics of mothers

	Rest of India					North-East				
Explanatory variables	Coef.	*p*-value	AOR	Lower limit	Upper limit	Coef.	*p*-value	AOR	Lower limit	Upper limit
Res	−0.131	0.000	0.877	0.851	0.904	−0.042	0.359	0.959	0.878	1.048
Sex	−0.012	0.463	0.988	0.956	1.021	0.015	0.707	1.015	0.939	1.097
WI	0.058	0.000	1.060	1.030	1.090	0.052	0.171	1.053	0.978	1.134
HH size	−0.035	0.089	0.965	0.926	1.005	0.155	0.000	1.167	1.073	1.270
Religion	−0.037	0.181	0.963	0.912	1.018	−0.114	0.015	0.892	0.814	0.978
ST	0.081	0.000	1.084	1.040	1.131	−0.043	0.362	0.958	0.875	1.050
BMI group	−0.205	0.000	0.814	0.791	0.839	−0.139	0.005	0.870	0.788	0.960
Newspaper	−0.028	0.052	0.973	0.946	1.000	0.039	0.312	1.039	0.964	1.120
TV	0.075	0.000	1.078	1.047	1.109	0.014	0.702	1.014	0.944	1.090
Literate	0.186	0.000	1.205	1.169	1.241	0.110	0.012	1.116	1.025	1.215
Anemia	0.022	0.064	1.022	0.999	1.047	0.047	0.135	1.049	0.985	1.116
Health insurance	−0.001	0.948	0.999	0.973	1.026	0.059	0.068	1.060	0.996	1.130
Tet_Inj_Pregnancy	0.251	0.000	1.285	1.213	1.362	0.273	0.000	1.314	1.162	1.487
Breastfeeding month	1.220	0.000	3.388	3.294	3.484	1.308	0.000	3.699	3.381	4.045
Antenatal visit	0.339	0.000	1.404	1.330	1.482	0.376	0.000	1.457	1.302	1.629
Place of delivery	0.448	0.000	1.565	1.502	1.630	0.618	0.000	1.855	1.708	2.014
Who decides	−0.004	0.855	0.996	0.956	1.038	0.041	0.422	1.042	0.943	1.151
Beating justified	−0.038	0.172	0.962	0.911	1.017	−0.079	0.340	0.924	0.785	1.087
Age_35	−0.614	0.000	0.541	0.520	0.564	−0.452	0.000	0.636	0.586	0.691

Child Vaccination is taken as 1 if the number of vaccination is at least 8 and 0 otherwise
AOR adjusted odds ratio

9.6 Discussion

Despite proportions of poor, female headed, and ST households are more in North-East India, and lack of infrastructure; overall healthcare conditions of mother and under-5 children are better in North-East India. Higher literacy rate and more empowerment of women in North-East India make them more aware about the care of mother and children who in general do not discriminate among male and female children as well. Marginally lower proportion of mothers not reading newspaper or watching television in North-East India does not matter much in this accomplishment for the societal cohesion, organized campaign, and other sources of information like various social media. Empowerment of women is therefore very crucial through education and their control over resources to better manage not only family but for the nurturing of children.

9.7 Concluding Remarks

Educated mothers learn to take necessary measures for baby or childcare and nurturing techniques going against all social inhibitions in many cases. The role of mother, who is empowered socially and economically and hailed from a wealthy family, can take care of a child in a much better way.

The findings of the analysis suggest that in comparison to women in other parts of the country, being more literate, and having more social empowerment as evidenced from the indicators, women in North-East India take some extra care by extended breast feeding and maintaining mothers' health so that healthy baby is born and they need not go for a higher number of vaccinations of children apart from basic immunizations provided by the government free of cost.

Therefore, it suggests that mothers' health is more important for a baby's health in the beginning, irrespective of the place of birth (hospital or at another place). Again, mothers' level of empowerment in all respects (mental, physical, and economical) is much important for their healthcare, which puts North-Eastern region a little ahead in many respects, despite having lesser wealth and lack of some healthcare infrastructure in the region.

Acknowledgement The authors are thankful to the reviewers for their valuable comments which helped in the improvement of this paper substantially.

References

Alderman H, Behrman JR, Hoddinott J (2007) Economic and nutritional analyses offer substantial synergies for understanding human nutrition. J Nutr 137(3):537–544. https://doi.org/10.1093/jn/137.3.537

Behrman JR, Rosenzweig MR (2002) Does increasing women's schooling raise the schooling of the next generation? Am Econ Rev 92(1):323–334

Bharati P, Pal M, Bharati S (2012) Can mother's education and family welfare reduce undernutrition of pre-school children in India? Hum Biol Rev 1(2):207–221

Braveman MMDH, Gottlieb MMDH (2014) The social determinants of health: it's time to consider the causes of the causes. Public Health Rep 129(Suppl 2):19–31. https://doi.org/10.1177/00333549141291S206

Compte MV, Burrola-Méndez S, Lozano-Marrufo A, Ferré-Eguiluz I, Flores D, Gaitán-Rossi P, Teruel G, Pérez-Escamilla R (2021) Urban poverty and nutrition challenges associated with accessibility to a healthy diet: a global systematic literature review. Int J Equity Health 20:40. Retrieved from https://equityhealthj.biomedcentral.com/articles/10.1186/s12939-020-01330-0 (29-07-2023)

Craig L (2006) Does father care mean fathers share? A comparison of how mothers and fathers in intact families spend time with children. Gend Soc 20:259–281

De UK, Ghosh BN (2011) Empowerment of rural women in backward region of India: a comparative study of Jharkhand, Tripura and Meghalaya. In: De UK, Ghosh BN (eds) Gender deprivation and empowerment of women: an Indian perspective. Lambert Academic Publishing, Germany, pp 111–146

De UK, Lyngdoh S (2020) Road connectivity on access to healthcare in rural Meghalaya: a case study. J Rural Dev 43(1):1–35. BARD, Comilla, Bangladesh

Finley GE, Mira SD, Schwartz SJ (2008) Perceived paternal and maternal involvement: factor structures, mean differences, and parental roles. Fathering 6(1):62–82

Gežová KC (2015) Father's and mother's roles and their particularities in raising children. Acta Technologica Dubnicae 5(1):45–50

Ghosh BN, De UK (2007) Process of empowerment of women: a comparative study of Tripura and Meghalaya. In: Ray AK, Dutta Ray B (eds) Women emancipation, focus north-East India. OM Publication, New Delhi, pp 265–288

Gragnolati M, Shekar S, Dasgupta M (2005) India's undernourished children: a call for reform and action. World Bank, Washington, DC

Jerrim J, Micklewright J (2011) Children's cognitive ability and parents' education: distinguishing the impact of mothers and fathers, chapter 9. In: Smeeding T, Erikson R, Jantti M (eds) Persistence, privilege and parenting: the comparative study of intergenerational mobility. Russell Sage Foundation, New York, pp 261–286

Korupp SE, Ganzeboom HBG, Van Der Lippe T (2002) Do mothers matter? A comparison of models of the influence of mothers' and fathers' educational and occupational status on children's educational attainment. Qual Quant 36:17–42

National Nutrition Monitoring Bureau (NNMB) (2006) 1979–2006 NNMB reports. National Institute of Nutrition, Hyderabad

Pal M, De UK, Bharati P, Bharati S (2021) Unequal effect of parents' education on child health and health care. Int J Stat Sci 21(1):55–74

Radhakrishna R, Ravi C (2004) Malnutrition in India: trends and determinants. Econ Polit Wkly 39:671–676

Ramchandran P (2007) Poverty nutrition linkage. Indian J Med Res 126:249–261

Rohner RP (2016) Introduction to interpersonal acceptance-rejection theory (IPARTheory) and evidence. Online Readings in Psychology and Culture, 6(1). https://doi.org/10.9707/2307-0919.1055

Veneziano RA (2003) The importance of paternal warmth. Cross Cult Res 37(3):265–281

WHO Multicentre Growth Reference Study Group (2006) WHO Child Growth Standards: length/height-for-age, weight-for-age, weight-for length, weight-for-height and body mass index-for-age: methods and development. Geneva: WHO, https://www.who.int/publications/i/item/924154693X

Zgourides G (2000) Developmental psychology, by IDG Books Worldwide, Inc., NY

Health-Seeking Behavior and Social Contract: A Qualitative Study on Manipuri People's Perception of Health and Healthcare System

10

Hanjala Bin Rostum Ms Zannatul Mawa Shin

10.1 Introduction

The Manipuri community, which is in Kamalganj, Sylhet, Bangladesh, has a strong cultural legacy and a unique healthcare system that is firmly based on their customs and beliefs.

This article's goal is to present a thorough examination of the healthcare system and the difficulties the Manipuri population in Kamalganj, Sylhet, has to deal with because there are no traditional healers there. The challenges faced by various ethnic communities, including the Manipuri community, in accessing healthcare services in rural Tripura, India, identify barriers related to language, cultural practices, geographical remoteness, and socioeconomic factors, providing insights into the specific challenges encountered by the Manipuri community (Chakraborty et al. 2020). This study intends to shed light on the effects and consequences of this shift on the community's health and well-being by assessing the community's dependence on scientific medicine and the conventional healthcare system. The health-seeking behavior of Manipuri mothers in rural Tripura, India, identifies the challenges they face in accessing healthcare services. The findings shed light on barriers such as language differences, cultural beliefs, and limited availability of healthcare facilities in the region (Roy et al. 2019). The Manipuri community has historically placed a lot of trust in traditional healers who use a variety of healing techniques, including the utilization of rituals, medicinal plants, and spiritual beliefs, to treat illnesses and preserve health. Traditional healthcare practices and medicinal plant knowledge among the Manipuri community in Bangladesh explore their traditional healing methods, including the use of medicinal plants, rituals, and traditional healers. The research provides insights into the traditional healthcare

H. B. R. M. Z. M. Shin (✉)
Department of Anthropology, University of Rajshahi, Rajshahi, Bangladesh
e-mail: s2010149151@ru.ac.bd

M. Pal et al. (eds.), *Public Health and Nutrition*,
https://doi.org/10.1007/978-981-97-7890-4_10

knowledge and practices within the community (Ahmed and Uddin 2020). However, there has been a reduction in the number of community-based traditional healers in recent years.

The Manipuri community today mainly relies on the scientific medicine offered by the mainstream healthcare system because there are no traditional healers left. This change offers both opportunities and difficulties. On the one hand, it gives residents of the neighborhood access to cutting-edge medical procedures, diagnostic tools, and specialized care. In the parts that follow, we'll go into detail about the research methods used, the results of the field study, and a thorough examination of the difficulties the Manipuri community had when seeking treatment. This study offers insightful information on the healthcare system and difficulties the Manipuri community in Kamalganj, Sylhet, Bangladesh, faces. Modern medical science has advanced, but traditional medical systems have been passed down through generations. In Bangladesh, different minority groups have different knowledge and usage rules. While articles and books focus on traditional medicine, the Manipuri community of India is given more priority. Most discussions focus on herbal plant medicines or medical systems, without mentioning medical pluralism.

By calling society and culture modern based on current information technology, we can call conventional and universally accepted medical systems modern medicine. The utilization of modern healthcare services among the Manipuri people in India, focuses on their reliance on scientific medicine. The research explores factors influencing their healthcare-seeking behavior, including access to healthcare facilities, cultural beliefs, and perceptions of traditional and modern medicine (Singh and Rajkumari 2018). New technologies are being added to the medical system with time. The immune system is also more complicated than before. We set out this study to find out the available medical systems and practices among Manipuri community in Sylhet area of Bangladesh. The field of public health is concerned with promoting and protecting health and well-being, which is related to SDG 2030 goal No. 3. It focuses on disease prevention and improving quality of life in communities and society. This study intends to shed light on the effects and consequences of this shift on the community's health and well-being by assessing the community's dependence on scientific medicine and the conventional healthcare system.

10.2 Objectives of the Study

In the context of Kamalganj region of Sylhet, we may research with some objectives to know the available healing system of tribal Manipuri community.

- To understand their perception about different health problems among the Manipuri people.
- To identify available healthcare options and their images in the locality.
- To investigate why they choose particular or multiple healthcare options.

Challenges faced by the Manipuri community in accessing healthcare services:

Ahmed et al. (2021) in "Barriers to accessing healthcare services among ethnic minority communities in Bangladesh: A qualitative study," explores the barriers to accessing healthcare services among ethnic minority communities in Bangladesh, including the Manipuri community. The research highlights issues such as language barriers, cultural differences, lack of health awareness, and discrimination as major challenges faced by these communities in seeking healthcare.

Bhowmik et al. (2020) investigate the healthcare-seeking behavior and challenges faced by indigenous communities in Bangladesh, including the Manipuri community. It examines the impact of socioeconomic factors, cultural beliefs, language barriers, and limited access to healthcare facilities on healthcare utilization among these communities.

The reliance of the Manipuri community on scientific medicine and the mainstream healthcare system:

Influence of Socio-Economic Status:

Alam et al. (2017) in the article entitled "Socio economic status of the ethnic Community in Bangladesh: An analysis using socio economic index" argued that the presence of indigenous ethnic groups in Bangladesh and highlights their cultural diversity, language variations, and distinct practices. It emphasizes the significance of these indigenous communities and their contributions to the country's culture and heritage. The main ethnic groups in the Sylhet region are identified as the Khasi and Manipuri, with each group having unique linguistic and cultural traditions. The socio-economic conditions of the Manipuri people in Kamalganj are examined, indicating that their economic situation varies, with some facing challenges of poverty. Despite these challenges, the Manipuri people value education, although higher education rates are not satisfactory. However, their literacy rates surpass national statistics.

Knowledge on Healthcare Practices

Yasmin et al. (2019) investigate indigenous knowledge and healthcare practices among the Manipuri community in Bangladesh. It explores their traditional beliefs, healing rituals, and healthcare-seeking behavior. The study sheds light on the traditional healthcare practices and cultural beliefs related to health and well-being within the Manipuri community.

10.3 Research Methods and Techniques

In order to fully examine the research issues, this qualitative study uses a multimethod approach that includes semi-structured interviews, a case study, and key informant interviews.

Participants were carefully chosen for the study based on their applicability to the subject matter and their capability to contribute insightful information. To ensure a comprehensive understanding, the sample contains people from a variety of backgrounds and experiences.

Open-ended questions were used to encourage participants to freely express their opinions and experiences. Participants were given the opportunity to elaborate on their answers because these interviews were done in a conversational style.

A single instance was picked to represent the research context. An extensive amount of information was gathered to give a thorough picture of the case, including documents, observations, and interviews.

To get deeper insights and validate information from various sources, people with particular knowledge or expertise in the research field were found and interviewed. On the other hand, there were some limitations.

We used both primary and secondary data, and we were constrained by those data's restrictions. Important variables like incurable illnesses, political variables, national circumstances, and statistical standing were not taken into account in this study. One of the major drawbacks of this research is time constraints, along with a lack of funding. Clearly, additional research is needed to understand how the Manipuri population in Bangladesh seeks out healthcare and how practices have changed.

10.3.1 Data Analysis

Thematic analysis was used to examine the interview data that had been transcribed. Initial codes were developed after becoming comfortable with the data, and then reoccurring motifs were found. Iterative review was used to improve the themes' relevancy and cohesion. In order to contextualize the research's findings and support its developing themes, journal articles and existing literature on the subject were evaluated. This process strengthened the study's reliability by triangulating the data.

By presenting preliminary findings to participants and taking into account their feedback, member checking was carried out to increase trustworthiness. Colleagues also participated in peer debriefing sessions to get a variety of viewpoints on the analysis. To enable potential transferability to related situations, comprehensive descriptions of the research methodology, sampling criteria, and data collection methodologies were supplied. To ensure transparency and dependability of the results, the study procedure—including judgments made during data analysis—was painstakingly documented. There are also semistructured interviews, case studies, and key informant interviews were used in this study's qualitative methodology, which was backed up by a theme analysis and literature review. The study concerns were thoroughly explored while upholding ethical rigor and methodological openness thanks to the approach.

10.3.2 Nature of Research

The subject of our research is the healthcare system of the Manipuri community in the context of Sylhet Kamalganj region. We asked them about what kind of healthcare methods are prevalent among the studied population, i.e., Manipuri tribals, the use of traditional medical methods, their effectiveness, the diversity of medical methods based on age, gender, different reasons for using these medical methods, their beliefs about such medical methods and various customs.

To find out whether there is variation in their use of this treatment by age and gender and their belief systems and practices related to this method. By analyzing the information received from them, we found my niche. Since in this study we have investigated various aspects of healthcare practices of Manipuri tribals, my study is an exploratory study.

In this qualitative study, informants, who had full independence regarding healthcare system and practices, express their opinions. This enabled me to get clear information which made our research logical. In my research, we were able to present the research in an unbiased way through this auditory approach, by prioritizing the views and experiences of the informants rather than our ideas and opinions.

10.3.3 Selection of Research Area

The objective of this study is to know about the various aspects of their medical practices existing among the Manipuri community of Kamalganj region of Sylhet. So, we had to interview people from the Manipuri community. We have selected Madhabpur and Adampur villages of Vanugach Thana of Kamalganj Upazila of Maulavibazar District as the research area for our research keeping in mind the purpose of our research.

10.3.4 Sampling and Sample Size

Sampling is basically a method by which some units are selected from the population to collect data for research purposes. In our research, we mainly adopted purposive, random, and snowball sampling. In purposive sampling, the researcher uses his judgment to form the sample by collecting the required number of sample units in accordance with the objective. That is, in this sampling, there is a specific objective with which to proceed. Again, global sampling research begins with a small population of people known to the researcher and expands the sample by identifying others who should participate in the study by asking this initial participant population. That is, after identifying an acquaintance and interviewing him, he can provide information about his acquaintance and the purpose of the study. A sample unit is collected by identifying such individuals in globular samples. To carry out the study, we collected data from about 30 informants. Completed 10 KIIs and about 20 in-depth interviews.

10.4 Findings and Results

According to the conceptual framework, there are main two factors based on what the Manipuri healthcare system will be discussed with the core ideas of findings that came from the fieldwork.

10.4.1 Modern Medicine as Healthcare System

In order to diagnose, treat, and prevent a wide range of illnesses and health disorders, modern medicine is a complete healthcare system that combines medical research, technology, and evidence-based practices. It covers a broad spectrum of medical professions and disciplines, such as general medicine, surgery, pediatrics, obstetrics and gynecology, cardiology, cancer, neurology, and many others. The healthcare utilization patterns and challenges faced by indigenous communities in India, including the Manipuri community, explore the extent of reliance on scientific medicine and the mainstream healthcare system and identify barriers such as language barriers, cultural practices, and limited accessibility to healthcare services (Lyngdoh and Choudhury 2021). As a healthcare system, modern medicine possesses the following salient features:

Scientific Approach: The foundation of contemporary medicine is evidence-based medicine and scientific research. The effectiveness and safety of medical therapies are evaluated using rigorous scientific research, clinical trials, and systematic reviews.

Diagnostic Methods: A key element of contemporary medicine is the use of advanced diagnostic methods. These comprise laboratory tests, genetic screening, and imaging modalities like X-rays, CT scans, MRI scans, and ultrasound. These devices aid in the proper diagnosis of diseases and ailments by doctors. Treatment Options: There are many different diseases and conditions that modern medicine can address. These include medical procedures, radiation therapy, chemotherapy, physical therapy, and rehabilitation in addition to pharmaceutical interventions (medications). The particular ailment and how severe it is determining the therapy option.

Modern medicine places a strong emphasis on preventive care in order to lower the prevalence of disease. This includes vaccinations, health screenings, lifestyle modifications (such as exercise and healthy diet), and counseling on risk factors like smoking and excessive alcohol consumption. The healthcare utilization patterns among the Manipuri community in Imphal East district, Manipur, India. It assesses the extent to which the community relies on scientific medicine and the mainstream healthcare system and identifies factors influencing their healthcare-seeking behavior, including socioeconomic status, education, and accessibility to healthcare facilities (Singh and Singh 2019). Healthcare should be provided using a multidisciplinary approach, according to modern medicine. The delivery of comprehensive and integrated treatment involves collaboration between medical practitioners from diverse professions. Primary care doctors, specialists, surgeons, nurses, pharmacists, therapists, and other medical personnel may be involved in this.

Patient-Centered Care: The practice of modern medicine must be patient-centered. Healthcare professionals work hard to respect patients' autonomy, involve them in decision-making, and take their values and preferences into account. To secure the best results, emphasis is placed on effective communication and shared decision-making.

Continuous Medical Education: Through CME, healthcare practitioners in contemporary medicine continually update their knowledge and abilities. As a result, they are kept abreast of the most recent developments, studies, and best practices in their specialized sectors.

Technological Progress: The quick development of technology has benefited modern medicine. Medical technology, robots, telemedicine, electronic health records, artificial intelligence, and machine learning are all included in this. The efficiency and patient outcomes are improved by the use of these technological tools in diagnosis, treatment, and healthcare delivery.

Ethical and Legal Frameworks: The ethical and legal frameworks within which modern medicine is practiced. Medical practitioners follow moral precepts including justice, autonomy, beneficence, and non-maleficence. To guarantee high-quality care and patient safety, regulatory agencies and professional groups set rules and standards.

While modern medicine has made significant advancements, it is not without limitations. Affordability, access to healthcare, healthcare disparities, and overreliance on technology are some of the challenges that need to be addressed to ensure equitable and effective healthcare delivery.

According to the conceptual framework of this research, there are two main healthcare services that Manipuri community people get when they are sick based on their demographic situation as well as transportation situation. The findings related to two major categories:

1. Pharmacy.
2. Clinic/hospital.

The objective is to find out when and why these healthcare services are received and based on what factors this healthcare system varies from time to time. Here are four main factors to consider in terms of receiving healthcare services. They are

1. Transportation situation.
2. Availability.
3. Financial condition.
4. Family decision.

Based on these factors the findings of both types of services are discussed below:

10.4.1.1 Pharmacy Healthcare Services

The younger generation's attitude is changing and they are becoming more familiar with modern medical facilities and their use. But rural Manipuri villages isolated from urban centers where hospitals and medical centers are located (Ahmmed and Singh 2007). Manipuri people normally go to pharmacy when they are in need of small medicines like paracetamol, gastric, pain killers, etc. But there are differences between those who are economically vulnerable, they go to pharmacy for every sickness whether it is severe or not. In maximum time poor people cannot go to clinic or hospital due to the lack of money and transportation cost. On the other hand, those who are busy at work and don't have time to go too far away hospital and they usually buy medicine without a prescription from a local pharmacy. There is another scenario, where underage girls and boys do not go to the pharmacy or to the clinic alone, they always go with their parents. At the same time, whether the person is poor or reach, he goes to a pharmacy first when gets sick. The cause of this tendency is pharmacies are available in every short distance and the medicines are available all the time to everyone at a reasonable rate.

10.4.1.2 Hospital/Clinic Healthcare Services

In terms of Manipuri people, they go to clinic less than they go to pharmacy, the main reason behind that can be transportation situation which means that clinics and hospitals are far from villages and local communities. On the other hand, the vaccination procedure for all age groups is done in primary and secondary schools because clinics or hospitals are not available in near distances. The Manipuri people only go to hospital when someone is in a huge accident or death bed. So, availability and transportation along with financial expenses play an important role in receiving healthcare services in Manipuri community.

Other factors that are important to mention in the case of healthcare services in Manipuri community.

- Maternity is always considered crucial and important in this community. So, almost 100% of babies are born in the hospital. Average mother goes for checkup three times during pregnancy and the rate of mother and child death is almost 0% within my sample. So, it can be said that the modern healthcare system is considered the most popular system among the mothers of Manipuri community.
- Child vaccination procedure is popular and known to all along with the families as well as in the community. So, almost every child gets vaccinated in the accurate time.
- Adolescence vaccination procedure is also maintained strictly in this community. Every vaccination follows the same procedure; at first there will be an announcement of vaccination and then everyone will gather to the destined place for vaccination then the vaccination will be done. Thus, every government aid reaches out to the Manipuri people without any hassle.

So, from the above discussion, it can be argued that all the factors that influence healthcare system along with the healthcare system itself are very important to understand for getting the right scenario of the Manipuri community's health-related situation.

10.4.2 Herbal Medicine as Cultural Healthcare System

Manipuri tribals use domestic plants as source in their daily medicine and also their belief about cured with herbal medicine is full of varieties. The sources used in this treatment are sometimes used directly and sometimes processed in various ways. Different diseases use these sources and substances differently. Sometimes only plants, medicinal plants treat them, sometimes as drinks, etc.

Past sources include

Plants and plant parts, and

Other sources include

Religious customs, beliefs, and practices, and there are both past and passive sources.

10.4.3 Reasons for Using Herbal Medicine (Domestic Herbs and Condiments)

They have shown the belief they received from their parents as the reason behind using traditional medical methods. In addition, according to them, the distance of their location from modern medical centers is also the reason behind adopting domestic herbal treatment methods.

He explains that they resort to traditional treatment here as they are unable to take modern treatment for the distance. Negi and Singh in their article "Tribal Health and Health Care Beliefs in India" write,

> Their reliance on herbal medicine is due to non-availability of healthcare in and around villages and their belief in centuries-old plants 42/49. (Negi and Singh 2018)

Other ingredients and methods used in their daily life treatment like herbal ingredients are also used by them to cure their various diseases due to centuries of belief. Besides, they say that they are cured by it and it costs less, so they also use traditional treatment methods. Another reason for its use is that they believe that their food habits have spiritual powers, so food can be used in order to prevent diseases. It should be noted here that they feel that their source of traditional medicine is on the verge of extinction. These sources are now decreasing due to various reasons including deforestation. Because of this, many people in their society are willing to turn to modern medicine, So, though their traditional methods are effective, but modern medicine is accepted by them all as the main healthcare system.

10.5 Discussion

The Manipuri community continues to rely on modern medicine for their healthcare needs. The Manipuri community resides in areas with bio-diverse flora, and over 80% of them depend on medicinal plants for their primary healthcare. The community has strong traditional knowledge of medicinal plants and their uses, which are still utilized today. However, the Manipuri community still faces various illnesses such as diarrhea, infections, diabetes, colds, coughs, and fevers. To address these challenges and to provide comprehensive healthcare services, it is essential to establish a well-organized modern medical service system in the Manipuri community. The government's investment in community clinics has been a landmark step toward the provision of quality healthcare services, especially to rural and disadvantaged populations. The Community clinics are playing a significant role in providing healthcare services to the Manipuri community. Furthermore, the rehabilitation medicine should be considered as an integral part of the modern medical service system in Bangladesh. In conclusion, the Manipuri community in Bangladesh has a unique culture with rich traditional knowledge of medicinal plants. However, to address the healthcare needs of the community comprehensively, a well-organized modern medical service system is essential.

Other factors that are important to mention in the case of healthcare services in Manipuri community:

- Maternity is always considered crucial and important in this community. So, almost 100% of babies are born in the hospital. Average mother goes for checkup three times during pregnancy and the rate of mother and child death is almost 0% within my sample. So, it can be said that modern healthcare system is considered the most popular system among the mothers of Manipuri community.
- Child vaccination procedure is popular and known to all along with the families as well as in the community too. So, almost every child gets vaccinated in the accurate time.
- Adolescence vaccination procedure is also maintained strictly in this community. Every vaccination follows the same procedure; at first there will be an announcement of vaccination and then everyone will gather to the destined place for vaccination then the vaccination will be done. Thus, every government aid reaches out to the Manipuri people without any hassle.

10.6 Conclusion

Among my studied indigenous Manipuri population, traditional medicine is adopted as other ethnic communities, but acceptance of modern medicine is higher among them than other medical methods. They prefer scientific methods of treatment for most physical and mental problems.

The main reason for this is their higher education and awareness. Among the cultural beliefs, herbal medicines like domestic plant use and spice/condiment use are prominent for simple sickness. The result of globalization encourages them to adopt modern medical methods, through which they can know about the cure and prevention of various diseases which are created by the combination of scientific and modern invention. We found that they were not motivated to receive treatment from outside of renowned medical or doctors. They do not have faith in quacks like traditional healers, a Manipuri woman says.

Though the knowledge-experiences received from the ancestors and their belief systems are important and acceptable by them and can be seen in the application of daily life in dresses, food and other lifestyle, they are properly aware about healthcare system and modern medicine is their main healthcare system at present time.

The findings showed that non-existence of traditional healing was caused by unfaithfulness toward traditional healing practices and the reason of this are some visible factors in the society:

- Social capital
- Education
- Transportation system
- Family decision
- Economic condition

Though the invisible social contract formation for the present healthcare system is the main finding of this paper. On the other hand, the findings also indicate that traditional medicine is not a practicing healthcare system there rather the modern healthcare system is the system that they think is the best option for seeking healthcare services.

However, it is worth noting that more research is needed to fully understand the effectiveness, benefits, and risks of the healthcare system among Manipuri community of Bangladesh.

References

Ahmed R, Uddin MJ (2020) Traditional healthcare practices and medicinal plant knowledge among the Manipuri community in Bangladesh. J Ethnobiol Ethnomed 16(1):1–15

Ahmed S, Sultana N, Alam MF (2021) Barriers to accessing healthcare services among ethnic minority communities in Bangladesh: a qualitative study. Int J Environ Res Public Health 18(5):2709

Ahmmed MF, Singh L (2007) State of the rural Manipuris in Bangladesh. Ethnic Community Development Organization, Sylhet

Alam M et al (2017) Socio economic status of the ethnic community in Bangladesh: an analysis using socio economic index. IOSR J Econ Finance 8:92–97

Bhowmik P, Paul A, Hasan MN (2020) Healthcare-seeking behavior and challenges faced by indigenous communities in Bangladesh. J Health Res Rev 7(2):65–71

Chakraborty P, Paul B, Ganguly A (2020) Challenges faced by ethnic communities in accessing healthcare in rural Tripura, India. J Soc Sci Hum Res 8(2):250–260

Lyngdoh MM, Choudhury B (2021) Healthcare utilization and challenges among indigenous communities in India: a study of the Khasi and Manipuri communities. Indian J Public Health Res Dev 12(5):694–699

Negi DP, Singh MM (2018) Tribal health and health care veners in India: a systematic review. Int J Res Soc Sci 5(1):219–224

Roy B, Sarkar S, Sultana S (2019) Health-seeking behavior and challenges faced by Manipuri mothers in rural Tripura, India. J Midwif Reprod Health 7(2):1634–1643

Singh YN, Singh SM (2019) Healthcare utilization among the Manipuri community in Imphal East district of Manipur, India. J Med Soc 33(1):44–47

Yasmin MR, Hoque N, Rahman MT, Biswas BK (2019) Indigenous knowledge and healthcare practices among the Manipuri community in Bangladesh. J Med Sci 28(2):149–155

A Qualitative Study on Health and Socio-demographic Facilities of Brothels' Children in Bangladesh

11

Sheikh Moin Uddin, Md. Masud Rana,
and Md. Golam Hossain

11.1 Introduction

Brothel-based female sex workers are the most at-risk group and threat to public health (Ngo et al. 2007). Living conditions are very poor. Most of the rooms are made with concrete and corrugated iron roofs—mostly narrow and only one room where they cook, live with children, with no cross-ventilation, window, sunlight can never enter in to the room, only one door, no sanitization, no renovation, damped room, no option discard for used condoms, and no water facilities available in the room. The room is full of semen and human excreta. The common toilet is also very dirty and there is no chance to clean it regularly (Saini 2020). Children of brothel-based female sex workers are more vulnerable because of their childhood spent in street and pavement (Kara 2013). Sex trade per week in brothels is higher than street-based, residential-based, and hotel-based sex trade in Bangladesh (Uddin et al. 2014). In the present situation, researchers found that from focus group discussions total of 11 registered brothels are now in Bangladesh. Shapla Mohila Sangstha (SMS), Mukti Mohila Sangstha (MMS), and Karmajibi Kallyan Sanstha (KKS) prepared mother list of brothel-based female sex workers and their children individually for their own project purpose. It is estimated that from these three sources, the total number of brothel-based female sex workers is 3837, where brothel is 3276 in Daulatdia, 379 in Rotkhola, and 182 in C&B Ghat. The total number of estimated children of brothel-based female sex workers is 806 where the brothel is 478 in

S. M. Uddin (✉)
TB and Leprosy Control Project Faridpur, Damien Foundation, Faridpur, Bangladesh

M. M. Rana
Institute of Water and Flood Management (IWFM), Bangladesh University of Engineering and Technology (BUET), Dhaka, Bangladesh

M. G. Hossain
Department of Statistics, University of Rajshahi, Rajshahi, Bangladesh

M. Pal et al. (eds.), *Public Health and Nutrition*,
https://doi.org/10.1007/978-981-97-7890-4_11

Daulatdia, 186 in Rotkhola, and 142 in C&B Ghat. Rothkhola brothel is in the heart of the city, C& B Ghat brothel is by the side of the river Padma, and Daulatdia brothel is by the side of the river Padma, Goalanda Upazila under Rajbari district. The research purpose of a qualitative study was to form nine focus groups from SMS, MMS, and KKS, which are three NGOs that deal with brothel-based female sex workers. We developed nine focus groups from these three NGOs, which included NGO personnel, brothel-based female sex workers, and children over the age of 10 years. In each group, there were three NGO employees, three brothel-based female sex workers, and three children over the age of ten. It is observed that an estimated 806 children are living with their mothers in three brothels (Roth Khola Brothel-Faridpur, C&B Ghat Brothel-Faridpur, and Doulotdia Ghat Brothel-Rajbari district), where several children are growing in different shelter homes, but another valued number of children are living with their mothers inside brothels or relatives' houses. These children were always subjected to physical, mental, emotional, social, cultural, and sexual abuse by their mothers and societies. Most mothers do not care about their daughters' education; their only concern is to force them into prostitution to earn money. There are no children retained with their mothers or frequentation in brothels before the age of 4 years of the children—section 9 under clause 77/1 of the Children Act 2013 (https://www.unicef.org/bangladesh/). Recent evidence-based reported data are not available about the absolute number of brothel-based female sex workers and their children in Faridpur and Rajbari districts. In this qualitative study, we used data from the grant proposal of three local NGOs funded by national and international donor agencies for directly implanting HIV/AIDS and STI control program and also social well-being of brothel-based female sex workers and their children. It was observed from the focus group discussion that most of the brothel-based children have experienced their mother's sexual intercourse with every unknown person causing psychological and emotional pressures. Ultimately, children become vulnerable and a threat to society.

11.2 Methodology

A qualitative study was used to acquire in-depth knowledge and information to identify gaps in the threats to the health and fundamental rights of brothel-based female sex workers' children through focus group discussions with mothers of these children and other stakeholders who were engaged to provide minimum ensured services. In March and April 2023, focus groups were conducted in Faridpur and Rajbari districts. In this study, a group of open-ended questions were used which focused on (1) learning about health care, (2) investigating educational facilities, (3) seeing sleeping facilities, (4) examining caring facilities, (5) looking at nursing facilities, (6) refreshment and restroom facilities, and (7) violence encountered by the children of female sex workers at the brothel. With the support of SMS, MMS, and KKS of these three local NGOs' management those who are directly implementing HIV/AIDS and Sexually Transmitted Disease control program, we selected a total of 27 Peer educators, Outreach Workers, and Volunteers. Individually, these three NGOs gave us a great opportunity to discuss our objectives with their Peer educators, Outreach Workers, and Volunteers during their weekly and monthly meetings. After successful orientation, training, and discussion, these 27 Peer educators, Outreach Workers, and Volunteers introduced us to 27 brothel-based female sex workers and 27 children over the age of 10 years. We formed nine focus groups with a total of 87 participants, and in each focus group, there were three NGO employees, three brothel-based female sex workers, and three children over the age of 10 years (Ma et al. 2017).

11.3 Data Analysis

After the focus group discussion, we analyzed the data considered including interview data, notes, physiological, psychological, body language, and eye-to-eye contact of each and individual focus group member. Only narrative data were included (Uddin et al. 2014). We emphasized the meaning of full words, phrases, or sentences. For critical understanding, we used common sense for interpretation. In this qualitative study, data were analyzed to ensure the accuracy, credibility, and validity of the results. All focus group members were invited to review the analyzed data and the interpretation for the accuracy of data.

11.4 Results

The socioeconomic profile of selected respondents was 18–40 years old (100%) and their children were over 10 years old (100%). Female sex workers in brothels are marginalized and stigmatized for their occupation, and they are alienated from their familial bonds (Vandepitte et al. 2006). Other sex workers were witnessed having sex with their sons who were verbally, physically, and sexually assaulted. Their way of life and vocations are not tolerated in this culture. Most of the children of brothel-based female sex workers do not have a national identity and hence do not have access to essential rights such as health, education, work, housing, legal assistance, family, and community support. Brothel-based female sex workers are marginalized and stigmatized for their profession and separated from their family bondage (Vandepitte et al. 2006; Todd et al. 2006). This society does not allow their lifestyle and professions. Most of the sex workers and their children did not get to identify nationally, resulting in not getting access to basic rights, that is, health, education, employment, housing, legal aid, family and community support, and safety net program support (Beattie et al. 2010). Mainstreaming brothel-based female sex workers through realizing their rights is not only a necessity to support them but also will benefit society in general by contributing better human rights realization. In this situation, it is needed to strengthen their rights and capacity and form a self-help group to the realization of human rights and dignity of life (Vandepitte et al. 2006; Sex Workers Network (SWN), Bangladesh and Sex Workers and Allies in South Asia (SWASA) 2016).

Table 11.1 showed that the focus group of socioeconomic profile was 18–40 years old the distribution of Focus group age 54 (66.7)% and 10–17 years old of Focus group age 27 (33.3)% where Peer educators 9 (11.1)%, Outreach Workers 9 (11.1)%, and Volunteers 9 (11.1)%, brothel-based female sex workers 27 (33.3)% and 10–17 years old respondents (33.4) where 10–17 years old respondents were Male 11 (40.75)% and Female 16 (59.25)%. Most of the respondents were born 48 (59.25)% in Dhaka, Barisal 23 (28.39)%, Khulna 6 (7.40)%, divisions and 4 (4.93)% was not specified. No education of the respondents was 5 (6.17)%, Pre-primary education 9 (11.11)%, Primary education of the respondents were 46 (56.79)%, secondary education 21 (25.92)%.

Tables 11.2 and 11.3 show that the selected respondents responded that 73 (90.12%) health care facilities were not adequate, whereas 8 (9.87)% had no response. In educational facilities, 69 (85.18)% were not adequate, whereas 12 (14.81)% had no response. In sleeping facilities, 73 (90.12)% were not adequate, whereas 8 (9.87)% had no response. In caring facilities, 79 (97.53)% were not adequate, whereas 2 (2.46)% had no response. In nursing facilities, 76 (93.82)% were

Table 11.1 Frequency distribution and socio-demographic factors of focus group discussion

Selected variables	Frequency ($n = 81$)	Percentage (%)
Focus group age		
18–40 years old	54	66.7
10–17 years old	27	33.3
Total	81	100
Focus group professional identity		
Peer educators	9	11.1
Outreach workers	9	11.1
Volunteers	9	11.1
Brothel-based female sex workers	27	33.3
10–17-year-old respondents	27	33.4
Total	81	100
10–17-year-old age focus group		
10–17-year-old respondents age male	11	40.75
10–17-year-old respondents age female	16	59.25
Total	27	100
Focus group birthplace division-wise		
Dhaka division	48	59.25
Barisal division	23	28.39
Khulna division	6	7.4
Not specified	4	4.93
Total	81	100
Focus group educational status		
No education	5	6.17
Pre-primary education	9	11.11
Primary education	46	56.79
Secondary education	21	25.92
Total	81	100

Table 11.2 Examples of meaning units, summarized meaning units, sub-theme, and theme of health and socio-demographic facilities of brothels children in Bangladesh: a qualitative study

Meaning unit	Summarized meaning unit	Sub-theme	Theme
Health care facilities	Not adequate	Suggest for better health care services	Experience of embarrassing
Educational facilities	Not adequate	Suggest for better educational facilities	Experience of stigma
Sleeping facilities	Not adequate	Suggest for better sleeping facilities	Experience of embarrassing
Caring Facilities	Not adequate	Suggest for better caring facilities	Experience of embarrassing
Nursing facilities	Not adequate	Suggest for better nursing facilities	Experience of embarrassing
Refreshment and restroom Facilities	Not adequate	Suggest for better refreshment and restroom facilities	Experience of stigma
Violence encountered by the children of female sex workers at the brothel	Very commonly	Suggest for preventing violence encountered by the children of female sex workers at the brothel	Experience of stigma

Table 11.3 Focus group discussion status

Selected variables	Frequency ($n = 81$)	Percentage (%)
Health care facilities at brothel		
Not adequate	73	90.12
No response	8	9.87
Total	81	100
Educational facilities at brothel		
Not adequate	69	85.18
No response	12	14.81
Sleeping facilities at brothel		
Not adequate	73	90.12
No response	8	9.87
Total	81	100
Caring facilities at brothel		
Not adequate	79	97.53
No response	2	2.46
Total	81	100
Nursing facilities at brothel		
Not adequate	76	93.82
No response	5	6.17
Total	81	100
Refreshment and restroom at brothel		
Not adequate	72	88.88
No response	9	11.11
Total	81	100
Violence encountered by the children of female sex workers at the brothel		
Very commonly	79	97.53
Not specified	2	2.46
Total	81	100

not adequate, whereas 5 (6.17)% had no response. In refreshment and restroom facilities, 72 (88.88)% were not adequate, whereas 9 (11.11)% had no response. Violence encountered by the children of female sex workers at the brothel occurred very commonly 79 (97.53)%, whereas 2 (2.46)% had no specific. In this qualitative study, the form of a table was identified including meaning unit, summarized meaning unit, sub-theme, and theme to understand transparent scenarios and clear interpretation from focus group discussion.

11.5 Discussion

In Bangladesh context, environment of brothels is not suitable for brothel-based female sex workers and their children—very congestive single rooms where they live with children and have sexual intercourse with clients, in the presence of children. Almost zero facilities in brothels room (Adhikari 2013). Brothel owners have no intention to improve living facilities for sex workers. Sex workers paid room rent on a daily basis. Fundamental rights in brothels are very negligible (Comte 2014). Health, safety, and rights outcomes for sex workers in brothels are always challenging issues. They always face violence and stigma (Shannon and Csete 2010). Every day and every moment, there is violence at brothels in many ways from clients and agents (musclemen) of the owners of brothels. Sex workers are always reporting to avoid more physical assault by agents (musclemen) (Pitpitan et al. 2013). Brothels suitable environment leads to reduced health and socio-demographic risks for children of brothel-based female sex workers (Project Report 2009). The study aimed to investigate themes of the study through focus group discussions about health care, education, caring, nursing facilities, and violence encountered by the children of female sex workers at brothels.

11.6 Health Care Facilities

The focus group did not openly disclose their personal health hazards and general health conditions and was not interested in going outside to seek doctors and good health service providers, because they did not have enough time, money, and opportunity. They suggested regular health screenings and services, management of STIs, HIV, cervical cancer, tuberculosis, contraceptive methods, safe abortions, post-abortion care, ante natal care, postnatal care, and neo natal care in brothels.

11.7 Educational Facilities

The focus group discussed that, in brothels, there are no educational facilities even restricted to children's education. Brothel-based female sex workers' children have equal rights without discrimination. They need good care and proper education in a healthy and playful environment. They need good education in brothels to be good citizens with fundamental human rights. Vocational and skilled development training are also needed. They need their children to mainstream in society.

11.8 Caring Facilities

Most commonly physical and psychological occurred to suppress both brothels based female sex workers and their children in brothels by brothel agents (muscle men). Girls of brothel-based female sex workers in brothel follow their mothers into sex work. They think and realize that this is their life and real society and social status. Sometimes, they help their mother with household work and engage with their mother's client's refreshment. On the contrary, boys are involved with all anti-social activities and become muscle men of brothel-based agents and brokers of brothel-based female sex workers.

11.9 Nursing Facilities

No nursing facilities are available in brothels in Bangladesh. There are no available management facilities for STIs, HIV, cervical cancer, tuberculosis, contraceptive methods, safe abortions, post-abortion care, ante natal care, post natal care, and neo natal care in brothels. Even for those who are drug users, there is no scope for harm reduction procedures. Day by day, drug users are increasing rapidly. Steroidal and non-steroidal drugs are used massively without caution and without the prescription of doctors.

11.10 Violence Encountered by the Children of Female Sex Workers at Brothel

The focus group discussed that Physical and sexual violence is a common experience in brothels. Gender-based violence is the most common. Sex workers are suffering from depression, anxiety, irritability, and distrust stress disorder. Physical violence results in cuts, injuries, and fractures. They think that violence from various parts of the job and there was nothing to be done about it.

11.11 Observations

In this qualitative study, we observed that SMS, MMS, and KKS are working for the social well-being of a small number of brothel-based female sex workers and their children with the limited scale with the support of international donor agencies as a project for a certain time with limited objectives. The limited facilities are available in brothels are very limited access. Some NGOs operate Drop-in

Centers at brothels with very small-scale health services. Many studies showed that female sex workers' HIV/AIDS, STI/STD, condom use status, harm reduction, prevention and control of communicable diseases but the living conditions in brothels with their children are very poorly documented. There was no evidence-based data reported in the recent study about living conditions in brothels for brothel-based female sex workers and their children at brothels in Bangladesh.

11.12 Limitation of the Study

The qualitative study was conducted in three brothels situated in Faridpur and Rajbari districts. A small number of participants were included in the focus group discussion because most of the female sex workers do not have enough time. They are always busy with income money, sex trade, and negotiation with clients for sex. More research is required to explore all brothels all over Bangladesh to identify the gap and access to need for the social well-being of brothel-based female sex workers and their children at brothels.

11.13 Ethical Considerations

With the cordial support of three NGOs SMS, MMS, and KKS, focus group discussion was very carefully with respect to societies cutler and norms. These three NGOs with the support of researchers briefed the focus group that this study is only for research purposes to identify the gap in better living conditions of brothel-based female sex workers and their children at brothels. Also ensure that the personal identity of focus group participants should never be used and it will be strictly prohibited. In this qualitative study, focus group participants' personal identities were strictly and completely excluded.

11.14 Recommendation

The government should take the initiative for social well-being and ensure fundamental rights for brothel-based female sex workers and their children. Society should support to government to stop becoming sex workers of brothel-based female sex workers girls and to stop boys from becoming anti-social activists.

11.15 Conclusions

This qualitative study investigated the status of health care, education, caring, nursing facilities, and violence encountered by the children of female sex workers at brothels with brothel-based female sex workers and their children with focus group discussion. It is also observed brothel facilities in the present time. It is high time to take the initiative and policy and implementation of policy to adopt brothel-based female sex workers children in the mainstream of society to reduce social crimes and terrorist activities.

Acknowledgments The authors would like to thank SMS, MMS, and KKS authorities, focus group discussion members including peer educators, outreach workers, volunteers, brothel-based female sex workers, and their children. We are grate ful to all members of the focus group because they have spent valuable time, energy, and experience for the purpose of this qualitative study.

Conflict of Interests None declared.

References

Adhikari H (2013) Beyond generational representation of children of female sex workers (FSWs) in sex trade (a stigmatized hidden profession): a desparate self-strategy of FSWs. Int J Sociol Anthropol 5(6):219–225. https://doi.org/10.5897/ijsa12.069

Beattie TSH, Bhattacharjee P, Ramesh BM, Gurnani V, Anthony J, Isac S, Moses S (2010) Violence against female sex workers in Karnataka state, south India: impact on health, and reductions in violence following an intervention program. BMC Public Health 10:476. https://doi.org/10.1186/1471-2458-10-476

Comte J (2014) Decriminalization of sex work: feminist discourses in light of research. Sex Cult 18(1):196–217. https://www.researchgate.net/publication/257771229_Decriminalization_of_Sex_Work_Feminist_Discourses_in_Light_of_Research

Kara S (2013) Zero traffick: eliminating sex trafficking in India, DASRA. https://cup.columbia.edu/book/sex-trafficking/9780231180337

Ma PH, Chan ZC, Loke AY (2017) The socio-ecological model approach to understanding barriers and facilitators to the accessing of health services by sex workers: a systematic review. AIDS Behav 21(8):2412–2438. https://pubmed.ncbi.nlm.nih.gov/28631228/

Ngo AD, McCurdy SA, Ross MW, Markham C, Ratliff EA, Pham HT (2007) The lives of female sex workers in Vietnam: findings from a qualitative study. Cult Health Sex 9(6):555–570. https://pubmed.ncbi.nlm.nih.gov/17963096/

Pitpitan EV, Kalichman SC, Eaton LA, Strathdee SA, Patterson TL (2013) HIV/STI risk among venue-based female sex workers across the globe: a look back and the way forward. Curr HIV/AIDS Rep 10(1):65–78. https://www.ncbi.nlm.nih.gov/pmc/articles/PMC3567216/

Project Report (2009) Safe home program for girls, Rajbari. https://oro.open.ac.uk/36227/2/7567BC5B.pdf. Accessed 15 July 2012

Saini M (2020) Dwindling protections for India's sex workers. Int Soc Public Policy. https://www.sbhambriadvocates.com/post/study-on-lives-of-children-in-brothels

Sex Workers Network (SWN), Bangladesh and Sex Workers and Allies in South Asia (SWASA) (2016) Bangladesh Chapter submission on the status of sex workers in Bangladesh to the United Nations Committee on the elimination of discrimination againt women 65th session. https://www.nswp.org/sites/default/files/cedaw_report_bangladesh_swasa_-_2016.pdf

Shannon K, Csete J (2010) Violence, condom negotiation, and HIV/STI risk among sex workers. JAMA 304(5):573–574. https://pubmed.ncbi.nlm.nih.gov/20682941/

Todd CS, Alibayeva G, Sanchez JL, Bautista CT, Carr JK, Earhart KC (2006) Utilization of contraception and abortion and its relationship to HIV infection among female sex workers in Tashkent, Uzbekistan. Contraception 74(4):318–323

Uddin S et al (2014) High risk behaviour of HIV/AIDS among female sex workers in Bangladesh: survey in Rayshahi City. Jpn J Infect Dis 67:191–196. https://pubmed.ncbi.nlm.nih.gov/24858608/

Vandepitte J, Lyerla R, Dallabetta G, Crabbé F, Alary M, Buvé. (2006) Estimates of the number of female sex workers in different regions of the world. Sex Transm Infect 82(Suppl 3):iii18–iii25. https://www.ncbi.nlm.nih.gov/pmc/articles/PMC2576726/

An Insight Into the Healthcare Facility and Accessibility in Assam

12

Nazneen Ara Hoque, Saddam Hussain,
and Utpal Kumar De

12.1 Introduction

In today's society, health care is an essential service that helps to enhance people's quality of life and social welfare. Access to healthcare refers to the procedures of governing people and demographic groups' entrance into the healthcare delivery system. One of the most important amenities for the whole population of a country is access to healthcare, which is largely influenced by the accessibility and expense of services. There are five dimensions that can be used to categorize accessibility: availability (appropriateness of the provision of health services), accessibility (travel barrier between the patients and service providers), accommodation (appropriateness and suitability of health services), affordability (costs of using healthcare), and acceptability (the adherence and satisfaction with health services) (Penchansky and Thomas 1981). However, the ability and desire to utilize healthcare are connected to the degree of accessibility to healthcare (Andersen 1995; Sloan 1977).

Since independence, India has witnessed a considerable and consistent decrease in mortality and a rise in life expectancy due to improved access to treatments, medications, and growing technologies. The average Indian citizen's life expectancy was roughly 32 years at the time of independence in 1947 and that has been increased to 70.42 years in 2023. The death rate of infants declined from 146 per 1000 in 1951 to 70 per 1000 in 2001, which further decreased to 26.62 deaths per 1000 in 2023 (Visaria et al. 2004). The average Indian citizen's life expectancy was roughly 32 years at the time of independence in 1947 (Visaria et al. 2004) and that

N. A. Hoque (✉)
Department of Economics, Damdama College, Kamrup, Assam, India

S. Hussain · U. K. De
Department of Economics, North-Eastern Hill University, Shillong, India

M. Pal et al. (eds.), *Public Health and Nutrition*,
https://doi.org/10.1007/978-981-97-7890-4_12

has been increased to 70.42 years in 2023. The death rate of infants declined from 146 per 1000 in 1951 to 70 per 1000 in 2001, which further decreased to 26.62 deaths per 1000 in 2023 (MacroTrends 2023).

The government of India has implemented several initiatives and programs to strengthen the country's post-independence healthcare facilities like the National Health Mission (NHM) (2005), the National Rural Health Mission (NRHM) (2005), Janani Suraksha Yojana (JSY) (2005), Janani Shishu Suraksha Karyakram (JSSK) (2011), and Pradhan Mantri Surakshit Matrutva Abhiyan (PMSMA) (2016), National Urban Health Mission (2013), the biggest government-funded health assurance/insurance program in the world, that is, Ayushman Bharat Pradhan Mantri Jan Arogya Yojana (AB PM-JAY) (2017), and so on (Press Information Bureau 2023).

Despite their intention to provide high-quality public health services, these institutions were unable to do so due to the lack of healthcare infrastructure, professionals, and personnel, and thus the child health concerns and maternal mortality remain too high in India post-independence, indicating an ineffective healthcare system (Baru et al. 2010; Horton and Das 2011; Sengupta and Prasad 2011; Ministry of Health and Family Welfare 2023). The majority of Indian states have very poor health outcomes as a result of the low level of funding for public health care, for instance, states such as Assam, Bihar, Madhya Pradesh, and Odisha perform like some of the less developed countries with very low health results in terms of infant mortality rates (Datta 2020).

Assam, which is in India's North-Eastern region, occupies around 2.4% of the country's total land area. There are some notable progresses in the healthcare sector as evidenced by the establishment of the National Rural Health Mission (NRHM) in 2005 to deliver quality, affordable, equitable, and accessible healthcare facilities, and then in 2010, it became the first state in the country to guarantee the right to healthcare to all of its residents; Assam Arogya Nidhi (AAN) mission of 2013 to serve underprivileged sections of society, especially BPL families. Furthermore, Assam has the highest number of medical colleges (six) among all the Northeastern states, accounting for 2.44% of all medical colleges in India. The state had 4401 government doctors in 2014 (0.14 per 1000 population), which went up to 6082 in 2017 (0.19 per 1000 population). As per NHP 2018, there has also been increased number of registered nurses and midwives from 18,506 in 2014 (0.59 per 1000 population) to 22,388 in 2018 (0.71 per 1000 population). The number of pharmacists has increased from 2429 in 2014 (0.077 per 1000 population) to 15,462 (0.49 per 1000 population) in 2019 (NHP 2015, 2019).

However, Assam has been showing poor performance in the case of IMR, life expectancy, and MMR. The IMR has been higher than the national average since 2011 and life expectancy has been lower than the national's average since 1971 (Statistical Handbook, Assam, 2022, #United Nations—World Population Prospects, 2022, +SRS, ^NFHS 5). Furthermore, since 2014–2016 to 2017–2019, the state's MMR has been higher than the nation's average MMR. According to the National

Family Health Survey-5 (2019–2021), 32% of women get married before the legal minimum age in Assam, whereas 25% of women aged 18–29 years married before the minimum age required by law nationwide. Approximately 60% of women suffer from anemia in eight Indian states, including Assam and Tripura (Ministry of Health and Family Welfare 2023).

Further recent data shows that there is a significant shortfall of health facilities such as sub-centers (29%), PHCs (14%), and CHCs (36%) in the rural areas of Assam (Rural Health Statistics 2021). The shortfall of sub-centers is more than the nation's average. However, for the urban area, the shortfall in PHCs is around 18%. Moreover, according to the Economic Survey 2021, there are only five allopathic and Ayush physicians, 15 nurses, and midwives for every 10,000 people in Assam, indicating a lopsided skill mix ratio between doctors and nurses. Furthermore, Economic Survey, Assam 2022–2023 revealed that life expectancy in the state is the lowest in the country, that is, 63.9 years only. In addition to the government statistics, some of the empirical studies have also shown the healthcare status of the state. For instance, Assam performs less satisfactorily than the national level standard, as per Sarma and Sharma (2014) analysis of the influence of human development indicators on human development rank, in terms of health indicators including sanitization services, institutional births in public facilities, and women giving birth or conceiving at that age of 15–19 years vary significantly throughout Assam's districts (Paul et al. 2019). However, there is still a need for inquiry into healthcare facilities and accessibility links, as well as people's preference for opting them.

In addition to the government statistics, some of the empirical studies have also shown the healthcare status of the state. For instance, the government only allocates 1.3% of GDP for public healthcare, resulting in a severe doctor shortage and high medical expenditure in both rural and urban hospitals of Assam (Das et al. 2005). Moreover, Assam performs less satisfactorily than the national level standard, as per Sarma and Sharma (2014) analysis of the influence of human development indicators on human development rank, in terms of health indicators including sanitization facilities, institutional births in public facilities, and women giving birth or becoming pregnant at the age of 15–19 years vary significantly throughout Assam's districts (Paul et al. 2019). There are still so many challenges in the form of inadequate access to free medicines, quality doctors, and sufficient government hospitals, resulting in poor health indicators like infant mortality and life expectancy (Gogoi et al. 2021; Neog 2023). Hence, inquiry into healthcare facilities and accessibility links, as well as people's preferences for them, is necessary.

Objectives of the Study

- To explore inter-district variation among different districts based on healthcare facilities
- To explore inter-district variation in healthcare facilities
- To investigate people's preferences regarding accessibility of healthcare facilities

12.2 Methodology

12.2.1 First Objective

12.2.1.1 Data Source

It is examined on the basis of Rural Health Statistics (2021), Statistical Handbook Assam (2022), and NFHS (2020) data. The initial part of the objective uses information related to No. of sub-centers, PHCs, CHCs, sub-divisional hospitals, district hospitals, and medical colleges and their bed availability, district-wise health centers, and available doctors, nurses, pharmacists, and so on.

12.2.2 Area of the Study and Sampling Design

Assam, located in India's North-East region, is bordered by seven states—Arunachal Pradesh, Manipur, Meghalaya, Mizoram, Nagaland, Tripura, and West Bengal—and two South Asian countries, including Bhutan and Bangladesh. It comprises 2.4% of the country's total area of 78,523 km^2 Assam, a state with a diverse population, has a population of 312.05 lakh, with 159.39 lakh males and 152.66 lakh females, as per the 2011 Census of India.

There are several Indian states such as Assam, Bihar, Madhya Pradesh, and Odisha which are experiencing poor health outcomes due to low public healthcare spending, similar to less developed countries with high infant mortality rates (Datta 2020). Based on this information, the state Assam has been selected purposively in the first step, while, in the next step, all 33 districts (31 March 2022) of Assam have been considered for the analysis.

12.2.2.1 Analysis

Analysis has been conducted by using the one-way ANOVA method to highlight the significant differences among districts of Assam. Districts have been arranged in five groups as per current district divisions of Assam, that is, Upper, North, Lower, Central, and Barak Valley. Here the ***hypothesis*** tested is whether there is any significant difference in health parameters across various district divisions or not.

For the inter-district variation analysis, the following health parameters (NFHS-5) have been considered:

- Women aged 15–19 years who were already mothers or pregnant at the time of the survey (%)
- Households using improved sanitation facility (%)[1]
- Institutional births in public facilities (%)

[1] Flush to piped sewer system, flush to septic tank, flush to pit latrine, flush to do not know where, ventilated improved pit {VIP}/biogas latrine, pit latrine with slab, twin pit/composting toilet, which is not shared with any other household. This indicator does not signify complete access to toilet facility.

- Children aged 12–23 months fully vaccinated based on information from either vaccination card or mother's recall[2] (%)
- Households with any usual member covered under a health insurance/financing scheme (%)

12.2.3 Second Objective

12.2.3.1 Data Source

It is mainly based on primary data, which explores preferences regarding accessibility of healthcare facilities. Data have been collected through household surveys through structured schedules.

12.2.3.2 Area of the Study and Sampling Design

This part of the study adopts a Multistage sampling technique. In the ***first stage***, a semi-urban area (Azara) has been selected purposively near the capital (Dispur) of Assam. Azara is a small town in the northwestern section of Guwahati, Assam. It is around 5 km (3.1 miles) from Guwahati Airport and is surrounded by the Borjhar and Jalukbari areas. It is in Assam's Kamalpur subdivision of the Kamrup district. The total land area is 173.61 hectares. The literacy rate of the area is 83.17%, with 89.05% men and 76.75% females being literate as per census 2011. The ***second stage*** involves the identification of the total households and the calculation of no. of sample households. A total of 927 households has been found as per census 2011, and only 10% of it has been chosen (approximately 92) as sample households due to resource and time constraints. The ***third stage*** involves data collection, which has been collected through structured schedules from the randomly selected households. Focus group discussions have also been conducted. The study was conducted between May and June 2023.

12.2.3.3 Analysis

The factors influencing the preference of the respondents to access healthcare facilities available in their locality have been analyzed through a ***Binary Probit Regression*** model. The model comprises the dependent and independent variables identified from various literatures.

Dependent Variable

Preference for the access of healthcare facilities available at their locality (i.e., 1 if there is Preference to Access Healthcare Facility and 0 otherwise).

[2] Vaccinated with BCG, measles-containing vaccine {MCV}/MR/MMR/Measles, and three doses each of polio (excluding polio vaccine given at birth) and DPT or Penta vaccine.

Independent Variables

Variables	Definition	Expected effects
Age	Respondents age in years	+/−
Gender	1 if male, 0 otherwise	+/−
Education	(1 = illiterate, 2 = primary, 3 = secondary, 4 = graduate and above)	+/−
Family income	Actual INR per year	+/−
Household size	Number of family members	+/−
Distance from PHC	In km	+/−

Model Specification

Let U*PAHL = Expected utility while preferring access to healthcare at their locality and U*NPAHL = Expected utility while not preferring access to healthcare at their locality.

$$\text{Preference to Access healthcare at their locality} = 1 \quad \text{if} \quad U*PAHL - U*NPAHL > 0$$
$$0 \quad \text{if} \quad U*PAHL - U*NPAHL \leq 0$$

The binary choice of preference to access healthcare at their locality is assumed to be generated by a linear latent variable model (Y*):

$$\text{Preference to access healthcare at their locality}: Y_i = 1, \quad y^*_i > 0\left(\text{where}, Y^* = \text{latent variable}\right)$$
$$0, \quad y^*_i \leq 0$$

$$Y*_i = X_i\beta + u_i, \qquad u_i|x_i - N\left(0,\sigma^2\right)$$

$$P\left(Y_i = 1|X_i\right) = P\left(Y*_I > 0|x_i\right) = P\left(X_i\beta + u_i > 0|x_i\right)$$

$$= P\left(u_i > -X_i\beta|X_i\right) = P\left(u_i/\sigma > -X_i\beta/\sigma|x_i\right) = 1 - \Phi\left(-X_i\beta/\sigma\right) = \Phi\left(X_i\beta/\sigma\right)$$

y^*_i = net utility received to the respondent by accessing healthcare facility available at their locality, x = independent variables, and u = random term.

Finally, marginal effects have been calculated for each explanatory factor (Mutlu and Gracia 2006; Yen and Su 1995), to demonstrate the degree to which the variables influence their choice decision.

12.3 Results

Recent data from Rural Health Statistics (2021) as presented in Table 12.1 shows that there is a significant shortfall of health facilities like sub-centers (29%), PHCs (14%), and CHCs (36%) in the rural parts of Assam. The shortfall of sub-centers is more than the nation's average. However, for the urban area, the shortfall in PHCs is around 18%. Moreover, according to the Economic Survey 2021, there are only

Table 12.1 Shortfall in health facilities in rural and urban areas of Assam and India

Shortfall in health facilities as per mid-year population (as of 1 July 2022) in rural areas

State/ UT	Estimated mid-year population for rural areas	Estimated mid-year population for tribal areas	Sub centers				PHCs				CHCs			
			R	*P*	*S*	%Sf	*R*	*P*	*S*	%S	*R*	*P*	*S*	%Sf
Assam	29,996,000	4,101,442	6546	4667	1879	29	1068	920	148	14	267	172	95	36
All India/ total	898,870,000	101,657,344	193,310	157,935	48,060	25	31,640	24,935	9742	31	7894	5480	2852	36

Shortfall in primary health centers as per mid-year population (as of July 1, 2022) in urban areas

State/ UT	Estimated mid-year population for urban areas (as of July 1, 2022)	PHCs			
		Required	In position	Shortfall	% of shortfall
		R	P	S	
Assam	5,494,000	110	90	20	18
All India	480,880,000	9618	6118	3822	39.7

The required number of PHCs is rounded to the nearest integer and is based on population norms of 50,000. *R* required, *P* in position, *S* shortfall, *Surplus, *Sf shortfall

Source: Rural Health Statistics (2021)

five allopathic and Ayush physicians, 15 nurses, and midwives for every 10,000 people in Assam, indicating a lopsided skill mix ratio between doctors and nurses. Furthermore, Economic Survey, Assam 2022–2023 revealed that life expectancy in the state is the lowest in the country, that is, 63.9 years only.

Inter-District Variation This section presents variations among different districts of Assam in terms of different healthcare facilities. The total number of functional health centers of rural and urban areas as of 31 March 2022, in Assam (33 districts) is 5951 (16.42 per lakh population). The availability of district-wise healthcare centers per lakh population is presented in Table 12.2, which shows that Biswanath (*newly created district in 2015*) has the highest and West Karbi Anglong (*newly created district in 2016*) has the lowest health centers per lakh population.

The availability of district-wise doctors, pharmacists, and nurses (in no.'s) is presented in Figs. 12.1 and 12.2, which show that the highest numbers of rural and urban doctors were found in the districts of Kamrup and Kamrup Metro, respectively, whereas the highest numbers of ANM workers (rural) were found in Cachar district.

ANOVA: Table 12.3 indicates the mean score for all the health parameters for five divisions. Results have been analyzed using the SPSS software. The mean score of the Upper Assam group has been found to be the highest in comparison to the other groups in the case of three parameters (Sl. No. 2, 3, and 4). However, for Sl. No. 1, the Lower Assam group scores the highest mean relative to other groups. Likewise, for Sl. No. 5, the North Assam group has the highest mean value relative to the other groups.

ANOVA has been carried out using the SPSS 16 software. Table 12.3 indicates the mean score for all the health parameters for the five divisions. The Upper Assam group has the highest mean score in three parameters (Sl. No. 2, 3, and 4), while the Lower Assam group scores the highest mean in Sl. No. 1 and the North Assam group has the highest mean value in Sl. No. 5.

From Table 12.3, it is observed that there is a statistically significant difference in households with improved sanitation facilities and fully vaccinated children of age group (12–23 months) among various district divisions. However, for the other parameters like already mothers or pregnant at the age group (15–19), institutional births at public facility, and households with health insurance, there is no significant difference across district divisions. Hence, in this case, the alternate hypothesis cannot be supported.

As two of the parameters, that is, households with improved sanitation facility and fully vaccinated children of age group (12–23 months), show statistically significant differences, a post hoc test (Tukey HSD (honest significant difference)) for the two has been used to assess multiple comparisons among different divisions of the district (Table 12.4).

When the null hypothesis is rejected on the ground that there are significant differences, the question of "which particular means are different" arises. This is why the test has been used to seek further information after test results.

Table 12.2 District-wise availability of health centers per lakh population, Assam

Name of the district	Total no. of functional health centers	Total population (estimated, 2022)	Health centers per lakh population
Baksa	201	1,254,099	16.03
Barpeta	327	2,235,582	14.63
Biswanath	170	82,980	204.87
Bongaigaon	142	975,222	14.56
Cachar	313	2,060,000	15.19
Charaideo	92	505,384	18.20
Chirang	116	636,454	18.23
Darrang	201	1,225,620	16.40
Dhemaji	127	905,696	14.02
Dhubri	235	2,573,021	9.13
Dibrugarh	275	1,470,000	18.71
Dima Hasao	92	282,615	32.55
Goalpara	200	1,330,802	15.03
Golaghat	193	1,190,000	16.22
Hailakandi	125	791,500	15.79
Hojai	107	292,518	36.58
Joraht	153	1,441,778	10.61
Kamrup	360	1,730,000	20.81
Kamrup Metro	102	1,460,000	6.99
Karbi Anglong	145	1,262,334	11.48
Karimganj	269	1,480,000	18.18
Kokrajhar	211	1,171,028	18.02
Lakhimpur	188	1,375,621	13.67
Majuli	45	126,025	35.71
Marigaon	163	1,166,700	13.97
Nagaon	344	3,400,000	10.11
Nalbari	180	1,018,564	17.67
Sivasagar	181	1,519,386	11.91
Sonitpur	182	2,200,000	8.27
South Salmara	61	153,884	39.64
Tinsukia	198	1,510,000	13.11
Udalguri	182	1,097,802	16.57
West Karbi Anglong	71	1,262,334	5.63

Source: Rural Health Statistics (2021)

Part A of Table 12.4 indicates that Barak Valley has significant differences with Upper Assam and North Assam in terms of households with improved sanitation facility. Conversely, however, Part B shows that Upper Assam has significant differences with North, Lower, and Central Assam in terms of fully vaccinated children of age group (12–23 months), while the rest of them have no significant difference.

Case study on factors influencing respondents' preference to access healthcare facilities: In order to determine people's preference to access locally available

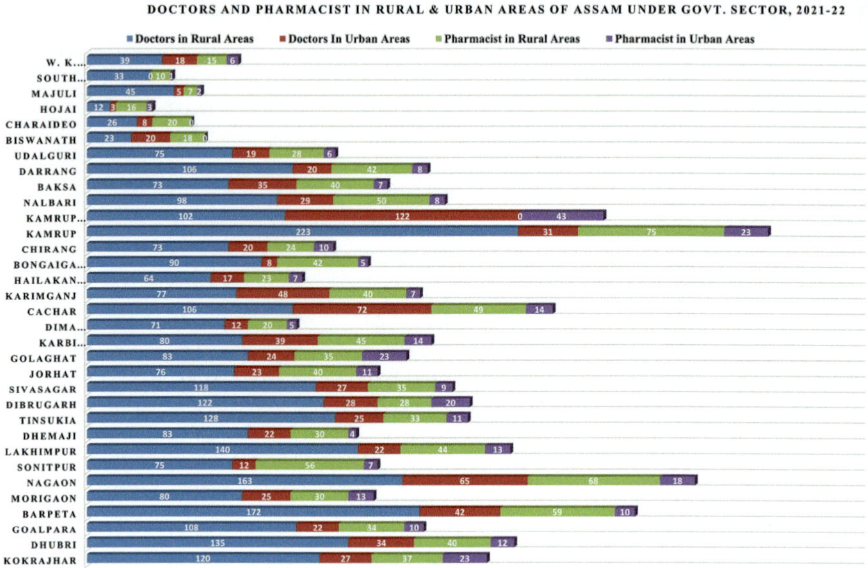

Fig. 12.1 No. of doctors and pharmacists in rural and urban areas, Assam. Source: Statistical Handbook Assam (2022)

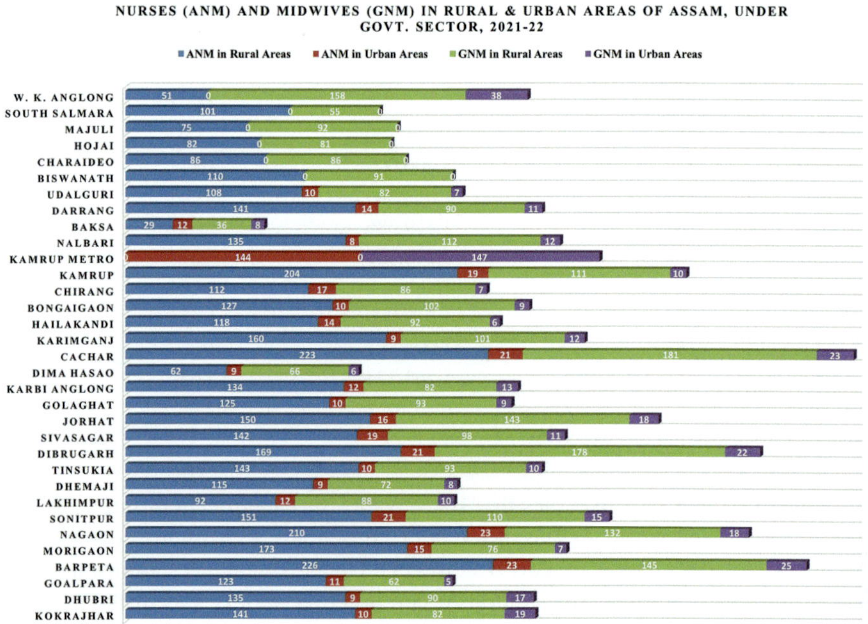

Fig. 12.2 No. of nurses and midwives in rural and urban areas, Assam. Source: Statistical Handbook Assam (2022)

Table 12.3 Result of ANOVA

Sl. No.	Health parameters	District division	No. of districts	Mean	Std. deviation	*F*	Sig.
1	Already mothers or pregnant at the age group (15–19)	Upper Assam	9	8.81	3.326	0.991	0.429
		North Assam	4	9.08	5.004		
		Lower Assam	11	**25.34**	35.974		
		Central Assam	6	10.45	4.374		
		Barak Valley	3	9.6	0.985		
		Total	33	14.72	21.703		
2	Households with improved sanitation facility	Upper Assam	9	**73.81**	5.588	3.616	**0.017**
		North Assam	4	72.62	3.637		
		Lower Assam	11	68.41	5.65		
		Central Assam	6	71.2	8.67		
		Barak Valley	3	59.7	1.967		
		Total	33	70.11	6.858		
3	Institutional births at public facility	Upper Assam	9	**78.72**	7.783	0.836	0.514
		North Assam	4	76.68	3.779		
		Lower Assam	11	72.81	9.236		
		Central Assam	6	73.05	9.455		
		Barak Valley	3	73.27	3.004		
		Total	33	74.98	8.035		
4	Fully vaccinated children of age group (12–23 months)	Upper Assam	9	**76.59**	6.782	5.493	**0.002**
		North Assam	4	58.12	14.405		
		Lower Assam	11	64.15	7.574		
		Central Assam	6	60.48	8.712		
		Barak Valley	3	71.37	3.356		
		Total	33	66.8	10.472		
5	Households with health insurance	Upper Assam	9	63.16	3.852	1.155	0.352
		North Assam	4	**64.9**	7.62		
		Lower Assam	11	58.26	8.828		
		Central Assam	6	61.4	4.419		
		Barak Valley	3	58.63	5.437		
		Total	33	61.01	6.689		

Source: Authors' own calculation

Bold values less than or equal to 0.05 (5% level of significance) are considered to be significant here and values above are considered as insignificant.

Table 12.4 Post hoc analysis

(1) Division of districts	(2) Division of districts	Mean difference (1–2)	Sig.
Part A: Multiple comparisons for households with improved sanitation facility			
Upper Assam	North Assam	1.186	0.997
	Lower Assam	5.402	0.283
	Central Assam	2.611	0.918
	Barak Valley	**14.111***	**0.011**
North Assam	Upper Assam	−1.186	0.997
	Lower Assam	4.216	0.744
	Central Assam	1.425	0.996
	Barak Valley	**12.925***	**0.058**
Lower Assam	Upper Assam	−5.402	0.283
	North Assam	−4.216	0.744
	Central Assam	−2.791	0.885
	Barak Valley	8.709	0.193
Central Assam	Upper Assam	−2.611	0.918
	North Assam	−1.425	0.996
	Lower Assam	2.791	0.885
	Barak Valley	11.500	0.074
Barak valley	Upper Assam	**−14.111***	**0.011**
	North Assam	**−12.925***	**0.058**
	Lower Assam	−8.709	0.193
	Central Assam	−11.500	0.074
Part B: Multiple comparisons for fully vaccinated children of age group (12–23 months)			
Upper Assam	North Assam	**18.464***	**0.008**
	Lower Assam	**12.443***	**0.020**
	Central Assam	**16.106***	**0.009**
	Barak Valley	5.222	0.881
North Assam	Upper Assam	**−18.464***	**0.008**
	Lower Assam	−6.020	0.734
	Central Assam	−2.358	0.992
	Barak Valley	−13.242	0.261
Lower Assam	Upper Assam	**−12.443***	**0.020**
	North Assam	6.020	0.734
	Central Assam	3.662	0.909
	Barak Valley	−7.221	0.680
Central Assam	Upper Assam	**−16.106***	**0.009**
	North Assam	2.358	0.992
	Lower Assam	−3.662	0.909
	Barak Valley	−10.883	0.374
Barak Valley	Upper Assam	−5.222	0.881
	North Assam	13.242	0.261
	Lower Assam	7.221	0.680
	Central Assam	10.883	0.374

Source: Authors own calculation (*the mean difference is significant at the 0.05 level)
Bold values less than or equal to 0.05 (5% level of significance) are considered to be significant here and values above are considered as insignificant

healthcare facilities, information related to the number of PHCs and its facilities has been gathered. One 30-bed PHC, namely, Azara PHC, is also an FRU *(First Referral Unit)* of Kamrup district. The PHC has gynecologists, anesthesiologists, and so on, except doctors in medicine. The availability of facilities there are listed in Table 12.5.

The available facilities and infrastructures of the PHC were discussed with the respondents before their response on willingness to access healthcare facilities. Approximately 79% of the respondents had full information on the available healthcare facilities at the PHC, while the rest had partial information. Though the PHC has various facilities, whether people choose to access them or not is analyzed below by using a binary probit regression model. Table 12.6 displays the result of the model that regresses the probability of respondents' preference to access healthcare facilities available in their locality. STATA software has been used to analyze the data.

Here the model converged at the fourth iteration. The table shows that all the observations (92) were used in the analysis with a p-value of 0.0487 indicating that the model is statistically significant. The result shows that factors such as age,

Table 12.5 Facilities available at Azara PHC

Facilities	Available
Doctors (both male and female)	Yes
Nurses	Yes
Laboratory technician	Yes
Pharmacist	Yes
Accountant	Yes
Fourth-grade worker	Yes
Sweeper	Yes
Quarter for doctors and nurses	Yes
Treatment rooms	Yes
Delivery rooms	Yes
Mobile van	Yes
Indoor bed	Yes
OT	Yes
OPD	Yes
Blood test facilities	Yes
Urine test and stool test	Yes
X-ray machine	Yes
Ultrasonography	Yes
Computer facility	Yes
24-h electricity supply	Yes
Running water	Yes
Wheel chair	Yes
Stretcher	Yes
Saline stand	Yes
24-h emergency and delivery service	Yes
Antenatal care	Yes
Immunization	Yes

Source: Survey data

Table 12.6 Marginal effect estimates of factors influencing preferences for accessing healthcare facilities available at their locality (probit model)

Variables				
Willingness to access health care facilities	Marginal effects	Robust std. errors	Z	$P > \|Z\|$
Age	0.002937	0.0034941	0.84	0.401
Gender	0.1124747	0.0927573	1.21	0.225
Education	–0.0701404	0.0339544	–2.07	**0.039****
Family income	-6.04×10^{-6}	2.39×10^{-6}	–2.53	**0.009*****
Household size	–0.0136762	0.0153188	–0.89	0.372
Distance from the PHC	–0.0305977	0.0342128	–0.89	0.371

Note: $N = 92$, Log pseudo-likelihood = –53.72685; Wald chi² (6) = 12.66, Prob > chi² = 0.0487, Pseudo $R^2 = 0.1209$. ***, ** specify significance at 1% and 5% level
Source: Survey data

gender, household size, and distance from PHC have no influence on the respondent's preference to access locally available healthcare facilities. However, ***educational level*** has a significant influence on the respondent's preference. The marginal effect estimation shows that respondents' preference to access locally available healthcare facilities decreases by –0.0701404 percentage points as the education level goes up. This result is similar to the findings of Ghosh (2014) which shows that individuals with higher educational levels tend to seek healthcare from private health centers with improved infrastructures. Furthermore, the marginal effect of ***Family income*** indicates that as the income of the family increases, their preference to access healthcare available locally decreases by -6.04×10^{-6} percentage points. This outcome is similar to the result of Uchendu et al. (2013) and Ghosh (2014), who found a negative relation between increasing income and accessing services from public healthcare providers.

12.4 Discussion and Concluding Remarks

The *first part* of the paper deals with the status of health conditions in Assam as compared with India's average and its inter-district variations. While investigating the health condition of the state and its districts, we have found some improved scenarios like the number of government doctors and nurses and midwives from 2014 to 2018 increased by about 38% and 17%, respectively, and there was also a 536.56% increase in the number of registered pharmacists during 2014–2019 (NHP 2015). On the contrary, shortfalls of healthcare facilities such as sub-center, PHC, and CHC at rural and urban levels have also been observed (Table 12.1). Furthermore, from the result of ANOVA, we can see that there are significant differences in terms of health parameters like households with improved sanitation facilities and full vaccination of children in the age group (12–23 months). In the *second part* of the chapter, the result of the probit model pointed out that households with higher educational levels and high family income do not prefer to access facilities in their locality. On average, there is a huge ***inflow*** of patients per month from outside, that is, approximately 4500 above, and currently, there is no Doctor of Medicine that might lead people to go for another option. As the area is situated near Guwahati city, where Guwahati Medical College and other reputed hospitals are available with sophisticated facilities; it might be a reason for the educated ones to give less preference to the facilities available at their locality. Furthermore, there is a tendency that households with more family income would likely to go for private facilities rather than depending on the government facilities with so many inadequacies.

The result is similar to the studies of Ghosh (2014) who also found a negative correlation between education and household income with the preference for opting of public health facilities for treatment. Furthermore, some of the studies like Uchendu et al. (2013) and Ghosh (2014) display a negative correlation between income growth and the use of public health care services, suggesting that individuals tend to access private healthcare services more as their income increases. Our study also found a similar outcome. However, regarding the age parameter, studies have different opinions; some indicate that elders are more likely to use public health facilities, while some say that private health facilities are more commonly used by the elders (Kang et al. 1993; Doghaither et al. 2003; Manzambi et al. 2000). The result of our study shows a positive association but non-significant. Likewise, in the case of gender, our study shows similar results to the study of Doghaither et al. (2003) and Keene and Li (2005) which show that males are more likely to use private hospitals. However, it contradicts the study of Ghosh (2014) who found that women are more likely to visit better private facilities compared with men.

From the above discussion, the following suggestions can be made. As the state has a higher MMR than other states, it requires greater investment in the healthcare industry. Furthermore, in the ANOVA analysis, we have found significant differences in two of the health parameters namely, households with improved sanitation facilities and full vaccination of children of age group (12–23 months), the concerned authorities may take proper steps to provide awareness to improve these health parameters so that the inter-district differences of the state can be minimized and overall development of the health sector can be achieved. As poor sanitation facilities are one of the root causes of 7% of total illness burden and 19% of child mortality worldwide (Pruss-Ustun 2008), improving sanitation awareness can be effective in minimizing these problems. Moreover, increasing vaccination awareness also helps to protect children from infectious illnesses including hepatitis, diphtheria, tetanus, pertussis (whooping cough), measles, and polio. Furthermore, measures can be taken to improve infrastructural facilities at government hospitals to minimize the hardships of the patients. If people prefer private health care facilities, the concerned authorities should also ensure an acceptable standard.

References

Andersen RM (1995) Revisiting the behavioural model and access to medical care: does it matter? J Health Soc Behav 36:1–10

Baru R, Acharya A, Acharya S, Kumar AS, Nagaraj K (2010) Inequities in access to health services in India: caste, class, and region. Econ Polit Wkly 45(38):49–58

Das C, Valley T, Bhowal A (2005) Efficiency and performance of sub-centres on selected maternal and child healthcare services: a case study of Hailakandi District in Assam. Life 43(63):67–63

Datta S (2020) Political competition and public healthcare expenditure: evidence from Indian states. Soc Sci Med 244:112429

Ghosh S (2014) Health sector reforms and changes in prevalence of untreated morbidity, choice of healthcare providers among the poor and rural population in India. Int J Health Policy Manag 2(3):125

Gogoi M, Sarat Hazarika KKP, Gogoi P (2021) Rural healthcare infrastructure of North-East India and its challenges. Int J Cur Res Rev 13(13):56

Horton R, Das P (2011) Indian health: the path from crisis to progress. Lancet 377(9761):181–183

Kang JT, Chen CF, Chou P (1993) Factors related to the choice of different hospitals providing Chinese traditional medicine. Chin Med J 51(6):448–456

Keene J, Li X (2005) Age and gender differences in health service utilization. J Public Health 27(1):74–79

MacroTrends (2023) India infant mortality rate 1950-2024

Manzambi JK, Tellier V, Bertrand F, Albert A, Reginster JY, Van Balen EH (2000) The behavioral determinants for health centers in health districts of urban Africa: results of a survey of households in Kinshasa, Congo. Trop Med Int Health 5(8):563–570

Ministry of Health and Family Welfare (2023) Ministry of Health and Family Welfare 2012, Govt. of India

Mutlu S, Gracia A (2006) Spanish food expenditure away from home (FAFH): by type of meal. Appl Econ 38(9):1037–1047

Neog N (2023) An inter district analysis of public healthcare infrastructure disparities in Assam. Online J Health Allied Sci 22(1):1

NFHS (2020) NFHS-5 report 2019–2020. https://rchiips.org/nfhs/NFHS-5Reports/NFHS-5_INDIA_REPORT.pdf. Accessed 18 May 2023

NHP (2015) National Health Profile (NHP) of India - 2015: Central Bureau of Health Intelligence. https://cbhidghs.nic.in. Accessed 9 June 2023

NHP (2019) National Health Profile (NHP) of India-2019. Ministry of Health and Family Welfare. https://cbhidghs.nic.in. Accessed 9 June 2023

Paul KP, Jana KS, Maiti A (2019) An analysis of health status of the state of Assam, India Research Review International Journal of Multidisciplinary 04(03):1179–1187

Penchansky R, Thomas JW (1981) The concept of access: definition and relationship to consumer satisfaction. Med Care 19:127–140

Press Information Bureau (2023). https://pib.gov.in/PressReleasePage.aspx?PRID=1926803. Accessed 18 June 2023

Pruss-Ustun A (2008) Safer water, better health: costs, benefits and sustainability of interventions to protect and promote health. World Health Organization, Geneva

Rural Health Statistics (2021) Ministry of Health & Family Welfare, Govt. of India. https://main.mohfw.gov.in/sites/default/files/RHS2021-22_2.pdf. Accessed 10 June 2023

Sarma A, Sharma PS (2014) Impact of social sector expenditure on human resource development: a look into the education and health sector. International Journal of Business and Management 3(12):18–26.

Sengupta A, Prasad V (2011) Towards a truly universal Indian health system. Lancet 377(9767):702–703

Sloan FA (1977) Access to medical care and the local supply of physicians. Med Care 15(4):338–346

Statistical Handbook Assam (2022) Statistical handbook | Directorate of Economics and Statistics | Government of Assam, India

Uchendu OC, Ilesanmi OS, Olumide AE (2013) Factors influencing the choice of health care providing facility among workers in a local government secretariat in south western Nigeria. Ann Ibadan Postgrad Med 11(2):87–95

United Nations (2022) World population prospects - population division. United Nations, New York

Visaria L, Ramachandran V, Ganatra B, Kalyanwala S (2004) Abortion in India: emerging issues from qualitative studies. Econ Polit Wkly 39:5044–5052

Yen ST, Su SJ (1995) Modeling US butter consumption with zero observations. J Agric Resour Econ 24:47–55

Part III

Morbidity

Status of Morbidity in SAARC Countries: Analysis with Panel Data 13

Utpal Kumar De, Premananda Bharati, and Manoranjan Pal

13.1 Introduction

There are several studies where the impacts of investment in human capital on economic growth and development have been examined in developing countries (Kim and Lane 2013; Romer 1994). Based on the endogenous growth model, the status of health and healthcare can be identified as an important component to affect the development of human capital (Romer 1994). It is also inherent in Grossman's human capital model (Somi et al. 2009). In this context, it has been seen that there is a significant effect of health status on the present and future well-being of households (Novignon et al. 2012).

Many researchers working in health economics have examined the relationship between healthcare expenditure and the status of health (Bokhari et al. 2007; Bradley et al. 2011; Kim and Lane 2013; Poullier et al. 2002). The role of public expenditure in improving health outcomes has emerged as an important issue (Bhalotra 2007; Gani 2009). Findings of many studies emphasized the need to increase public health expenditure towards providing primary healthcare and ameliorate the effect of diseases on the productive span of life of individuals (Verhoeven et al. 1999). Using panel data for the period 1993–2012 from the seven South Asian Association for Regional Cooperation (SAARC) nations, Mohapatra (2022) found a significant influence of health expenditure in improving health outcomes in these countries.

U. K. De (✉)
Department of Economics, North-Eastern Hill University, Shillong, India

P. Bharati
Biological Anthropology Unit, Indian Statistical Unit (ISI),
Kolkata, West Bengal, India

M. Pal
Economic Research Unit, Indian Statistical Unit (ISI), Kolkata, West Bengal, India

M. Pal et al. (eds.), *Public Health and Nutrition*,
https://doi.org/10.1007/978-981-97-7890-4_13

The SAARC region is one of the poorest regions in the world in terms of health indicators. The largest number of people in the world have micronutrient deficiencies, and diabetes is found in this region. Also, about 40% of the world's tuberculosis burden and high burden of cardiovascular diseases as well as worst cases of reproductive health are found here (Nishtar 2002). Moreover, health-related risks posed by close animal contact are very much in existence in this region.

The SAARC is an association of eight countries situated in the southern part of Asia that includes Nepal, Afghanistan, Maldives, Bangladesh, Pakistan, Bhutan, India, and Sri Lanka. It is an economic as well as a political organization. The organization aims to promote the welfare of people and achieve overall social progress and cultural development in the region. These would be achieved by utilizing the full potential of the people, strengthening collective self-reliance among the member countries, and building mutual trust and understanding through socio-economic, cultural, technical, and scientific collaborations.

Deficiency in nutrition among women is common in developing countries, particularly in the South Asian region (Bhandari et al. 2016). Over three and a half million women succumb to death each year in developing countries due to a lack of nutritional intake (Black et al. 2008). Almost 50% of the world's malnourished women live in this Indian sub-continent, the three neighboring developing countries: India, Bangladesh, and Pakistan (Ali et al. 2020). The proportion of malnourished women is decreasing but is still very high across Bangladesh, India, and Nepal. Waghmare et al. (2022) observed that over 16% of women were underweight in these three countries of south Asia belonging to SAARC. Only in Pakistan, the percentage of underweight women is less than 8. The proportion of underweight women in reproductive age has decreased from 36% in 1999 to 33% in 2006 (Chaparro et al. 2014).

Despite having modest economic growth in South Asia in the recent past, malnutrition and lack of food security continued to prevail in the region. The proportion of the population suffering from severe food insecurity rose from 13.5% in 2017 to 19.9% in 2020. The incidence of poverty among the working population in South and Southwest Asia is 25.4% among men, whereas it is 30.9% among women, which is the highest rate in the Asia-Pacific region (Suri and Ashok 2022).

Regional culture may be responsible for excessive neglect of maternal nutrition, which leads to the high prevalence of child malnutrition in South Asia. The women in South Asia suffer from excessive stress in their reproductive life and that has profound implications toward their overall nutritional status (Osmani and Bhargava 1998).

This chapter tries to analyze the progress of health status and the healthcare indicators since 2000 in SAARC countries and the impacts of various measures on health status by using pooled data.

13.2 Data and Methodology

Data on various health indicators and healthcare-related variables of eight SAARC countries have been collected from the world development indicators for the period 2000–2020. To be very precise, the source is https://databank.worldbank.org/source/world-development-indicators, updated as of February 2024. Many of the variables had to be discarded because of too many missing values. We had to use imputation methods to fill up the few gaps that we had in the database to make the data balanced.

Since our objective is to see the pattern and extent of various morbidity in the SAARC countries, we focused on the morbidity variables, namely, overall "prevalence of undernutrition", overall "incidence of tuberculosis", "prevalence of stunting" among under-5 children, "anemia among pregnant women," overall "incidence of malaria," "anemia among under-5 children," and "anemia among women." The explanatory variables taken for this purpose are total "fertility rate," "immunization against tetanus," people "practicing open defecation," "hand washing facility," "basic sanitation practice," "number of Physicians," "immunization for DPT," and "safe drinking water." It should be noted here that some more appealing variables could not be taken because of too many missing values. A list of these variables and their detailed descriptions are made in Table 13.1.

We shall see later that some of the explanatory variables could not be utilized in the regression analysis due to the problem of multicollinearity problem. Thus, the results of the subsequent analysis are shown only for the variables supported by the regression analysis.

We first carried out the analysis of variance (ANOVA) separately for the morbidity variables across countries to see whether the variations of means across countries are significant. Also, we see the variations of means over time to ascertain whether fixed effect model should be taken for the time variable also. Usually, panel data analysis does not take time as a potential component to explain the variations in the concerned variables.

After examining the comparative picture of growth of various health indicators across the SAARC countries and time, we compute bivariate correlations of each health indicator with the healthcare variables for each year. Based on the correlations, a panel data regression has been carried out in order to estimate the impacts of various healthcare indicators on the health outcome variables. The Hausman specification test has been applied in order to ascertain which model is appropriate between random effect and fixed effect models. The test suggested the appropriateness of the fixed effect model in almost all the cases. The fixed effect model can be written as

$$Y_{\mathrm{ikt}} = \beta_0 + \Sigma \beta_m X_{\mathrm{mkt}} + \Sigma \gamma_j D_{\mathrm{jt}} + \Sigma \delta_k D_k + u_{\mathrm{it}},$$

Table 13.1 The list along with the detailed descriptions of variables proposed to be used in the analysis

Name of the variable	Definition	Explanation
Prevalence of undernutrition	Percentage of undernourished people	Morbidity variable
Incidence of tuberculosis	Incidence of tuberculosis per lakh population	Morbidity variable
Prevalence of stunting	"Prevalence of stunting is the percentage of children under age 5 whose height for age is greater than two standard deviations below the median for the international reference population aged 0–59 months"	Morbidity variable
anemia among pregnant women	Percentage of pregnant women who are anemic, i.e., having hemoglobin level <110 g/L	Morbidity variable
Incidence of malaria	Number of new cases of malaria in a year per 1000 population	Morbidity variable
Anemia among under-5 children	Percentage of children ages 6–59 months whose hemoglobin level is less than 110 g/L	Morbidity variable
Anemia among women	Percentage of women ages 15–49 years with hemoglobin levels below 12 g/dL	Morbidity variable
Fertility rate	"Total fertility rate is the number of children that would be born to a woman if she were to live to the end of her childbearing years and bear children in accordance with age-specific fertility rates of the specified year"	Explanatory variable
Immunization against tetanus	Percentage of newborn babies given Tetanus	Explanatory variable
Practice of open defecation	Percentage of people practicing open defecation	Explanatory variable
Hand washing facility	Percentage of people with basic handwashing facilities including soap and water	Explanatory variable
Basic sanitation practice	Percentage of people using basic sanitation facilities which include "flush/pour flush to piped sewer systems, septic tanks or pit latrines; ventilated improved pit latrines, compositing toilets or pit latrines with slabs" and are not shared with other households	Explanatory variable
Number of physicians	Number of physicians per 1000 population	Explanatory variable
Immunization for DPT	Percentage of children ages 12–23 months immunized for DPT	Explanatory variable
Safe drinking water	Percentage of people who use safe drinking water	Explanatory variable

Source: World Bank

where Y_{ikt} is the value of the ith dependent variable of the kth country in the year t, X_{mkt} is the value of the mth explanatory variable of the kth country in the year t, D_{jt} represents the dummy variable for the tth year, and D_k is the dummy for the kth country.

Table 13.2 Mean values over the years 2000–2020 of different morbidity status across countries

Countries→ Variables↓	AFG	BGD	BTN	IND	LKA	MDV	NPL	PAK
Undernutrition	28.89	14.21	10.43	16.55	11.74	17.90	12.19	15.61
Incidence of tuberculosis	188.76	221.00	189.00	269.67	65.43	42.00	315.33	272.38
Prevalence of stunting	46.57	41.97	33.36	42.97	17.40	21.05	43.05	42.37
Anemia among pregnant women	39.71	44.63	42.46	51.85	34.27	48.18	45.83	46.86
Incidence of malaria	31.14	4.35	3.25	14.01	3.69	0.00	3.52	5.33
Prevalence of anemia children	45.23	47.53	73.47	60.22	27.27	36.52	49.60	57.88
Prevalence of anemia women	37.80	35.89	41.15	53.50	35.10	47.02	38.18	41.81

13.3 Results

Table 13.2 shows the mean values over the years 2000–2020 of different morbidity variables across countries.

The first thing to be noted from this table is that Sri Lanka has the minimum value in four (prevalence of stunting, anemia among pregnant women, prevalence of anemia among children, and prevalence of anemic women) out of seven cases. Afghanistan tops with maximum value in three cases (undernutrition, stunting, and malaria). India takes the mid position except in the case of prevalence of anemia among women. Bangladesh and Pakistan are the only two countries neither positioned at the top nor at the bottom. Maldives is the only country that is free of Malaria. The incidence of tuberculosis is also the lowest in that country. Note that the average rates are much higher compared with developed countries.

The ANOVA table corresponding to these mean values is shown in Table 13.3. As ANOVA tests show significant F-ratios for all the morbidity variables, we can conclude that there are considerable variations across countries for all the variables, which confirms that the panel data analysis for these data is a must.

Mean morbidity rates can also be computed for each year aggregating countries. The same is given in Table 13.4.

The rates are decreasing on average except for extent of anemia among women. Incidence of stunting, prevalence of anemia among pregnant women, and prevalence of anemia among children decreased but not much. There is no considerable variation in the morbidity rates across time. The ANOVA, thus, shows a mixed picture (Table 13.5).

There have been significant variations in the mean values over time with respect to prevalence of undernutrition in the population and stunting among under-5 children only. Other morbidity statuses do not vary much over time. So far as incidence of tuberculosis and prevalence of anemia among women are concerned, the values varied little compared between countries. However, the analysis of variation does not show how the mean values moved over time. This only shows that the panel data

Table 13.3 Results of ANOVA of different morbidity status across countries

Variable		Sum of squares	df	Mean square	*F*	Sig.
ANOVA among countries						
Undernutrition	Between countries	4977.08	7	711.01	26.66	0.000
	Within countries	4267.74	160	26.67		
	Total	9244.82	167			
Incidence of tuberculosis	Between countries	1,406,792.28	7	200,970.32	265.07	0.000
	Within countries	121,307.24	160	758.17		
	Total	1,528,099.52	167			
Prevalence of stunting	Between countries	18,108.38	7	2586.91	64.19	0.000
	Within countries	6447.86	160	40.30		
	Total	24,556.24	167			
Anemia among pregnant women	Between countries	4325.34	7	617.90	153.76	0.000
	Within countries	642.99	160	4.02		
	Total	4968.33	167			
Incidence of malaria	Between countries	15,052.35	7	2150.33	18.68	0.000
	Within countries	18,417.49	160	115.11		
	Total	33,469.835	167			
Prevalence of anemia among children	Between countries	29,820.245	7	4260.03	4.61	0.000
	Within countries	146,668.49	159	922.44		
	Total	176,488.74	166			
Prevalence of anemia among women	Between countries	5664.19	7	809.17	188.62	0.000
	Within countries	682.10	159	4.29		
	Total	6346.29	166			

model should incorporate country as well as time in both the fixed effect and random effect models. However, the R-package does not have any in-built statement for random effect over time.

The mean values show that the values of the variables decrease over time which is expected. However, to get a clear picture, we must draw the line diagram as shown in Fig. 13.1.

Figure 13.1 clearly shows that incidence of tuberculosis decreases fast registering the maximum negative slope. However, it does not guarantee that it will have a maximum negative growth rate. One can ascertain the significance of the growth rate by regressing each variable on time (Year) taking the usual growth curve. In fact, one of the main uses of taking mean values for each year aggregating over countries is that we can find the overall growth rate for each variable. The outcomes for the same are displayed in Table 13.6. For completeness of results, growth rates of explanatory variables are also given along with other growth rates.

All the growth rates are significant except prevalence of anemia among women. As expected, all the morbidity rates have negative growth rates, and the maximum negative growth rate is for incidence of malaria. This shows that the SAARC has improved a lot in controlling malaria. However, the journey is on till the incidence of malaria becomes zero. Maldives has long back achieved it. Among the explanatory variables, the rate of open defecation has also decreased a lot. The

Table 13.4 Mean values of morbidity rates in the SAARC region

Year	Under-nourishment	Incidence of tuberculosis	Prevalence of stunting	Anemia among pregnant	Incidence of malaria	Prevalence of anemia among children	Prevalence of anemia among women
2000	23.51	224.13	44.19	47.26	23.62	55.75	42.98
2001	23.01	219.13	43.61	46.85	19.53	54.34	42.51
2002	22.29	217.13	43.08	46.49	18.99	53.08	42.14
2003	21.28	213.88	42.46	46.18	15.41	51.95	41.86
2004	20.09	209.50	41.79	45.85	10.31	50.91	41.63
2005	18.95	207.63	41.14	45.54	8.93	49.98	41.43
2006	17.71	201.88	40.40	45.21	7.16	49.08	41.23
2007	16.50	202.38	39.53	44.89	7.48	48.24	41.05
2008	15.20	198.75	38.53	44.53	6.78	47.44	40.85
2009	14.75	199.00	37.43	44.21	5.88	46.73	40.66
2010	14.45	200.38	36.28	43.90	5.95	46.10	40.53
2011	14.28	195.88	35.15	43.68	5.90	45.51	40.50
2012	13.99	191.75	34.06	43.43	4.19	45.01	40.49
2013	13.43	187.75	33.06	43.19	3.83	44.58	40.50
2014	12.83	185.13	32.15	42.98	3.91	44.21	40.63
2015	12.33	181.75	31.31	42.80	3.98	43.94	40.78
2016	11.95	182.75	30.46	42.65	5.56	43.71	40.98
2017	11.55	173.50	29.59	42.53	5.32	43.54	41.23
2018	11.58	171.50	28.75	42.35	4.00	43.40	41.54
2019	12.19	172.13	27.89	42.18	2.83	43.33	41.84
2020	12.88	168.50	27.06	42.05	1.82	43.30	43.10
Overall	15.94	195.45	36.09	44.22	8.16	49.85	41.34

Table 13.5 ANOVA of morbidity rates over time

Morbidities		Sum of squares	df	Mean square	*F*	Sig.
Prevalence of undernutrition	Between years	2587.05	20	129.35	2.856	0.000
	Within years	6657.77	147	45.29		
	Total	9244.82	167			
Incidence of tuberculosis	Between years	44,233.39	20	2211.67	0.219	1.000
	Within years	1,483,866.12	147	10,094.33		
	Total	1,528,099.52	167			
Prevalence of stunting	Between years	5093.82	20	254.69	1.924	0.015
	Within years	19,462.42	147	132.40		
	Total	24,556.24	167			
Anemia among pregnant women	Between years	435.54	20	21.78	0.706	0.815
	Within years	4532.79	147	30.83		
	Total	4968.33	167			
Incidence of malaria	Between years	5861.46	20	293.07	1.560	0.070
	Within years	27,608.38	147	187.81		
	Total	33,469.83	167			
Prevalence of anemia among children	Between years	22,759.10	20	1137.95	1.081	0.376
	Within years	153,729.64	146	1052.94		
	Total	176,488.74	166			
Prevalence of anemia among women	Between years	100.94	20	5.05	0.118	1.000
	Within years	6245.35	146	42.78		
	Total	6346.29	166			

explanatory variables, namely, percentage of children protected through tetanus injection, percentage of people observing basic sanitation facilities, number of physicians, and rate of immunization of children through DPT have naturally increased. The line diagrams of the explanatory variables may throw some light and thus are given in Fig. 13.2.

As the line diagrams show, the SAARC countries are improving at a steady pace. The incidence of open defecation shows a steady downward trend. The fertility rate is possibly decreasing. All other variables are increasing. All the trends are in favorable directions.

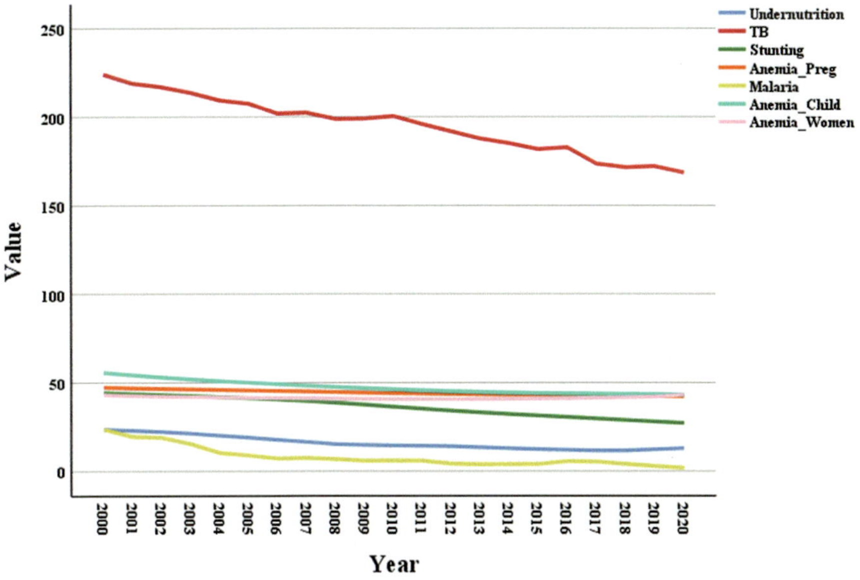

Fig. 13.1 Line diagrams of morbidity rates: years 2000–2020

Table 13.6 Growth rates of morbidity rates and explanatory variables

Name of the variable	Growth rate	R square	Sig.
Undernutrition	–0.037	0.920	<0.001
TB	–0.014	0.979	<0.001
Stunting	–0.026	0.987	<0.001
Anemia of pregnant women	–0.006	0.982	<0.001
Malaria	–0.099	0.861	<0.001
Anemia child	–0.013	0.936	<0.001
Anemia women	–0.001	0.069	0.250
Fertility rate	–0.024	0.994	<0.001
Tetanus	0.004	0.401	0.002
Open defecation	–0.082	0.967	<0.001
Basic sanitation	0.034	0.993	<0.001
Physicians	0.041	0.974	<0.001
DPT	0.010	0.920	<0.001

Let us take this opportunity to compute the correlation coefficient of yearly mean data as given in Tables 13.7 and 13.8.

All the pairs of variables in Table 13.7 are positively correlated excepting the prevalence of anemia among the under-5 children. However, the striking feature is that prevalence of undernutrition, stunting among under-5 children, anemia among pregnant women, and incidence of Malaria form a group with a strong correlation (more than 0.8) with each other. However, prevalence of anemia among under-5 children and prevalence of anemia among women have comparatively low

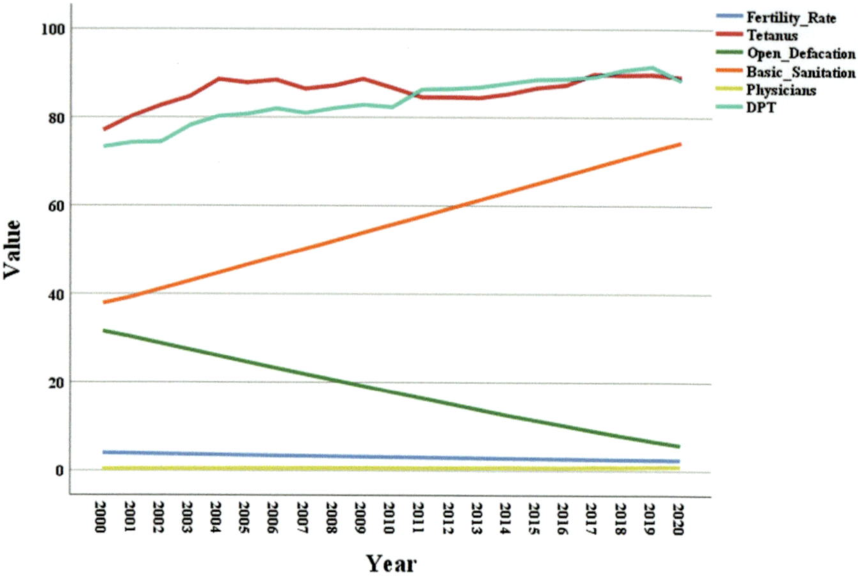

Fig. 13.2 Line diagrams of explanatory variables: years 2000–2020

Table 13.7 Correlation coefficients between pair of mean morbidity values of Table 13.4

	TB	Stunting	Anemia_preg	Malaria	Anemia_child	Anemia_women
Undernutrition	0.932**	0.929**	0.978**	0.929**	0.131	0.543*
TB		0.984**	0.975**	0.857**	−0.085	0.237
Stunting			0.982**	0.820**	−0.081	0.233
Anemia_preg				0.904**	0.001	0.395
Malaria					0.050	0.584**
Anemia_child						0.671**

Note: ***, ** and * indicate that the coefficient is significant at .001, .01 and .05 level of significance by two-tailed test

correlations with these four variables, but a reasonably high correlation (0.67) between them. Thus, anemia among pregnant women has a special status in the sense that it has a very high correlation with the other three in the group and a low correlation with the other two anemia groups.

All the explanatory variables in Table 13.8 have a very high correlation among themselves, except Child immunization by Tetanus which is also reasonably high. Observe that Tetanus, Basic Sanitation, and Physician are expected to improve the morbidity rates by lowering these values, whereas Open Defecation has just the opposite effect. Thus, Open Defecation is likely to have a negative correlation with Tetanus, Basic Sanitation, and Physician, which is reflected by the sample correlation values. The role of Fertility Rate is not clear. However, looking at the values of the correlations with other variables, it becomes clear that Fertility Rate should be

Table 13.8 Correlation coefficients between pair of mean morbidity values of Table 13.10

	Tetanus	Open defecation	Basic sanitation	Physicians	DPT
Fertility_rate	−0.664**	0.999**	−0.996**	−0.977**	−0.975**
Tetanus		−0.637**	0.629**	0.636**	0.689**
Open_ defecation			−0.999**	−0.980**	−0.970**
Basic_sanitation				0.984**	0.962**
Physicians					0.929**

Note: ***, ** and * indicate that the coefficient is significant at .001, .01 and .05 level of significance by two-tailed test

Table 13.9 Correlation coefficients between pair of mean morbidity values of Table 13.4

	TB	Stunting	Anemia among pregnant	Malaria	Anemia among children	Anemia among women
Undernutrition	−0.070	0.366	−0.010	0.863**	−0.193	0.083
TB		0.877**	0.458	0.184	0.626	0.090
Stunting			0.395	0.545	0.552	0.056
Anemia among pregnant women				−0.142	0.459	0.793*
Malaria					0.035	0.014
Anemia among children						0.352

Note: ***, ** and * indicate that the coefficient is significant at .001, .01 and .05 level of significance by two-tailed test

grouped with Open Defecation. But the problem with high correlations among the explanatory variables regardless of whether positive or negative is that it may lead to multicollinearity problems as these variables are used as regressors.

Recall Table 13.2 in this chapter where the mean values of the variables were computed for each country. Thus, taking country as a unit, we can compute the correlation coefficients between a pair of variables (given in Table 13.9) which will obviously be different from the correlation coefficient computed in Table 13.7.

Now the numerical values of the correlation coefficient are much less. The pattern over time was similar, but the pattern over countries is not so. We have, however, some high values—malaria with undernutrition, stunting with TB, and anemia among pregnant women with anemia among all women. What it says is that the pair of values has the same relation over countries. In the earlier case, it says that the pair of values has the same relation over time.

For ready reference, we produce the mean values of the explanatory variable for each year aggregating over SAARC countries in Table 13.10.

Let us summarize what we have got so far. Though the status of health in SAARC countries does not show a comparatively healthy picture, the trends of the morbidity rates and the proposed associated explanatory variables show an encouraging picture. Morbidity patterns are steadily decreasing over time and the explanatory variables have the right kind of trend to improve the situation.

Table 13.10 Mean values of the explanatory variables in the SAARC region

Year	Fertility rate	Protected against tetanus	Open defecation	Basic sanitation services	Physicians	Immunization DPT
2000	3.9512	77.0000	31.5388	37.8700	0.3875	73.2500
2001	3.8488	80.2500	30.2613	39.2725	0.3950	74.2500
2002	3.7513	82.7500	28.8288	41.0863	0.4200	74.3750
2003	3.6525	84.7500	27.4113	42.9025	0.4350	78.1250
2004	3.5663	88.6250	26.0013	44.7213	0.4513	80.2500
2005	3.4725	87.8750	24.5975	46.5512	0.5050	80.7500
2006	3.3788	88.5000	23.2150	48.3663	0.5375	82.0000
2007	3.3138	86.5000	21.8488	50.1813	0.5750	81.0000
2008	3.2413	87.2500	20.4912	52.0188	0.5888	82.1250
2009	3.1600	88.7500	19.1438	53.8662	0.5912	82.8750
2010	3.0837	86.7500	17.8025	55.7200	0.6050	82.3750
2011	3.0138	84.6250	16.4700	57.5775	0.6200	86.3750
2012	2.9512	84.6250	15.1475	59.4438	0.6525	86.5000
2013	2.8900	84.5000	13.8325	61.3125	0.6850	86.8750
2014	2.8175	85.3750	12.5350	63.1888	0.7338	87.7500
2015	2.7500	86.7500	11.3525	65.0613	0.7050	88.6250
2016	2.6850	87.3750	10.1750	66.9288	0.7038	88.7500
2017	2.6100	89.8750	8.9975	68.7913	0.7963	89.2500
2018	2.5488	89.6250	7.8413	70.6438	0.8063	90.7500
2019	2.4913	89.7500	6.7425	72.5000	0.8825	91.5000
2020	2.4450	89.1250	5.7487	74.3225	0.9350	88.3750
Total	3.1249	86.2202	18.0944	55.8251	0.6196	83.6250

We have so far discussed the features of the mean values of the morbidity rates and the explanatory variables. We can, however, compute the correlation coefficients by taking unaggregated data also. However, here we shall compute the correlation table for each morbidity rate with the explanatory variables for each year taking country data as units. We produce these correlation tables in the Appendix and give the summary findings below.

Undernutrition is positively related to fertility rate and inversely related to immunization of children and tetanus of newborns (Table 13.13). It indicates that the country with a high fertility rate has a low nutritional level, while those having better immunization register improved nutrition. The incidence of Tuberculosis has a significant positive correlation with open defecation and a negative correlation with basic sanitation services (Table 13.14). Similarly, basic sanitation facilities and immunization are inversely related to stunted growth of children (Table 13.15). Anemia among pregnant women and anemia among working-aged women is also related to these variables but not significantly (Tables 13.16 and 13.19). Incidence of malaria has a significant positive correlation with fertility rate but a negative correlation with the immunization of DPT or tetanus of children (Table 13.17). A similar relation is also observed in the case of anemia among children (Table 13.18).

13.4 Panel Data Regression

The bivariate correlation analysis from Tables 13.13, 13.14, 13.15, 13.16, 13.17, 13.18, and 13.19 helps us to identify variables that can be included in the panel data regression of different health indicators. The results of ***random effect model*** of six health indicators on six morbidity variables are presented in Table 13.11.

It shows significant negative impacts of DPT immunization of children on all the morbidity rates except anemia among women. However, this is not significant. Tetanus protection of newborn babies also has a significant negative relation with undernutrition and incidence of malaria, and for other morbidity variables, no significant relation is found. Fertility rate has a significant positive impact on undernutrition and prevalence of anemia among pregnant women but a negative relation on anemia of children. How a higher fertility rate reduces anemia of children is not clear. Surprisingly, basic sanitation facilities are seen to increase undernutrition. However, it has the right sign with the other morbidity status whenever significant. The habit of open defecation is also significantly positively related to undernutrition but behaves properly with other morbidity variables.

The Hausman test (Chi Sq.) presented in the last row of Table 13.11 reveals that, except in the case of anemia, all other models are fit for the application of ***fixed effects model***. For anemia, any of the two models can be taken. Therefore, the fixed effect model has been applied to all the six variables and the results are presented in Table 13.12. Here, we introduce both year-wise time dummy and country dummy.

However, the overall impacts of fertility, immunization, lifestyle as reflected in open defecation, use of basic sanitation facilities, and safe drinking water on various health indicators remain more or less the same. The results of fixed effect model are like those of random effect model except in a few cases. First, contrary to the random effect model, open defecation is seen to have a negative relation with anemia of women in the fixed effect model which is compatible. Second, basic sanitation did not show any significant impact on anemia of women in the random effect model; here, it shows a significant impact with the right (negative) sign. Third, though the number of physicians shows the same negative sign with stunting in both cases, in fixed effect model, it is significant. Fourth, the effect of number of physicians on anemia of pregnant women was positive and significant in the random effect model; here, in the fixed effect model, it shows the right negative sign but is not significant. Finally, the effect of immunization through DPT on anemia of pregnant women is negative in both cases but significant in the random effect model. In short, except in the last case, the fixed effect model gives the right sign and/or significance in all other four cases clearly manifesting the superiority of the fixed effect model. Observe that, in the fixed effect model, we took intercept dummies for countries as well as time panel.

Table 13.11 Random effect model of different health indicators on healthcare variables

	Under-nourishment	Stunting	Malaria	Anemia pregnant	Anemia children	Anemia women
	Estimate	Estimate	Estimate	Estimate	Estimate	Estimate
Fertility rate	6.263***	0.8652	3.6064	2.301***	−13.648**	−1.0886
Newborns' tetanus	−0.0971***	0.0275	−0.4140***	0.0026	0.0902	−0.0305
Open defecation	0.3359***	−0.0397	−0.4949***	−0.0560*	−0.1356	0.1461**
Basic sanitation	0.4393***	−0.4731***	−0.2503	−0.1057***	−0.1318	0.0139
Physicians	−13.616***	−0.6722	3.232	1.0305**	−9.805	0.1992
Immunization DPT	−0.1355**	−0.0173	−0.7124***	−0.0013**	−1.089**	0.0445
Constant	−6.100	6.855	113.09	43.193***	191.55***	40.071***
R-squared						
Within	0.7243	0.8084	0.5909	0.8352	0.0292	0.1726
Between	0.4409	0.9548	0.6458	0.0038	0.4140	0.2593
Overall	0.4498	0.9142	0.5078	0.0066	0.0939	0.2498
Wald chi^2 (6)	373.42***	1095.67***	203.50***	729.27***	7.75	33.65***
Hausman Chi^2	24.57***	110.80***	17.97***	28.10***	7.51	61.72***

Note: ***, **, and * indicate that the coefficient is significant at 0.001, 0.01, and 0.05 levels of significance, respectively

Table 13.12 Fixed effect model of health status variables on various healthcare variables

	Under-nourishment	Stunting	Malaria	Anemia pregnant	Anemia children	Anemia women
	Estimate	Estimate	Estimate	Estimate	Estimate	Estimate
Fertility rate	7.592***	0.856	2.887	1.680***	−15.129	−2.979**
Newborns tetanus	−0.122**	0.031	−0.405***	−0.0003	0.160	−0.023
Open defecation	0.626**	−0.981***	−1.214*	−0.346***	0.876	−0.349*
Basic sanitation	0.860**	−1.454***	−1.016	−0.493***	0.512	−0.650***
Physicians	−13.474***	−9.621***	2.803	−1.207	−10.809	−2.764
Immunization DPT	−0.114*	−0.057	−0.775***	−0.019	−0.639	0.022
Factor (year) 2000	−38.782*	106.604***	145.267**	51.778***	140.629	83.257***
Factor (year) 2001	−38.297*	106.933***	143.419**	51.817***	138.269	83.031***
Factor (year) 2002	−38.287*	107.882***	144.299**	52.050***	135.809	83.170***
Factor (year) 2003	−38.349*	108.902***	144.808**	52.401***	135.744	83.294***
Factor (year) 2004	−38.628*	109.721***	143.275**	52.692***	134.622	83.579***
Factor (year) 2005	−39.057*	111.004***	142.251**	53.029***	133.580	83.920***
Factor (year) 2006	−39.620*	111.994***	142.044**	53.342***	132.595	84.216***
Factor (year) 2007	−40.896*	112.839***	141.047**	53.573***	131.128	84.629***
Factor (year) 2008	−41.970*	113.415***	141.917**	53.808***	130.229	84.965***
Factor (year) 2009	−42.245*	113.770***	142.680**	54.095***	128.790	85.293***
Factor (year) 2010	−42.835*	114.230***	141.986**	54.367***	127.386	85.667***
Factor (year) 2011	−42.841*	114.997***	144.607**	54.810***	129.016	86.080***
Factor (year) 2012	−42.978*	115.699***	143.375**	55.170***	128.206	86.721***
Factor (year) 2013	−43.392*	116.516***	143.640**	55.548***	127.649	87.386***
Factor (year) 2014	−43.378*	117.613***	145.153**	56.010***	127.313	88.198***
Factor (year) 2015	−44.354*	118.128***	147.209**	56.446***	126.124	88.886***
Factor (year) 2016	−45.030*	118.870***	149.801**	56.919***	124.958	89.702***
Factor (year) 2017	−44.115*	120.454***	151.382**	57.553***	124.648	90.834***

(continued)

Table 13.12 (continued)

	Under-nourishment	Stunting	Malaria	Anemia pregnant	Anemia children	Anemia women
	Estimate	Estimate	Estimate	Estimate	Estimate	Estimate
Factor (year) 2018	−44.218*	121.417***	151.747**	58.036***	124.756	91.754***
Factor (year) 2019	−42.948*	122.998***	151.719**	58.600***	125.108	92.904***
Factor (year) 2020	−42.572	124.233***	148.656*	59.109***	172.665	94.028***
Factor_ Bangladesh	24.933***	−2.100	12.013	10.625***	−25.240	−13.254***
Factor_ Bhutan	2.919	16.965***	28.173*	18.185***	−9.947	4.151
Factor_India	0.798	39.782***	50.764**	31.439***	−52.346	20.193***
Factor_ Maldives	7.577	53.761***	54.300	38.364***	−48.544	29.670***
Factor_Nepal	−2.457	33.694***	39.934**	23.459***	−52.221	2.576
Factor_ Pakistan	−4.464	27.118***	6.249	19.297***	−16.587	10.597***
Factor_ SriLanka	−5.643	36.615***	53.906*	21.407***	−62.162	13.021*

Note: ***, **, and * indicate that the coefficient is significant at 0.001, 0.01, and 0.05 levels of significance, respectively

13.5 Conclusion

The findings of the analysis reveal significant regional variation in different morbidity rates which, however, have decreased over the years but at different rates. The countries that are deficient in basic sanitation, have less drinking water facilities, and have a habit of open defecation suffer from various diseases more intensively. Furthermore, immunization of DPT and tetanus in children provides protection against different morbidities and enhances life expectancy. Thus, livelihood pattern, immunization of pregnant women, adequate number of physicians, and so on would provide the necessary impetus for the healthy life of citizens including women and children. The laggard nations like Afghanistan should give more emphasis to these healthcare measures to address the health issues in their own countries (Tables 13.13, 13.14, 13.15, 13.16, 13.17, 13.18, and 13.19).

Appendix

Table 13.13 Bivariate correlation with undernutrition

Year	Fertility rate	Protected against tetanus	Open defecation	Basic sanitation services	Physicians	Immunization DPT
2000	0.762*	−0.799*	0.021	−0.149	0.008	−0.669
2001	0.739*	−0.745*	0.056	−0.153	0.060	−0.620
2002	0.776*	−0.800*	0.111	−0.206	0.064	−0.658
2003	0.748*	−0.715*	0.158	−0.202	0.116	−0.703
2004	0.731*	0.488	0.176	−0.216	0.070	−0.704
2005	0.766*	0.631	0.211	−0.292	0.035	−0.629
2006	0.791*	0.510	0.199	−0.311	0.007	−0.621
2007	0.802*	−0.113	0.162	−0.316	0.043	−0.493
2008	0.803*	−0.273	0.177	−0.314	0.082	−0.533
2009	0.763*	0.164	0.097	−0.279	0.154	−0.527
2010	0.714*	−0.112	−0.001	−0.239	0.121	−0.392
2011	0.645	−0.418	−0.094	−0.221	0.076	−0.498
2012	0.742*	−0.540	−0.059	−0.339	−0.079	−0.585
2013	0.738*	−0.438	−0.013	−0.430	−0.151	−0.630
2014	0.737*	−0.345	0.056	−0.459	−0.120	−0.682
2015	0.730*	−0.390	0.070	−0.524	−0.289	−0.645
2016	0.730*	−0.424	0.069	−0.528	−0.404	−0.583
2017	0.749*	−0.650	0.102	−0.568	−0.392	−0.650
2018	0.779*	−0.719*	0.183	−0.583	−0.360	−0.694
2019	0.829*	−0.797*	0.336	−0.615	−0.371	−0.853**
2020	0.857**	−0.846**	0.482	−0.660	−0.407	−0.747*
	0.748**	−0.526**	0.303**	−0.467**	−0.244**	−0.656**

Note: ***, ** and * indicate that the coefficient is significant at .001, .01 and .05 level of significance by two-tailed test

Table 13.14 Bivariate correlation with incidence of tuberculosis

Year	Fertility rate	Protected against tetanus	Open defecation	Basic sanitation services	Physicians	Immunization DPT
2000	0.248	−0.293	0.818*	−0.860**	−0.521	−0.379
2001	0.247	−0.317	0.848**	−0.867**	−0.499	−0.479
2002	0.239	−0.119	0.837**	−0.868**	−0.520	−0.515
2003	0.238	−0.142	0.853**	−0.872**	−0.468	−0.484
2004	0.243	−0.480	0.854**	−0.877**	−0.444	−0.484
2005	0.231	−0.419	0.849**	−0.875**	−0.464	−0.653
2006	0.228	−0.574	0.851**	−0.879**	−0.482	−0.511
2007	0.205	−0.691	0.836**	−0.872**	−0.514	−0.620
2008	0.204	−0.831*	0.831*	−0.871**	−0.515	−0.609
2009	0.187	−0.874**	0.784*	−0.860**	−0.589	−0.491
2010	0.167	−0.467	0.730*	−0.834**	−0.627	−0.554
2011	0.187	−0.411	0.735*	−0.841**	−0.628	−0.445
2012	0.216	−0.432	0.744*	−0.847**	−0.594	−0.538

(continued)

Table 13.14 (continued)

Year	Fertility rate	Protected against tetanus	Open defecation	Basic sanitation services	Physicians	Immunization DPT
2013	0.246	−0.508	0.737*	−0.847**	−0.605	−0.496
2014	0.258	−0.547	0.732*	−0.845**	−0.623	−0.455
2015	0.296	−0.604	0.732*	−0.840**	−0.529	−0.483
2016	0.293	−0.570	0.658	−0.823*	−0.513	−0.501
2017	0.360	−0.462	0.681	−0.829*	−0.486	−0.523
2018	0.381	−0.450	0.638	−0.822*	−0.599	−0.539
2019	0.370	−0.462	0.586	−0.811*	−0.617	−0.441
2020	0.361	−0.401	0.558	−0.795*	−0.649	−0.542
	0.285**	−0.402**	0.761**	−0.815**	−0.539**	−0.523**

Note: ***, ** and * indicate that the coefficient is significant at .001, .01 and .05 level of significance by two-tailed test

Table 13.15 Bivariate correlation with prevalence of stunting

Year	Fertility rate	Protected against tetanus	Open defecation	Basic sanitation services	Physicians	Immunization DPT
2000	0.517	−0.523	0.538	−0.902**	−0.537	−0.595
2001	0.541	−0.565	0.553	−0.922**	−0.543	−0.653
2002	0.555	−0.465	0.567	−0.937**	−0.560	−0.715*
2003	0.570	−0.499	0.580	−0.951**	−0.565	−0.688
2004	0.585	−0.155	0.595	−0.964**	−0.585	−0.612
2005	0.585	−0.012	0.608	−0.973**	−0.546	−0.727*
2006	0.573	−0.203	0.619	−0.980**	−0.552	−0.640
2007	0.564	−0.641	0.629	−0.984**	−0.579	−0.687
2008	0.555	−0.804*	0.641	−0.985**	−0.617	−0.686
2009	0.548	−0.678	0.653	−0.983**	−0.635	−0.647
2010	0.546	−0.540	0.663	−0.980**	−0.634	−0.715*
2011	0.542	−0.679	0.673	−0.975**	−0.626	−0.679
2012	0.546	−0.682	0.684	−0.968**	−0.618	−0.755*
2013	0.556	−0.696	0.694	−0.961**	−0.618	−0.728*
2014	0.564	−0.693	0.706	−0.951**	−0.632	−0.716*
2015	0.583	−0.758*	0.710*	−0.940**	−0.596	−0.723*
2016	0.603	−0.744*	0.713*	−0.927**	−0.559	−0.753*
2017	0.612	−0.695	0.721*	−0.912**	−0.570	−0.744*
2018	0.629	−0.686	0.730*	−0.895**	−0.640	−0.767*
2019	0.636	−0.701	0.743*	−0.877**	−0.639	−0.720*
2020	0.644	−0.675	0.769*	−0.853**	−0.676	−0.797*
	0.623**	−0.536**	0.687**	−0.957**	−0.634**	−0.714**

Note: ***, ** and * indicate that the coefficient is significant at .001, .01 and .05 level of significance by two-tailed test

Table 13.16 Bivariate correlation with anemia among pregnant women

Year	Fertility rate	Protected against tetanus	Open defecation	Basic sanitation services	Physicians	Immunization DPT
2000	0.057	0.017	0.716*	−0.560	0.157	−0.205
2001	0.024	−0.004	0.705	−0.548	0.143	−0.254
2002	0.005	0.165	0.693	−0.543	0.148	−0.282
2003	−0.015	0.099	0.683	−0.531	0.169	−0.276
2004	−0.035	−0.368	0.670	−0.516	0.171	−0.286
2005	−0.061	−0.202	0.658	−0.495	0.234	−0.387
2006	−0.090	−0.368	0.645	−0.474	0.250	−0.330
2007	−0.098	−0.253	0.633	−0.448	0.246	−0.411
2008	−0.104	−0.307	0.623	−0.419	0.245	−0.358
2009	−0.103	−0.398	0.606	−0.387	0.233	−0.275
2010	−0.120	0.255	0.590	−0.347	0.245	−0.303
2011	−0.144	0.060	0.568	−0.302	0.281	−0.234
2012	−0.167	0.086	0.542	−0.247	0.329	−0.194
2013	−0.194	0.100	0.517	−0.193	0.348	−0.108
2014	−0.215	0.078	0.479	−0.130	0.386	−0.026
2015	−0.231	0.112	0.457	−0.068	0.414	0.022
2016	−0.241	0.189	0.435	−0.007	0.434	0.058
2017	−0.253	0.232	0.420	0.051	0.499	0.095
2018	−0.259	0.269	0.391	0.112	0.483	0.117
2019	−0.270	0.276	0.371	0.164	0.500	0.166
2020	−0.292	0.317	0.342	0.214	0.497	0.149
	−0.014	−0.004	0.609**	−0.392**	0.183*	−0.262**

Note: ***, ** and * indicate that the coefficient is significant at .001, .01 and .05 level of significance by two-tailed test

Table 13.17 Bivariate correlation with incidence of malaria

Year	Fertility rate	Protected against tetanus	Open defecation	Basic sanitation services	Physicians	Immunization DPT
2000	0.590	−0.685	−0.189	−0.042	−0.285	−0.584
2001	0.824*	−0.869**	−0.004	−0.335	−0.322	−0.768*
2002	0.854**	−0.946**	0.047	−0.399	−0.410	−0.786*
2003	0.873**	−0.912**	0.143	−0.485	−0.418	−0.828*
2004	0.800*	0.293	0.289	−0.581	−0.427	−0.827*
2005	0.712*	0.336	0.453	−0.661	−0.374	−0.759*
2006	0.698	0.150	0.518	−0.685	−0.392	−0.785*
2007	0.697	−0.283	0.494	−0.739*	−0.423	−0.658
2008	0.625	−0.421	0.529	−0.719*	−0.412	−0.590
2009	0.478	−0.342	0.668	−0.691	−0.345	−0.592
2010	0.554	−0.454	0.713*	−0.701	−0.311	−0.607

(continued)

Table 13.17 (continued)

Year	Fertility rate	Protected against tetanus	Open defecation	Basic sanitation services	Physicians	Immunization DPT
2011	0.743*	−0.743*	0.602	−0.693	−0.305	−0.820*
2012	0.633	−0.649	0.696	−0.642	−0.242	−0.835**
2013	0.803*	−0.730*	0.592	−0.670	−0.319	−0.888**
2014	0.761*	−0.583	0.511	−0.710*	−0.412	−0.818*
2015	0.794*	−0.685	0.532	−0.667	−0.434	−0.825*
2016	0.875**	−0.768*	0.385	−0.604	−0.524	−0.822*
2017	0.878**	−0.864**	0.335	−0.598	−0.478	−0.825*
2018	0.887**	−0.892**	0.376	−0.592	−0.467	−0.847**
2019	0.887**	−0.893**	0.458	−0.639	−0.486	−0.922**
2020	0.891**	−0.919**	0.585	−0.638	−0.499	−0.853**
	0.680**	−0.636**	0.300**	−0.495**	−0.353**	−0.696**

Note: ***, ** and * indicate that the coefficient is significant at .001, .01 and .05 level of significance by two-tailed test

Table 13.18 Bivariate correlation with prevalence of anemia among children

Year	Fertility rate	Protected against tetanus	Open defecation	Basic sanitation services	Physicians	Immunization DPT
2000	0.213	−0.130	0.602	−0.741*	−0.286	−0.325
2001	0.184	−0.177	0.596	−0.732*	−0.308	−0.389
2002	0.165	−0.028	0.591	−0.722*	−0.346	−0.428
2003	0.150	−0.137	0.586	−0.711*	−0.335	−0.365
2004	0.157	−0.661	0.583	−0.705	−0.337	−0.418
2005	0.157	−0.537	0.585	−0.699	−0.342	−0.507
2006	0.146	−0.684	0.587	−0.695	−0.362	−0.497
2007	0.155	−0.717*	0.593	−0.693	−0.394	−0.590
2008	0.167	−0.644	0.601	−0.694	−0.391	−0.575
2009	0.182	−0.677	0.610	−0.690	−0.400	−0.568
2010	0.197	−0.207	0.620	−0.688	−0.394	−0.623
2011	0.208	−0.359	0.629	−0.682	−0.373	−0.564
2012	0.224	−0.374	0.638	−0.679	−0.357	−0.584
2013	0.241	−0.482	0.648	−0.673	−0.357	−0.547
2014	0.253	−0.543	0.656	−0.665	−0.355	−0.488
2015	0.268	−0.524	0.659	−0.656	−0.325	−0.476
2016	0.284	−0.480	0.663	−0.643	−0.284	−0.488
2017	0.288	−0.467	0.672	−0.632	−0.297	−0.485
2018	0.299	−0.454	0.676	−0.620	−0.348	−0.515
2019	0.300	−0.466	0.684	−0.608	−0.354	−0.465
2020	−0.388	0.075	−0.414	0.132	−0.304	0.302
	0.009	−0.099	0.149	−0.178*	−0.161*	−0.132

Note: ***, ** and * indicate that the coefficient is significant at .001, .01 and .05 level of significance by two-tailed test

Table 13.19 Bivariate correlation with prevalence of anemia among women

Year	Fertility rate	Protected against tetanus	Open defecation	Basic sanitation services	Physicians	Immunization DPT
2000	−0.396	0.385	0.574	−0.044	0.364	0.189
2001	−0.393	0.345	0.569	−0.043	0.366	0.092
2002	−0.384	0.436	0.566	−0.051	0.379	0.051
2003	−0.362	0.336	0.560	−0.060	0.407	−0.009
2004	−0.330	−0.304	0.554	−0.066	0.407	−0.192
2005	−0.301	−0.252	0.543	−0.070	0.394	−0.200
2006	−0.273	−0.377	0.536	−0.073	0.374	−0.262
2007	−0.230	−0.125	0.533	−0.078	0.343	−0.335
2008	−0.185	−0.069	0.525	−0.077	0.346	−0.287
2009	−0.134	−0.205	0.509	−0.064	0.344	−0.273
2010	−0.102	0.231	0.498	−0.051	0.346	−0.214
2011	−0.078	0.058	0.482	−0.032	0.366	−0.262
2012	−0.064	0.049	0.459	0.000	0.388	−0.205
2013	−0.054	0.038	0.429	0.036	0.401	−0.187
2014	−0.045	0.000	0.398	0.069	0.411	−0.150
2015	−0.025	0.037	0.378	0.107	0.402	−0.125
2016	−0.007	0.054	0.364	0.135	0.360	−0.079
2017	−0.001	−0.020	0.357	0.159	0.390	−0.088
2018	0.012	−0.027	0.356	0.178	0.415	−0.097
2019	0.014	−0.041	0.362	0.189	0.402	−0.136
2020	−0.068	0.116	0.261	0.493	0.534	0.071
	−0.149	0.069	0.431**	−0.005	0.347**	−0.126

Note: ***, ** and * indicate that the coefficient is significant at .001, .01 and .05 level of significance by two-tailed test

References

Ali SA, Ali SA, Razzaq S, Tikmani SS, Allana A, Rizvi N, Saleem S (2020) Determinants of under-nutrition among women of reproductive age in Sindh, Pakistan: findings from Pakistan Demographic and Health Survey, 2012-2013. Popul Med 2:26

Bhalotra S (2007) Spending to save? State health expenditure and infant mortality in India. Health Econ 16(9):911–928

Bhandari S, Sayami JT, Thapa P, Sayami M, Kandel BP, Banjara MR (2016) Dietary intake patterns and nutritional status of women of reproductive age in Nepal: findings from a health survey. Arch Public Health 74(1):1–11

Black RE, Allen LH, Bhutta ZA, Caulfield LE, De Onis M, Ezzati M, Maternal and Child Undernutrition Study Group (2008) Maternal and child undernutrition: global and regional exposures and health consequences. Lancet 371(9608):243–260. https://doi.org/10.1016/S0140-6736(07)61690-0

Bokhari FA, Gai Y, Gottret P (2007) Government health expenditures and health outcomes. Health Econ 16(3):257–273

Bradley EH, Elkins BR, Herrin J, Elbel B (2011) Health and social services expenditures: associations with health outcomes. BMJ Qual Saf 20(10):826–831

Chaparro C, Oot L, Sethuraman K (2014) Overview of the nutrition situation in four countries in South and Central Asia. https://www.fantaproject.org/sites/default/files/download/South-and-Central-Asia-Nutrition-Overview-Mar2014.pdf

Gani A (2009) Health care financing and health outcomes in Pacific Island countries. Health Policy Plan 24(1):72–81

Kim TK, Lane SR (2013) Government health expenditure and public health outcomes: a comparative study among 17 countries and implications for US Health care reform. Am Int J Contemp Res 3(9):8–13

Mohapatra S (2022) Health expenditures, health infrastructure and health status in SAARC countries: a panel data analysis. J Decis Makers 47(3):205–216

Nishtar S (2002) Prevention of coronary heart disease in south Asia. Lancet 360:1015–1018

Novignon J, Olakojo SA, Nonvignon J (2012) The effects of public and private health care expenditure on health status in sub-Saharan Africa: new evidence from panel data analysis. Heal Econ Rev 2(1):22

Osmani S, Bhargava A (1998) Health and nutrition in emerging Asia. Asian Dev Rev 16(1):31–71

Poullier JP, Hernandez P, Kawabata K, Savedoff WD (2002) Patterns of global health expenditures: results for 191 countries. World Health Organization, Geneva

Romer PM (1994) The origins of endogenous growth. J Econ Perspect 8(1):3–22

Somi MF, Butler JR, Vahid F, Njau JD, Abdulla S (2009) Household responses to health risks and shocks: a study from rural Tanzania raises some methodological issues. J Int Dev 21(2):200–211

Suri S, Ashok S (2022) The role of women's nutrition literacy in food security in South Asia. ORF Issue Brief No. 601, December 2022, Observer Research Foundation

Verhoeven M, Gupta MS, Tiongson ME (1999) Does higher government spending buy better results in education and health care? International Monetary Fund, Washington

Waghmare H, Mondal NA, Prasad RD (2022) Determinants of nutritional status among women in South Asian countries: a cross-sectional study. Demogr India 51(2):100–110

Integrative Bioinformatics Analysis for Investigating Potential Genes of Prostate Cancer

14

Md. Amanat Ullah Arman, Muhammad Habibulla Alamin, Md. Selim Reza, Tasnia Akter Maya, and Md. Tofazzal Hossain

Abbreviations

BPH	Benign prostatic hyperplasia
cDEGs	Common differentially expressed genes
DEGs	Differentially expressed genes
FNA	Fine-needle aspiration
GEO	Gene expression omnibus
GLOBOCAN	Global cancer observatory
GO	Gene ontology
HubGs	Hub genes
KEGG	Kyoto encyclopedia of genes and genomes
KGs	Key genes
LIMMA	Linear models for microarray data
MCC	Maximal clique centrality
NCBI	National Center for Biotechnology Information
PCa	Prostate cancer
PPI	Protein–protein interaction
PSA	Prostate-specific antigen
TCGA	The Cancer Genome Atlas

M. A. U. Arman · M. H. Alamin · T. A. Maya · M. T. Hossain (✉)
Faculty of Science, Department of Statistics, Bangabandhu Sheikh Mujibur Rahman Science and Technology University, Gopalganj, Bangladesh

M. S. Reza
Division of Biomedical Informatics and Genomics, Tulane Center of Biomedical Informatics and Genomics, Deming Department of Medicine, School of Medicine, Tulane University, New Orleans, LA, USA
e-mail: mreza@tulane.edu

M. Pal et al. (eds.), *Public Health and Nutrition*,
https://doi.org/10.1007/978-981-97-7890-4_14

14.1 Introduction

Prostate cancer (PCa) is a high-incidence malignant cancer in the urinary system of men and ranks second most malignant cancer globally. The prostate is a little gland located in the pelvis that is found in men only. It is situated between the penis and the bladder, roughly the size of a walnut. The primary purpose of prostate is to aid in the creation of semen. The most common cancer (20%) in men is PCa, which also accounts for 6.8% of all cancer-related deaths in men worldwide. The World Cancer Survey Statistics (GLOBOCAN) estimates that, in 2020, there were around 1.41 million newly detected PCa cases and 375,000 new deaths from the disease (Sung et al. 2021; Ferlay et al. 2019). Especially in recent years, in Asian men, the PCa rate is increasing at an alarming rate. Bangladeshi men are also becoming victims of this fatal disease nowadays. In 2020, statistical data of GLOBOCAN calculated 2441 new PCa cases, resulting in 1289 deaths in Bangladeshi males. Due to population expansion and aging, it is anticipated that by 2040, there will be 2.43 million new cases of PCa worldwide, along with 740,000 new fatalities (Sung et al. 2021; Ferlay et al. 2019). Although the most frequently used screening tool for PCa detection is prostate-specific antigen (PSA) level, it is not an exact approach to forecast the malignancy of a disease. Additionally, there may be advantages to using genomic profiling for early PCa identification (Herget et al. 2016; Albertsen 2008). Early-stage PCa patients may benefit from surgery or radiation therapy, but it is not effective for severe or advanced-stage patients (Albertsen 2008; So et al. 2005). Therefore, it is critical to screen out molecular biomarkers to differentiate between the different phases of the disease and to aid in developing better treatment strategies for PCa.

Bioinformatics approaches and microarray technologies have also been extensively used to elucidate variations in gene expression that can aid in our understanding of the mechanisms of PCa (Huang et al. 2017). In this study, we analyzed three freely accessible gene expression profiles (GSE104749, GSE46602, and GSE55945) to investigate the putative biomarkers of PCa. We identified 458 common differentially expressed genes (cDEGs) from these three datasets and constructed a protein–protein interaction (PPI) network of these genes with the help of STRING database (Szklarczyk et al. 2019). The gene ontology (GO) term and Kyoto Encyclopedia of Genes and Genomes (KEGG) pathway analyses of the top 15 HubGs detected from the PPI network indicated that some HubGs exhibited enrichment in multiple significant biological processes, molecular mechanisms, cellular components, and pathways associated with PCa. The cancer genome atlas (TCGA) data also supported the expression of HubGs in PCa. We also found by survival analysis that the five genes BIRC5, CENPF, TK1, cell division cycle-associated (CDCA)5, and NUSAP1 were significantly associated with PCa.

14.2 Methods and Materials

14.2.1 Data Sources and Descriptions

We downloaded microarray profiles for PCa from the National Center for Biotechnology Information (NCBI) (http://www.ncbi.nlm.nih.gov/geo/) on 2 May 2023 with accession numbers GSE46602 (Mortensen et al. 2015), GSE55945 (Arredouani et al. 2009), and GSE104749 (Shan et al. 2017). The number of PCa tissues and the normal prostate tissues of the three datasets are, respectively, 34 and 14; 13 and 8; and 4 and 4.

14.2.2 Detecting cDEGs

We identified DEGs between two groups (normal vs. cancer) for each of the GSE46602, GSE55945, and GSE104749 datasets separately using the R package LIMMA (Smyth 2004). Then, we selected cDEGs from the three DEG sets of three datasets. The cut-off for defining statistically significant DEGs was considered as $|\text{Log2Fold Change}| > 1.0$ and $p\text{-value} < 0.05$.

14.2.3 Detection of HubGs From the PPI Network

The PPI network of the cDEGs was constructed with the help of the online database STRING (accessed 2 May 2023). To visualize and improve the quality of the network, we used Cytoscape (Shannon et al. 2003). The HubGs were detected using cytoHubba (Chin et al. 2014), a Cytoscape plugin. Using cytoHubba, a sub-network was created with the top 15 HubGs, and then the HubGs were taken out of the sub-network. Maximal Clique Centrality (MCC) was used in selecting HubGs.

14.2.4 Analysis of GO Terms and KEGG Pathways

To examine the enrichment of the HubGs in PCa-related biological processes, cellular components, and molecular functions, we performed the widely recognized GO analysis. Again, to assess the involvement or influence of the HubGs in PCa-associated pathways, we conducted a KEGG pathway analysis. The GO and KEGG pathway analyses were performed using the online tool DAVID (Huang et al. 2009). A threshold of $p\text{-value} < 0.05$ was employed to determine the statistically significant GO terms and pathways.

14.2.5 Study of Association Between Expression of HubGs and PCa

The expression of HubGs in PCa tissue samples was compared with normal tissue samples using the online tool GEPIA (Tang et al. 2019). The web-based application GEPIA compares the gene expression profiles of cancer and normal samples using the TCGA database. The survival analysis is also performed by GEPIA. The threshold log-rank $P < 0.05$ was considered to treat an association as statistically significant.

14.3 Result

14.3.1 Identification of cDEGs for PCa Patients

Volcano plots (Fig. 14.1a–c) were used to depict the DEGs that were found from the three datasets GSE104749, GSE55945, and GSE46602. In the first dataset, 4934 DEGs (2075 upregulated and 2859 downregulated) were identified; in the second dataset, 9445 DEGs (3787 upregulated and 5658 downregulated) were identified; and finally, in the third dataset, 2403 DEGs (794 upregulated and 1609 downregulated) were identified. Then, we found 458 cDEGs for PCa patients (Fig. 14.1d).

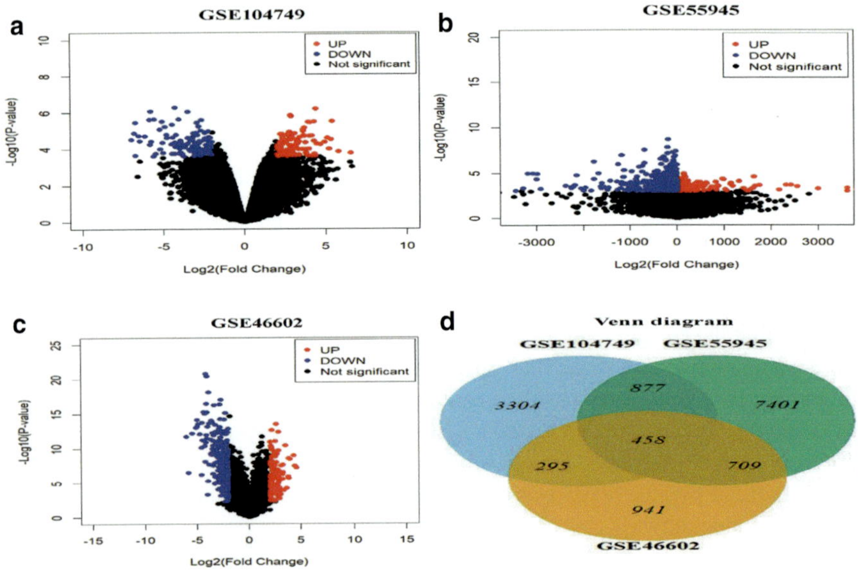

Fig. 14.1 Expressions of the identified genes. The volcano plots of the datasets (**a**) GSE104749, (**b**) GSE55945, and (b) GSE46602 are used to find out the DEGs. Red, blue, and black colors indicate upregulated, downregulated, and equally expressed genes, respectively. (**d**) Venn diagram of the identified DEGs is used to find the cDEGs

14.3.2 Identification of HubGs

Using STRING database, we constructed a PPI network with the cDEGs, which contained 238 nodes and 539 edges. Then, a sub-network (Fig. 14.2) was created with the top 15 HubGs {TOP2A, RRM2, NCAPG, BUB1B, CENPU, CENPF, AURKA, TPX2, MKI67, BIRC5, CDCA5, NUSAP1, EZH2, ECT2, and TK1} applying MCC topological measures. We used these 15 HubGs for further analysis.

14.3.3 PCa-Related GO Terms and KEGG Pathways

To investigate the functions of the HubGs, we conducted GO term and KEGG pathway analyses using the 15 HubGs identified from the PPI network. The investigation of the GO term "biological process" revealed that certain genes exhibited enrichment in several cellular activities, including cell division, mitotic cell cycle, mitotic chromosome condensation, mitotic spindle assembly, and checkpoint, among others. The examination of molecular function using GO terms revealed that some genes were found to be enriched in the function of microtubule binding, protein homodimerization activity, protein binding, chromatin binding, as well as protein C-terminus binding, among other functions. The examination of cellular components using GO terms revealed that some genes exhibited enrichment in several cellular locations, including nucleus, spindle, chromosome, centromeric region, kinetochore, and pronucleus, among others. The analysis of KEGG pathways revealed that several HubGs exhibited significant enrichment in the pyrimidine metabolism pathway. The outcomes of the noteworthy GO terms and KEGG pathways are presented in Table 14.1.

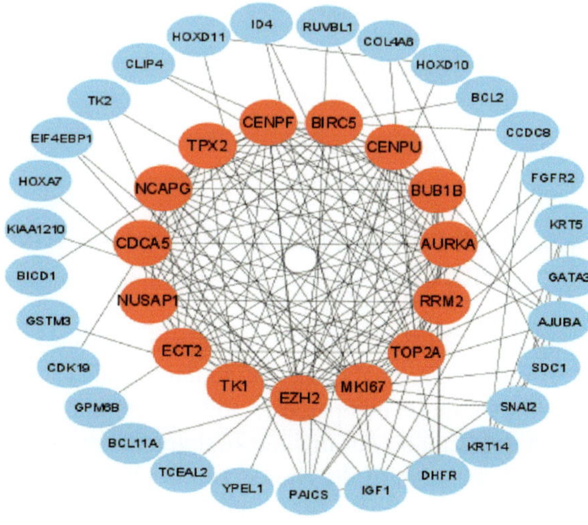

Fig. 14.2 Using cytoHubba, a sub-network was created comprising the top 15 HubGs and their associated genes. This sub-network was derived from a PPI network obtained after submitting 458 cDEGs to STRING database. The nodes with a deeper red color indicate a higher degree

Table 14.1 List of top significant GO terms and pathways obtained by submitting the 15 hub genes to DAVID database

GO term	Go name	Number of genes	*P*-value
Biological process			
GO:0051301	Cell division	7	1.54×10^{-7}
GO:0000278	Mitotic cell cycle	5	3.31×10^{-6}
GO:0007076	Mitotic chromosome condensation	3	7.34×10^{-5}
GO:0007094	Mitotic spindle assembly checkpoint	3	2.37×10^{-4}
GO:0000281	Mitotic cytokinesis	3	0.001039
GO:0007059	Chromosome segregation	3	0.001666
GO:0007049	Cell cycle	4	0.002009
GO:0031536	Positive regulation of exit from mitosis	2	0.00432
GO:0006915	Apoptotic process	4	0.00891
GO:0010389	Regulation of G2/M transition of mitotic cell cycle	2	0.010052
GO:0045840	Positive regulation of mitotic nuclear division	2	0.021425
Cellular component			
GO:0005634	Nucleus	15	3.32×10^{-8}
GO:0005819	Spindle	6	3.38×10^{-8}
GO:0000775	chromosome, centromeric region	5	9.35×10^{-8}
GO:0000776	Kinetochore	5	3.37×10^{-6}
GO:0045120	Pronucleus	3	4.27×10^{-6}
GO:0072686	Mitotic spindle	4	1.12×10^{-4}
GO:0000793	Condensed chromosome	3	1.60×10^{-4}
GO:0030496	Midbody	4	2.48×10^{-4}
GO:0005654	Nucleoplasm	10	3.17×10^{-4}
GO:0005829	Cytosol	11	6.95×10^{-4}
GO:0005874	Microtubule	4	0.001241
GO:0032133	Chromosome passenger complex	2	0.004067
Molecular function			
GO:0008017	Microtubule binding	4	8.69×10^{-4}
GO:0042803	Protein homodimerization activity	5	0.001656
GO:0005515	Protein binding	15	0.003486
GO:0003682	Chromatin binding	4	0.004477
GO:0008022	Protein C-terminus binding	3	0.008496
GO:0005524	ATP binding	5	0.022621
GO:0046982	Protein heterodimerization activity	3	0.030241
Pathway ID	Pathway description	Number of genes	*P*-value
hsa00240	Pyrimidine metabolism	2	0.047004

14.3.4 Validation of Expression and Association of HubGs with PCa

Using the GEPIA database, we examined how the 15 HubGs expressed in samples of prostate and normal tissue. We found that all 15 genes showed increased expression in PCa tissue compared to adjacent normal tissue (Fig. 14.3a–o). Therefore, TCGA data support our findings of upregulation of the 15 HubGs.

The association of the HubGs and the PCa was also investigated by the TCGA data, and we found that PCa patients with lower expression of the genes BIRC5, CDCA5, CENPF, NUSAP1, and TK1 had improved survival rates (Fig. 14.4a–e).

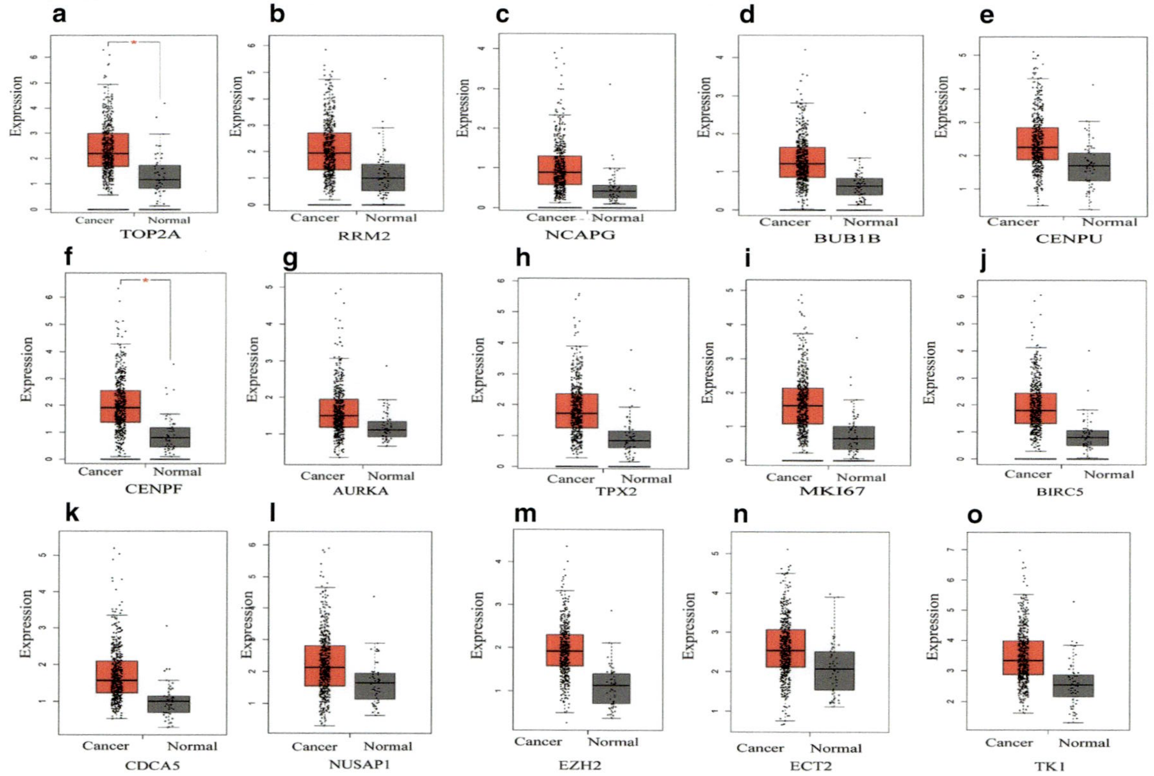

Fig. 14.3 Expression validation of 15 HubGs in PCa by TCGA data. Increased expression of the genes (**a**) TOP2A, (**b**) RRM2, (**c**) NCAPG, (**d**) BUB1B, (**e**) CENPU, (**f**) CENPF, (**g**) AURKA, (**h**) TPX2, (**i**) MKI67, (**j**) BIRC5, (**k**) CDCA5, (**l**) NUSAP1, (**m**) EZH2, (**n**) ECT2, and (**o**) TK1 was found in PCa tissues while comparing with normal tissues

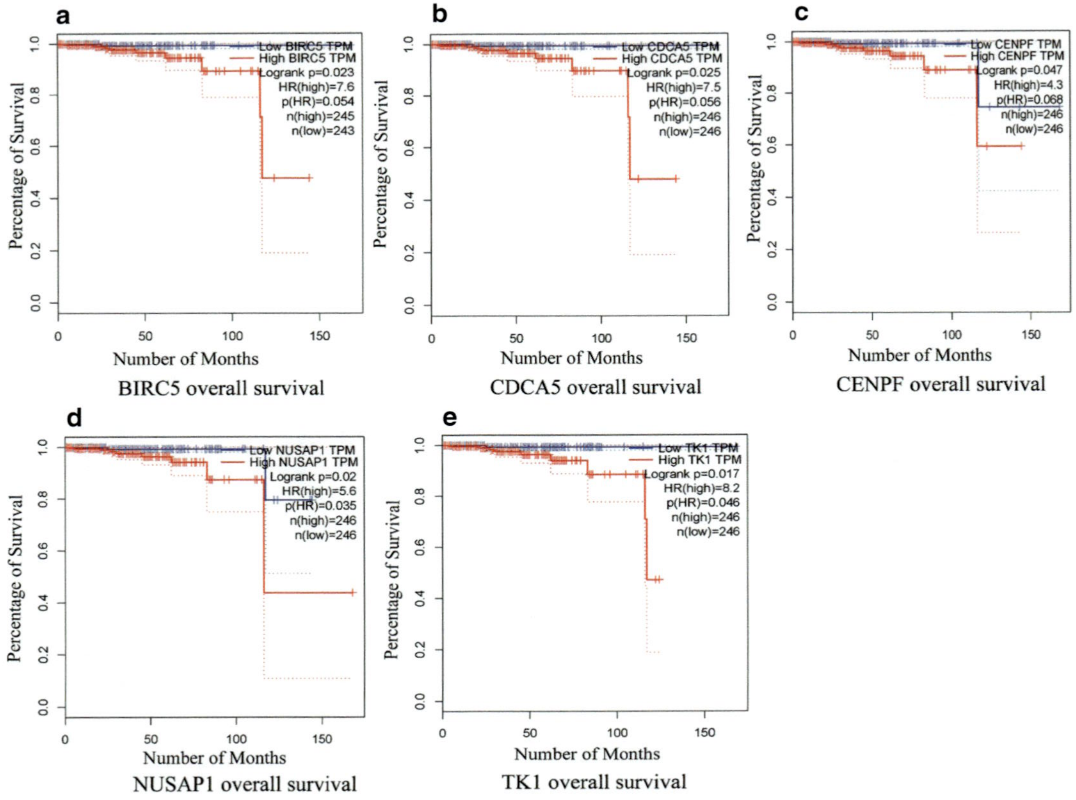

Fig. 14.4 The survival curves of the potential HubGs were analyzed in order to determine their overall impact on survival outcomes. Patients with lower expression levels of genes (**a**) BIRC5, (**b**) CDCA5 (**c**) CENPF, (**d**) NUSAP1, and (**e**) TK1 had better survival rates. Red and blue lines indicate higher and lower

14.4 Discussion

PCa is a malignant cancer affecting the urinary system in males. It ranks fifth in terms of male cancer-related mortality and is the most often diagnosed cancer in men globally. To examine the genetic impact of PCa infections, a total of 458 cDEGs were discovered. Fifteen HubGs, namely, TOP2A, RRM2, NCAPG, BUB1B, CENPU, CENPF, AURKA, TPX2, MKI67, BIRC5, CDCA5, NUSAP1, EZH2, ECT2, and TK1, were identified from the PPI network of cDEGs.

The GO term and KEGG pathway analyses were conducted for the 15 HubGs. The GO term analyses demonstrated that certain HubGs were shown to be enriched in a number of significant biological processes, molecular functions, and cellular components (Table 14.1). Previous research also showed that PCa-associated genes were enriched in the biological processes, namely, cell division, mitotic cell cycle, mitotic chromosome condensation, mitotic spindle assembly, and checkpoint; the molecular functions, namely, microtubule binding, protein homodimerization activity, protein binding, chromatin binding, as well as protein C-terminus binding; and the cellular components, namely, nucleus, spindle, chromosome, centromeric region, kinetochore, and pronucleus (He et al. 2019; Balk and Knudsen 2008; Coschi et al. 2010). The KEGG pathway analysis (Table 14.1) revealed that certain HubGs have an enrichment in signaling pathway pyrimidine metabolism relevant to PCa (Siddiqui and Ceppi 2020).

According to the survival study results, PCa patients who had lower expression levels of the genes TK1, NUSAP1, CENPF, BIRC5, and CDCA5 had higher survival rates (Fig. 14.4). Previous research identified these five genes as important biomarkers of PCa (Fig. 14.5). For example, BIRC5 is considered essential for PCa metastasis (Fan et al. 2018), is crucial for the development and spread of cancer (Altieri 2008), plays a vital role in colorectal cancer carcinogenesis (Wang et al. 2014), interacts with cell adhesion during microtubule-kinetochore attachment (Vitale et al. 2011), is significantly expressed in the majority of malignancies (Xu et al. 2021), and has increased expression in primary prostate tumors and metastases (Hennigs et al. 2020). It has been demonstrated that CENPF functions as a synergistic master moderator of PCa malignancy and is a prognostic marker for metastasis and poor survival (Aytes et al. 2014), (Mitrofanova et al. 2015). A number of cancers, including PCa, have aggressive tumor characteristics that are associated with CENPF overexpression (Göbel et al. 2018). Reduced CDCA5 expression stops PCa cell growth by blocking the ERK signaling pathway and hence might be a viable therapeutic target for PCa (Ji et al. 2021). Increased expression of CDCA5 in PCa tissues can be a major factor in the development of PCa (Gu et al. 2022). Upregulation of the CDCA protein family is found in PCa cell lines which has an essential role in cell division and proliferation (Zhang et al. 2020). In PCa, NUSAP1 increases invasion, cell migration, and metastasis (Gulzar et al. 2013). NSAP1 is present in prognostic gene sets linked to higher grades of PCa (Penney et al. 2011). It is reported that TK1 can be considered a prognostic marker for PCa (Zhang et al. 2022). According to recent research, intracellular TK1 plays a hallmark function in the proliferation of cancer cells and is associated with the invasion and spread of cancer

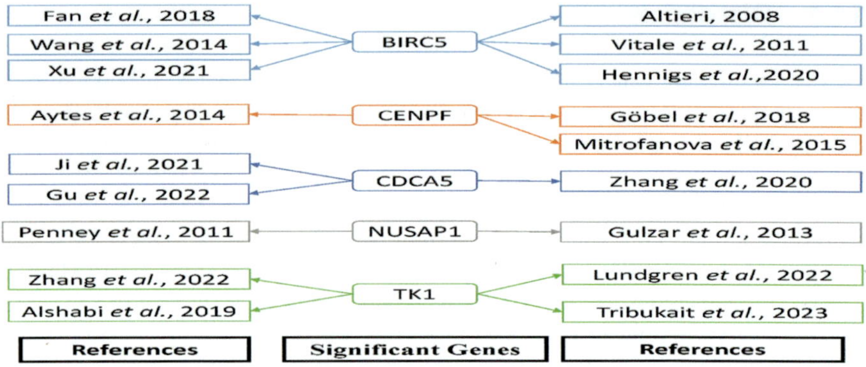

Fig. 14.5 Previous studies that support our identified genes as a potential biomarker for prostate cancer

cells (Alshabi et al. 2019). Baseline TK1 blood levels were linked to subsequent PCa-specific death (Lundgren et al. 2022). PSA and TK1 serum concentrations can be used to forecast PCa patients' long-term risk (Tribukait et al. 2023). Therefore, it is plausible that the above-mentioned genes, including BIRC5, CDCA5, CENPF, NUSAP1, and TK1, can potentially function as biomarkers for PCa. Additional wet lab experimental validation is required.

14.5 Conclusion

A total of 458 cDEGs were found in our study. Fifteen HubGs were identified through the investigation of the PPI network. Functional enrichment analysis demonstrated that several HubGs were shown to be enriched in a number of significant biological processes, molecular functions, cellular components, and PCa-related pathways. Using the TCGA data, the HubGs' expressions were verified. Survival analysis revealed a significant association between the PCa patients and the five genes, namely, BIRC5, CDCA5, CENPF, NUSAP1, and TK. These five genes might be regarded as potential biomarkers for PCa. The literature review provided additional support for the candidate genes as key players for PCa. Hence, the molecular biomarkers suggested in this study have merit for the prognosis of PCa.

References

Albertsen P (2008) Predicting survival for men with clinically localized prostate cancer. Cancer 112(1):1–3. https://doi.org/10.1002/cncr.23107

Alshabi AM, Vastrad B, Shaikh IA, Vastrad C (2019) Identification of important invasion and proliferation related genes in adrenocortical carcinoma. Med Oncol. https://doi.org/10.1007/s12032-019-1296-7

Altieri DC (2008) Survivin, cancer networks and pathway-directed drug discovery. Nat Rev Cancer. https://doi.org/10.1038/nrc2293

Arredouani MS et al (2009) Identification of the transcription factor single-minded homologue 2 as a potential biomarker and immunotherapy target in prostate cancer. Clin Cancer Res 15(18):5794–5802. https://doi.org/10.1158/1078-0432.CCR-09-0911

Aytes A et al (2014) Cross-species regulatory network analysis identifies a synergistic interaction between FOXM1 and CENPF that drives prostate cancer malignancy. Cancer Cell. https://doi.org/10.1016/j.ccr.2014.03.017

Balk SP, Knudsen KE (2008) AR, the cell cycle, and prostate cancer. Nucl Recept Signal. https://doi.org/10.1621/nrs.06001

Chin CH, Chen SH, Wu HH, Ho CW, Ko MT, Lin CY (2014) cytoHubba: identifying hub objects and sub-networks from complex interactome. BMC Syst Biol 8(4). https://doi.org/10.1186/1752-0509-8-S4-S11

Coschi CH et al (2010) Mitotic chromosome condensation mediated by the retinoblastoma protein is tumor-suppressive. Genes Dev. https://doi.org/10.1101/gad.1917610

Fan S et al (2018) Identification of the key genes and pathways in prostate cancer. Oncol Lett 16(5):6663–6669. https://doi.org/10.3892/ol.2018.9491

Ferlay J et al (2019) Estimating the global cancer incidence and mortality in 2018: GLOBOCAN sources and methods. Int J Cancer 144:1941–1953. https://doi.org/10.1002/ijc.31937

Göbel C et al (2018) Upregulation of centromere protein F is linked to aggressive prostate cancers. Cancer Manag Res. https://doi.org/10.2147/CMAR.S165630

Gu P, Yang D, Zhu J, Zhang M, He X, Mojumdar K (2022) Bioinformatics analysis of the clinical relevance of CDCA gene family in prostate cancer. Medicine. https://doi.org/10.1097/MD.0000000000028788

Gulzar ZG, Mckenney JK, Brooks JD (2013) Increased expression of NuSAP in recurrent prostate cancer is mediated by E2F1. Oncogene. https://doi.org/10.1038/onc.2012.27

He Z, Duan X, Zeng G (2019) Identification of potential biomarkers and pivotal biological pathways for prostate cancer using bioinformatics analysis methods. PeerJ. https://doi.org/10.7717/peerj.7872

Hennigs JK et al (2020) Subcellular compartmentalization of survivin is associated with biological aggressiveness and prognosis in prostate cancer. Sci Rep. https://doi.org/10.1038/s41598-020-60064-9

Herget KA, Patel DP, Hanson HA, Sweeney C, Lowrance WT (2016) Recent decline in prostate cancer incidence in the United States, by age, stage, and Gleason score. Cancer Med 5:136–141. https://doi.org/10.1002/cam4.549

Huang DW, Sherman BT, Lempicki RA (2009) Bioinformatics enrichment tools: paths toward the comprehensive functional analysis of large gene lists. Nucleic Acids Res 37(1):1–13. https://doi.org/10.1093/nar/gkn923

Huang H et al (2017) Identification of prognostic markers of high grade prostate cancer through an integrated bioinformatics approach. J Cancer Res Clin Oncol. https://doi.org/10.1007/s00432-017-2497-0

Ji J, Shen T, Li Y, Liu Y, Shang Z, Niu Y (2021) CDCA5 promotes the progression of prostate cancer by affecting the ERK signalling pathway. Oncol Rep. https://doi.org/10.3892/or.2021.7920

Lundgren PO, Tribukait B, Kjellman A, Norming U, Jagarlmudi K, Gustafsson O (2022) Serum thymidine kinase 1 concentration as a predictive biomarker in prostate cancer. Prostate. https://doi.org/10.1002/pros.24335

Mitrofanova A, Aytes A, Zou M, Shen MM, Abate-Shen C, Califano A (2015) Predicting drug response in human prostate cancer from preclinical analysis of in vivo mouse models. Cell Rep. https://doi.org/10.1016/j.celrep.2015.08.051

Mortensen MM et al (2015) Expression profiling of prostate cancer tissue delineates genes associated with recurrence after prostatectomy. Sci Rep 5:1–11. https://doi.org/10.1038/srep16018

Penney KL et al (2011) mRNA expression signature of gleason grade predicts lethal prostate cancer. J Clin Oncol. https://doi.org/10.1200/JCO.2010.32.6421

Shan M et al (2017) Molecular analyses of prostate tumors for diagnosis of malignancy on fine-needle aspiration biopsies. Oncotarget 8(62):104761–104771. https://doi.org/10.18632/oncotarget.22289

Shannon P et al (2003) Cytoscape: a software environment for integrated models of biomolecular interaction networks. Genome Res 13(11):2498–2504. https://doi.org/10.1101/gr.1239303

Siddiqui A, Ceppi P (2020) A non-proliferative role of pyrimidine metabolism in cancer. Mol Metabol. https://doi.org/10.1016/j.molmet.2020.02.005

Smyth GK (2004) Linear models and empirical bayes methods for assessing differential expression in microarray experiments. Stat Appl Genet Mol Biol 3(1):1027. https://doi.org/10.2202/1544-6115.1027

So A, Gleave M, Hurtado-Col A, Nelson C (2005) Mechanisms of the development of androgen independence in prostate cancer. World J Urol. https://doi.org/10.1007/s00345-004-0473-1

Sung H et al (2021) Global cancer statistics 2020: GLOBOCAN estimates of incidence and mortality worldwide for 36 cancers in 185 countries. CA Cancer J Clin 71(3):209–249. https://doi.org/10.3322/caac.21660

Szklarczyk D et al (2019) STRING v11: protein-protein association networks with increased coverage, supporting functional discovery in genome-wide experimental datasets. Nucleic Acids Res 47(D1):D607–D613. https://doi.org/10.1093/nar/gky1131

Tang Z, Kang B, Li C, Chen T, Zhang Z (2019) GEPIA2: an enhanced web server for large-scale expression profiling and interactive analysis. Nucleic Acids Res 47(W1):W556–W560. https://doi.org/10.1093/nar/gkz430

Tribukait B et al (2023) Prediction of overall survival by thymidine kinase 1 combined with prostate-specific antigen in men with prostate cancer. Int J Mol Sci. https://doi.org/10.3390/ijms24065160

Vitale I et al (2011) Illicit survival of cancer cells during polyploidization and depolyploidization. Cell Death Differ. https://doi.org/10.1038/cdd.2010.145

Wang H et al (2014) Investigation of cell free BIRC5 mRNA as a serum diagnostic and prognostic biomarker for colorectal cancer. J Surg Oncol. https://doi.org/10.1002/jso.23526

Xu L, Yu W, Xiao H, Lin K (2021) BIRC5 is a prognostic biomarker associated with tumor immune cell infiltration. Sci Rep. https://doi.org/10.1038/s41598-020-79736-7

Zhang Y et al (2020) CDCA2 inhibits apoptosis and promotes cell proliferation in prostate cancer and is directly regulated by HIF-1α pathway. Front Oncol. https://doi.org/10.3389/fonc.2020.00725

Zhang C, Ma S, Hao X, Wang Z, Sun Z (2022) Methylation status of TK1 correlated with immune infiltrates in prostate cancer. Front Genet. https://doi.org/10.3389/fgene.2022.899384

Prevalence and Associated Factors of Menstrual Disturbance Among University Students in Bangladesh

15

Shangida Khatun Eva, Abu Sayed Md. Al Mamun, Md. Nurul Islam, Md. Ripter Hossain, and Md. Golam Hossain

15.1 Introduction

Menstruation is a natural process where blood is discharged from the uterus through the vagina, happening at regular monthly intervals during a woman's reproductive years. It typically begins in girls aged 11–14 years and lasts up to 7 days, with a cycle length of 21–45 days and an average blood loss of 20–80 mL (Rafique and Al-Sheikh 2018). Some women experience pain before or during their periods, which usually starts a day or two before the bleeding and may continue for the first 2 days. This pain often affects young women in their teens and early twenties (Hossain et al. 2011). Epidemiologic studies estimate that about 5–35% of women of reproductive age experience some symptoms of menstrual disturbances (Kwak et al. 2019). These disturbances include dysmenorrhea (painful periods), premenstrual symptoms, heavy bleeding (menorrhagia), frequent periods (polymenorrhea), abnormal vaginal bleeding, missed periods (amenorrhea), infrequent periods (oligomenorrhea), and irregular menstruation. Many women of reproductive age have health issues related to their menstrual cycles. Menstrual patterns can be influenced by factors such as age, ethnicity, family history, smoking, physical activity, and diet. The menstrual cycle and its hormonal changes shape the reproductive life cycle. Any irregularities in this cycle can affect many aspects of women's lives. Mental health is closely linked to reproductive features, such as the phase of the menstrual cycle and the regularity of menstrual flow (Park and Jung 2021). Menstrual problems can significantly affect women's quality of life, leading to absenteeism and negatively impacting academic performance. Despite this, most women get their information about menstrual issues from family and friends, as they often do not consult professionals, thinking that their symptoms are normal or doubting that professionals can help. Many women prefer self-care methods, although these are not

S. K. Eva · A. S. M. Al Mamun · M. N. Islam · M. R. Hossain · M. G. Hossain (✉)
Department of Statistics, University of Rajshahi, Rajshahi, Bangladesh

M. Pal et al. (eds.), *Public Health and Nutrition*,
https://doi.org/10.1007/978-981-97-7890-4_15

always the best option. The main self-care strategy used is self-medication with non-steroidal anti-inflammatory drugs to relieve menstrual pain, which can be costly and have side effects. Additionally, up to 18% of women find that their pain does not respond to these medications (Fernández-Martínez et al. 2020). No studies have been done to determine the prevalence and factors associated with menstrual disturbances among university students in Bangladesh. Therefore, it is important to conduct a study to understand the prevalence and factors related to menstrual disturbances among these students. Therefore, the authors decided to research menstrual disturbance among female students at Rajshahi University (RU) in Bangladesh.

15.2 Materials and Methods

Materials: The study was conducted at RU, the second-largest public university in Bangladesh, attracting students from all over the country. RU has 18 residential halls: six for women, 11 for men, and one international dormitory. Female students studying at the University of Rajshahi were the population of the study. RU has around 38,000 students at a particular time among them around 10,000 are female students. Around 5000 female students are living in residential halls at University campuses. The data were collected from female students currently studying at RU and residing in their residential halls at campus who had no severe mental problems. The survey was conducted from September 2022 to November 2022.

Sample size determination: To calculate the sample size for our study of 5,000 students, we used the formula: $n = \frac{N}{1 + Nd^2}$ (Rana et al. 2015). Here, n is the required sample size, N is the population size (5000), and d is the margin of error (0.05). With a 95% confidence level, the formula showed that 371 samples were needed. However, we initially decided to include 500 samples to account for a 10% absence rate.

Sample selection procedures: At first, we gathered the information from RU administration about the number of total female students residing in different Halls. We also collected the number of students residing in a particular Hall from the respective Hall administration office. All the other necessary information for sampling was collected from the respective Hall office. We selected 500 female students from all-female residence Halls in RU using random sampling with proportional allocation technique. We discussed with our selected female students the objectives of our study, but 30 students did not agree to provide their information. Finally, 470 samples were considered for the present study. We had taken their written consent.

Outcome variables: The outcome variable in this study was menstrual disturbance, and it was measured by students' self-reported two major problems; (a) painful menstruation, it was measured by a question to the subjects, did you have painful menstruation before or during menstruation period? (1) Yes (code: 1), (2) No (code: 0); and (b) irregular menstruation, it was also measured by a question to the subjects, did you have irregular menstruation? (1) Yes (code: 1), (2) No (code: 0). Finally, the subjects were classified into three classes according to their number of problems, (1) no problem, (2) one problem (either painful or irregular menstruation), and (3) two problems (painful and irregular menstruation).

Independent variables: Several socio-economic, demographic, and health-related factors were considered as independent variables, as they were assumed to be associated with menstrual disturbances in young adult females. These independent variables are listed in Table 15.1.

Statistical Analysis: We used frequency distribution and descriptive statistics to calculate percentages for qualitative variables and mean ± SD for quantitative variables. Simple and multiple logistic regression models were used in the study. The simple (univariate) model helped select independent variables for the multiple model; variables with a p-value less than 0.2 were included. We tested the goodness of fit of the multiple logistic models using the Hosmer and Lemeshow test and Negelkerke R^2. Model accuracy was checked by looking at sensitivity, specificity, positive and negative predictive values, and the receiver operator characteristic (ROC) curve. We also checked for multicollinearity among the independent variables using variance inflation factors. Statistical significance was set at $p < 0.05$. The analysis was done using the SPSS software (IBM version 22).

15.3 Results

A total of 470 female students were considered as a sample for our present study to investigate the prevalence and associated factors of menstrual disturbance among University students in Bangladesh. It was observed that only 6.6% and 4.7% of fathers and mothers were uneducated, while 53.8% and 27.9% of fathers and mothers were higher educated, respectively. Most of the students (73.9%) came from middle-income families (32.6% from low-middle-income families; and 41.3% upper-middle-income families). We observed that 20.0% and 11.9% of female students were suffering from under and over-nutrition, respectively. Most of the students' mothers (86.2%) were housewives, and 64.2% fathers had business (32.3%) or jobs (31.9%). Notably, 54.3% and 45.7% of students came from rural and urban environments, respectively, and 82.6% came from nuclear families. Near to 50% of students had one to two siblings, 70.9% of students were born at first (36.4%) or second (34.5%) order the order of birth. Notably, 86.4% of students had experienced that the duration of staying menstruation was 4–7 days, and 15.3% of students reached menarche at 9–11 years of age (Table 15.1). The mean age at first menarche (year) and duration of menstruation flow (day) were 12.73 ± 1.23 [95% CI: 12.62–12.84] and 5.38 ± 1.64 [95% CI: 5.23–5.53], respectively (Table 15.1).

Menstrual disturbance: It was noted that 71.1% and 17.7% of students were suffering from painful and irregular menstruation, respectively, and 63.2% and 12.8% of students had at least one problem (either painful or irregular menstruation) and two problems (painful or irregular menstruation), respectively, while 24.0% students reported that they did not have any problem (Fig. 15.1).

Painful and irregular menstruation: After controlling the effect of other variables, the multiple logistic models demonstrated that students who had suffered from fever

Table 15.1 Frequency distribution of students by parents' educational level

Variable	*N* (%)	Variable	*N* (%)
Father's educational level		Mother's educational level	
Uneducated	31 (6.6)	Uneducated	22 (4.7)
Primary	62 (13.2)	Primary	89 (18.9)
Secondary	124 (26.4)	Secondary	228 (48.5)
Higher and above	253 (53.8)	Higher and above	131 (27.9)
Monthly family income (BDT) group		Nutritional status	
Less than 10,000	47 (10)	Undernutrition (BMI < 18.5)	94 (20.0)
10,000–20,000	153 (32.6)	Normal (18.5 ≤ BMI <25)	320 (68.1)
20,001–49,999	194 (41.3)	Overnutrition (BMI ≥25)	56 (11.9)
50,000 and above	76 (16.2)	Mother's occupation	
Residence		Housewife	405 (86.2)
Rural	255 (54.3)	Job	65 (13.8)
Urban	215 (45.7)	Type of family	
Father's occupation		Joint	82 (17.4)
Farmer	85 (18.1)	Nuclear	388 (82.6)
Job	150 (31.9)	Number of Siblings	
Business	152 (32.3)	1–2	230 (48.9)
Others	83 (17.7)	3	131 (27.9)
Order of birth		4≥	109 (23.2)
First	171 (36.4)	Duration of staying menstruation (menstrual flow)	
Second	162 (34.5)	Abnormal	53 (11.3)
Third or mode	137 (29.1)	Normal (4–7 days)	417 (88.7)
Age at menarche (years)		Fever during menstruation	
9–11	72 (15.3)	No	408 (86.8)
12–13	279 (59.4)	Yes	62 (13.2)

(continued)

Table 15.1 (continued)

Variable	*N* (%)	Variable	*N* (%)
14 and above	119 (25.3)		
Physical activities			
No	121 (25.7)		
Yes	349 (74.3)		

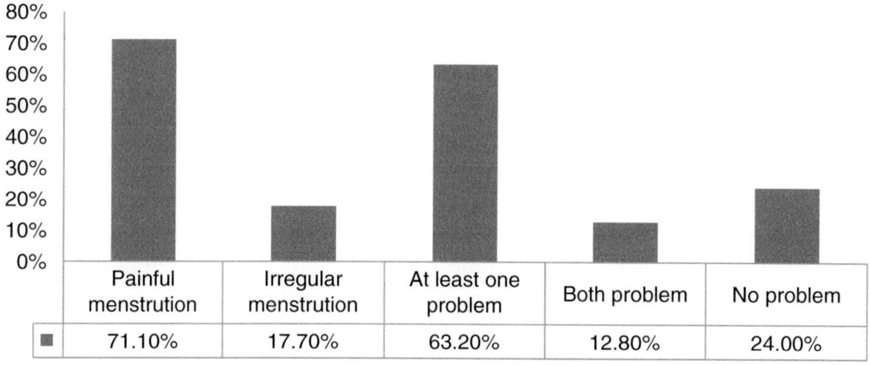

Fig. 15.1 Rate of female students suffering from different menstrual disturbance

during menstruation were more likely to get menstrual pain at 3.416 times higher compared with students who did not have fever [AOR = 3.416, 95% CI: 1.506–7.748; $p < 0.01$]. Students who preferred to consume Oily or fast food were more likely to experience painful menstruation [AOR = 3.586, 95% CI: 1.379–9.325; $p < 0.01$] compared who preferred to eat healthy and nutritious foods. On the contrary, students whose duration of menstrual flow was less than 4 days or more than 7 days were more likely to get irregular menstruation 2831 times higher than their counterparts [AOR = 2.83, 95% CI: 1.25–6.41; $p < 0.05$]. Students who did not engage in any physical activities were more likely to get irregular menstruation 2.23 times higher than the students who engaged in physical activities [AOR = 2.23, 95% CI: 1.07–4.63; $p < 0.05$] (Table 15.2). The overall accuracy of this model to predict the students having painful menstruation (with a predicted probability of 0.5 or greater) is 70%. The sensitivity was given by 8.10%, and the specificity was 95.20%. Positive predicted value (PPV) = 11/27 = 40.74% and negative predicted value (NPV) = 318/443 = 71.78% were observed. The accuracy was measured by the area under the ROC curve. The area of this curve of ROC was 0.638, by which we could say that, in almost 63.8% of all possible pairs of subjects, one suffered from painful menstruation and the other did not suffer from menstrual pain. The overall accuracy of this model to predict the students having irregular menstruation (with a predicted probability of 0.5 or greater) is 89.6%. The sensitivity was given by 375/387 = 96.90% and the specificity was 46/83 = 55.42%. PPV = 375/412 = 91.02% and NPV

Table 15.2 Impact of factors on painful and irregular menstruation of female students

Painful menstruation			Irregular menstruation		
Variable	AOR (95% CI: lower–upper)	*p*-value	Variable	AOR (95% CI: lower–upper)	*p*-value
Fever during menstruation			Duration of menstrual flow (days)		
Yes vs No[R]	3.416 (1.506–7.748)	0.003	Abnormal vs normal (4–7 days)[R]	2.83 (1.25–6.41)	0.013
Food type			Physical activities		
Oily or fast food vs nutrition and healthy[R]	3.586 (1.379–9.325)	0.009	No vs Yes[R]	2.23 (1.07–4.63)	0.032
Hosmer and Lemeshow test	χ^2-value = 5.30; *p*-value = 0.071	Nagelkerke $R^2 = 0.64$	Hosmer and Lemeshow test	χ^2-value = 1.86; *p*-value = 0.762	Nagelkerke $R^2 = 0.62$

[R] Reference case

= 46/58 = 79.31% were got. The area of this ROC was 0.92 which means that, in almost 92% of all possible pairs of subjects in which one had irregular menstruation and the other had regular menstruation, this model would assign a higher probability to the subject with irregular menstruation (Table 15.2).

15.4 Discussion

Menstrual disturbance is an important indicator of women. It is a common problem that affects daily activities. In developing and underdeveloped nations, it gets very little attention. This study was conducted to explore the prevalence and associated factors of menstrual disturbance among University students in Bangladesh. In this study, painful menstruation and irregular menstruation were considered menstrual disturbances.

Painful menstruation: Painful menstruation, known as dysmenorrhea, affects over half of women who have periods, causing pain for 1–2 days each month. While the pain is usually mild, some women experience severe pain that prevents them from doing their regular activities for several days. The present study showed that 71.1% of students reported menstrual pain. Similarly, a high prevalence of menstrual pain (72.3%) was found among female students at RU (Hossain et al. 2011), which is very close to our findings. Another study conducted in Rajshahi district among school-going girls reported that 77.50% of students suffered from menstrual pain. We found that fever during menstruation and food type were significantly associated with painful menstruation. These two factors were not found as significant associated factors of painful menstruation in the previous study conducted by Hossain et al. (2011); they found the duration of menstrual flow, birth order, age at first menarche, and family income were significantly associated with painful menstruation. However, the present study found that 70.9% of students with normal menstrual flow which was between 4 and 7 days experienced painful menstruation but not significantly also associated with birth order and age at first menarche were not significantly ($p > 0.05$) associated with painful menstruation. Our findings also supported the findings of the Japanese study (Yamamoto et al. 2009), Sweden study (Sundell et al. 1990), Nigerian study (Loto et al. 2008), Italian study (Balbi et al. 2000), and Spanish study (Bernis et al. 1999). In our study, we found that the nutritional status of students was not significantly associated with painful menstruation. However, different results were found in Spanish University women (Fernández-Martínez et al. 2020); they mentioned that a higher proportion of women with menstrual problems were obese, along the lines of previous research related to obesity with painful menstruation (Bajalan et al. 2019), also found in a previous study of Bangladesh by Hossain et al. (2011) that higher nutritional status of a girl experienced menstrual pain than others.

Irregular menstruation: Our study aimed to investigate menstrual irregularities among female students at RU. We found that 17.7% of students reported experiencing irregular periods, a higher prevalence compared with similar studies conducted in India (Sreelakshmi et al. 2019; Taheri et al. 2020; Singh and Wadhawan 2019). For instance, research on Indian teenagers showed that 11.2% of girls aged 10–19 years reported irregular periods (Maurya et al. 2022). Menstrual irregularity is known to signal both current and potential future health issues in women, impacting their daily lives significantly. A study conducted by (Hossain et al. 2011) mentioned only 12.90% of students experienced irregular menstruation. In the study, we found that duration of menstrual flow was associated with irregular menstruation. The multiple logistic regression analysis showed that students with menstrual flows of less than 4 days or more than 7 days were more likely to have irregular periods. Hossain et al. (2011) discovered a connection between menstrual flow duration and irregular periods among university students in Bangladesh. Similarly, Brooks-Gunn et al. (1985) observed this link among college students in New Jersey, and Cintio et al. (1997) found it in an Italian study. According to Hossain et al. (2011), early menarche, higher birth order, longer menstrual flow, and greater family income were the primary factors contributing to menstrual pain among Bangladeshi students. They also identified late menarche, longer menstrual flow, and higher BMI as causes of irregular periods. Both the age at menarche and the duration of menstrual flow influenced menstrual pain and irregular cycles among Bangladeshi students. Anai et al. (2001) similarly noted that delayed menarche was associated with irregular periods in young Japanese adults. Unlike the present study, females in Bangladesh were generally not conscious about their body weight. In this study, age at first menarche, birth order, family income, and BMI were not significantly linked to irregular menstruation ($p > 0.05$). However, in recent and previous studies among RU students, duration of menstrual flow was the common factor responsible for irregular menstruation. It was found that a lack of physical activity is also responsible for irregular menstruation. We found from multiple logistic regressions that students who did no physical activity were more likely to get irregular menstruation 2.23 times higher than their counterparts. Similarly, several studies in India found that a lack of physical activity and eating more junk food were linked to menstrual problems among adolescents. A previous study found that girls who did not exercise, smoked, or drank alcohol were much more likely to have irregular menstrual cycles compared with those who were physically active (Maurya et al. 2022).

Limitations of the study: This study has several limitations that need to be considered. Because it was conducted as a cross-sectional study, data were collected at a single point in time, which may not fully represent the overall situation accurately. Therefore, interpretations should be made cautiously. The use of self-reported questionnaires could introduce recall bias, as participants may not accurately remember or report their experiences. Additionally, relying on data provided by students might introduce bias, limiting how broadly the findings can be applied beyond this specific group.

To improve future research, larger samples from various universities across broader geographic areas should be included. This would help ensure that the results can be generalized to the entire population of the country. It is important to keep these limitations in mind when interpreting the findings of this study. Furthermore, the exposure variable of menstrual disturbance may be overestimated due to the use of self-reported data. More research is needed to better understand menstrual disturbances among adult females in Bangladesh. Addressing these limitations will be crucial for improving the accuracy and relevance of future studies on this topic.

15.5 Conclusions

A remarkable number of university female students were suffering from menstrual disturbance. This problem is one of the important causes of depression among adult female students which hamper their productivity and make it not possible to maintain their family properly. University female students are considered potential parts of a particular country, so efforts have to be made to improve their general health conditions. University female students deserve special attention because they can greatly influence their families and contribute significantly to the nation's workforce and productivity.

References

Anai T, Miyazaki F, Tomiyasu T, Matsuo T (2001) Risk of irregular menstrual cycles and low peak bone mass during early adulthood associated with age at menarche. Pediatr Int 43(5):483–488. https://doi.org/10.1046/j.1442-200x.2001.01442

Bajalan Z, Alimoradi Z, Moafi F (2019) Nutrition as a potential factor of primary dysmenorrhea: a systematic review of observational studies. Gynecol Obstet Investig 84:209–224

Balbi C, Musone R, Menditto A, Prisco LD, Cassese E, D'Ajello M, Ambrosio D, Cardone A (2000) Influence of menstrual factors and dietary habits on menstrual pain in adolescence age. Eur J Obstet Gynecol Reprod Biol 91:143–148

Bernis C, Montero P, Castro S (1999) Menstrual pain, menarcheal age and lifestyles in Spanish adolescents. Int J Anthropol 14:85–97

Brooks-Gunn J, Petersen AC, Eichorn (1985). The study of maturational timing effects in adolescence. J YouthAdolesc 14:149–161

Cintio E, Parazzini F, Tozzi L, Luchini L, Mezzopane R, Marchini M et al (1997) Dietary habits, reproductive and menstrual factors and risk of dysmenorrhoea. Eur J Epidemiol 13:925–930

Fernández-Martínez E, Fernández-Villa T, Amezcua-Prieto C, Suárez-Varela MM, Mateos-Campos R, Ayán-Pérez C, Molina de la Torre AJ, Ortíz-Moncada R, Almaraz A, Blázquez Abellán G, Delgado-Rodríguez M, Alonso-Molero J, Martínez-Ruíz V, Llopis-Morales A, Valero Juan LF, Cancela Carral JM, Martín-Peláez S, Alguacil J (2020) Menstrual problems and lifestyle among spanish university women. Int J Environ Res Public Health 17(20):7425. https://doi.org/10.3390/ijerph17207425. PMID: 33053847; PMCID: PMC7599672.

Hossain MG, Sabiruzzaman M, Islam S, Hisyam RZ, Lestrel PE, Kamarul T (2011) Influence of anthropometric measures and socio-demographic factors on menstrual pain and irregular menstrual cycles among University students in Bangladesh. Anthropol Sci 119(3):239–246

Kwak Y, Kim Y, Baek KA (2019) Prevalence of irregular menstruation according to socioeconomic status: a population-based nationwide cross-sectional study. PLoS One 14:1–12

Loto OM, Adewumi TA, Adewuya AO (2008) Prevalence and correlates of dysmenorrhea among Nigerian college women. Aust N Z J Obstet Gynaecol 48:442–444

Maurya P, Meher T, Muhammad T (2022) Relationship between depressive symptoms and self-reported menstrual irregularities during adolescence: evidence from UDAYA, 2016. BMC Public Health 22(1):758. https://doi.org/10.1186/s12889-022-13196-8. PMID: 35422014; PMCID: PMC9011997

Park M, Jung SJ (2021) Association between menstrual cycle irregularity and suicidal ideation among Korean women: Results from the Korea national health and nutrition examination survey (2010–2012). J Affect Disord 293:279–284

Rafique N, Al-Sheikh MH (2018) Prevalence of menstrual problems and their association with psychological stress in young female students studying health sciences. Saudi Med J 39(1):67–73. https://doi.org/10.15537/smj.2018.1.21438. PMID: 29332111; PMCID: PMC5885123

Rana M, Sayem A, Karim R, Islam N, Islam R, Zaman TK, Hossain G (2015) Assessment of knowledge regarding tuberculosis among non-medical university students in Bangladesh: a cross-sectional study. BMC Public Health,15:716. https://doi.org/10.1186/s12889-015-2071-0

Singh M, Wadhawan N (2019) Effect of dietary habits on menstrual problems in young girls. Int J Curr Microbiol App Sci 8:279–286

Sreelakshmi U, Tushara BV, Subhashini T, Saritha K (2019) Impact of dietary and lifestyle choices on menstrual patterns in medical students. Int J Reprod Contracept Obstet Gynecol 8:1271–1277

Sundell G, Milsom I, Andersch B (1990) Factors influencing the prevalence and severity of dysmenorrhoea in young women. Br J Obstet Gynaecol 97:588–594

Taheri R, Ardekani FM, Shahraki HR, Heidarzadeh-Esfahani N, Hajiahmadi S (2020) Nutritional status and anthropometric indices in relation to menstrual disorders: a crosssectional study. J Nutr Metab 2020:5980685

Yamamoto K, Okazaki A, Sakamoto Y, Funatsu M (2009) The relationship between premenstrual symptoms, menstrual pain, irregular menstrual cycles, and psychosocial stress among Japanese college students. J Physiol Anthropol 28:129–136

Factors Influencing Health-Related Quality of Life and Living Arrangements of the Ageing Population in the Northern Part of Bangladesh

16

Md. Abu Sayem, Md. Nurul Islam, and Md. Golam Hossain

16.1 Introduction

Health-related quality of life (HRQoL) metrics have become more widely used to assess the utility of health (Gold and Muennig 2002; Cooper et al. 2001). The introduction and development of more tools for measuring HRQoL have increased, although there is disagreement on whether one should be regarded as the gold standard (Guyatt 1997). The two main categories of health status tools are disease-specific and generic. The latter concentrated on the signs and effects of a particular illness or subpopulation on function, whereas the former was more generally thought to apply to illnesses or populations that were more widespread (Hahn 2007).

The physical abilities of elderly people have been proven to decline with age as a result of the reduction in muscle fibre size and number (Santanasto et al. 2015).

One in six individuals on the planet will be 60 or older by 2030. By this point, there will be 1.4 billion people over the age of 60 years, up from 1 billion in 2020. The number of individuals in the world who are 60 years or older will double (2.1 billion) by 2050. Between 2020 and 2050, the number of people 80 or older is projected to treble, reaching 426 million (WHO 2022).

In Bangladesh, as in other developing nations, the population is getting older (6.22% in 2001, 7.47% in 2011 and 9.25% in 2022). Bangladesh currently has 13 million persons over the age of 60 years, or 8% of the entire population (BBS 2022),

M. A. Sayem (✉)
EXIM Bank Agricultural University Bangladesh, Chapainawabganj, Bangladesh

Health Research Group, Department of Statistics, University of Rajshahi, Rajshahi, Bangladesh

M. N. Islam · M. G. Hossain
Health Research Group, Department of Statistics, University of Rajshahi, Rajshahi, Bangladesh

Department of Statistics, University of Rajshahi, Rajshahi, Bangladesh

M. Pal et al. (eds.), *Public Health and Nutrition*,
https://doi.org/10.1007/978-981-97-7890-4_16

and it is anticipated that this will rise in Bangladesh, reaching 11.5% (21.526 million) in 2030 and 21.5% (43.491 million) by 2050 (BBS 2022). The natural process of ageing is influenced by a variety of biological and psychological variables (Anil et al. 2016). Older persons' physical, mental and social well-being are all impacted by ageing (Russell et al. 1978). Quality of life, therefore, has become a major issue in several developed and developing countries, as well as developing countries such as Bangladesh.

Therefore, Bangladesh is not an exception to the global trend of an ageing population and healthcare providers must comprehend the quality of life and its associated factors because quality of life has an impact on a person's physical and mental health. To the best of our knowledge, there have been only a few studies that included quality of life and living arrangements in the quantitative analysis of factors influencing activity limitation in the Bangladeshi elderly population. Therefore, this study aimed to determine the factors influencing HRQoL and living arrangements of the ageing population in the northern part of Bangladesh. The findings from the current study may offer important information to help with the development of regional and national healthcare policy.

16.2 Materials and Methods

Study Area: North Bengal is a term used for the northwestern part of Bangladesh and the northern part of West Bengal. The Bangladesh part denotes the Rajshahi Division (Natore, Rajshahi, Sirajganj, Pabna, Bogura, Chapainawabganj, Naogaon, Joypurhat) and Rangpur Division (Dinajpur, Kurigram, Gaibandha, Lalmonirhat, Nilphamari, Panchagarh, Rangpur, Thakurgaon). Generally, it is the area lying west of Jamuna River and north of Padma River and includes the Barind Tract. The population of the region is 37,964,075 as per the 2022 census. The majority of the population follows Islam (90.04%), followed by Hinduism (9.32%), the largest minority and Others (0.64%) (BBS 2011).

Study Population: All elderly people aged 60 years and above were the population of our present study.

Sample Size Determination: The sample size was determined by using Cochran's (1977) sample size formula:

$$n = \frac{Z^2 pq}{d^2} = \frac{(1.96)^2 \times 0.64 \times 0.36}{(0.05)^2} = 354.04 \approx 355$$

where p is the estimated proportion of an attribute that is present in the population which is taken as 0.64 (Susanty et al. 2022), $q = 1—p = 1–0.64 = 0.36$, Z is the type I error at 5% level of significance = 1.96 and d is the absolute error = 0.05. However, we collected data from 540 participants because larger sample sizes give more reliable results with greater precision and power.

Sampling Technique: Multistage random sampling was used for selecting our sample from the population. In the first stage, two *Zilas* (Chapainawabganj and

Gaibandha) and two city corporations (Rajshahi and Rangpur) were randomly selected from the two divisions (Rajshahi and Rangpur). In the second stage, two *Upazilas* (Chapainawabganj Sadar and Shibganj *Upazila*) were randomly selected from five *Upazilas* of Chapainawabganj district and two wards (11 and 18) were randomly selected from Rajshahi City Corporation and two *Upazilas* (Gobindaganj and Sundarganj) were randomly selected from seven *Upazilas* of Gaibandha district and two wards (3 and 7) from Rangpur city corporation. In the third stage, four unions (Gobratola and Moharajpur from Chapainawabganj Sadar *Upazila* and Binodpur and Shahabajpur from Shibganj *Upazila*) were randomly selected and two mohallas (Malopara from 11 number ward and Shalbagan from 18 number ward) were randomly selected and four unions (Razahar and Mahimaganj from Gobindaganj Upazila and Haripur and Sreepur from Sundarganj *Upazila*) were randomly selected and two *mohallas* (Munsipara from 3 number ward and Babukhan from 7 number ward) were randomly selected. In the fourth stage, 376 (188 from the Rajshahi division and 188 from the Rangpur division) elderly women and men were randomly selected from each selected Union ($8 \times 47 = 376$) and 164 (82 from Rajshahi City Corporation and 82 from Rangpur City Corporation) elderly women and men were randomly selected from each selected ward ($4 \times 41 = 164$). All necessary information on elderly people was gathered from the respective Union Parishad office and ward council office.

Data Collection: We contacted our selected subjects and discussed the objectives of our present study. A total of 540 elderly people were considered as samples for the present study and their written consent was obtained. Twelve trained interviewers collected data from 540 elderly people using a standard questionnaire from 5 June 2022 to 18 August 2022.

Outcome Variable: HRQoL measured by EQ-5D-5L and living arrangements of elderly people was used as the dependent variable. The EQ-5D-5L has five dimensions—mobility, self-care, usual activities, pain/discomfort and anxiety/depression. There are five levels within each dimension, from 'no problems' to 'extreme problems'. The elderly completed the EQ-5D questionnaire based on their health status at that moment. The HK value set of EQ-5D-5L was developed by Wong from the JC School of Public Health and Primary Care (SPHPC). Then we dichotomized the EQ-5D-5L levels into 'no problems' (i.e. level 1) and 'problems' (i.e. levels 2–5), therefore changing the profile into frequencies of reported problems. In this study, the living arrangements of elderly people were categorized into two categories based on living with their children or not (Yes, living with children or spouse =1 or No, living alone or with others = 0).

Independent Variable: The survey questionnaire included gender, place of residence, religion, age, body mass index (BMI), marital status, schooling years, current occupation (After 60 years), previous occupation (Before 60 years), current family income (Tk.) (After 60 years), previous family income (Tk.) (Before 60 years), social benefits, family members, family support and self-rated health status as independent variables.

Statistical Analysis: Descriptive statistics was used to calculate the frequency distribution of categorical variables. Multiple binary logistic regression models were used to predict the risk factors for HRQoL and living arrangements of elderly people. Statistical significance was accepted at $p < 0.05$. Statistical analyses were carried out using the SPSS software (version IBM 25).

16.3 Results

Table 16.1 exemplifies the demographic characteristics of the ageing population in the northern part of Bangladesh. From the table, it is observed that a maximum (56.90%) of the ageing population was male and 43.10% of the ageing population was female. Most (69.60%) of the ageing population lived in rural areas and 30.40% of the ageing population lived in urban areas. Larger parts (65.70%) of the ageing population were Muslim and 14.30% of the ageing population were others (Hindu and Santal). The majority (23.00%) of the ageing population's aged were 60–70 years. Most (59.10%) of the ageing population's BMI was normal. Notably, 76.50% of the ageing population were married. A maximum (29.80%) of the ageing population were studied in high school. The majority (52.40%) of the ageing population were not working currently after 60 years. Before 60 years, most (38.30%) of the ageing population were homemakers. After 60 years, the maximum (59.10%) of the ageing population's current family income was Tk. 20,000 and less. Before 60 years, a majority (53.50%) of the ageing population‘s previous family income was Tk. 20,000 and less. A lion's share (65.70%) of the ageing population did not receive any allowance. Notably, 59.30% of the ageing population had less than five family members, 82.40% of the ageing population said that they got family support for care and 41.70% of the ageing population said that their self-rated health status was fair.

Table 16.2 represents the frequency of elderly people reporting levels 1–5 by dimension and by age group in the northern part of Bangladesh. From Table 16.2, it is explored that mobility, self-care, usual activities and pain/discomfort have significant associations with the age of the elderly in the northern part of Bangladesh.

Table 16.3 represents the association of demographic characteristics with mobility and self-care of the ageing population in the northern part of Bangladesh. From Table 16.3, it is seen that gender, place of residence, age, marital status, current occupation, family members, family support and self-rated health status were the associated factors of mobility of the ageing population in the northern part of Bangladesh. Place of residence, age, current occupation, family members and self-rated health status were the associated factors of self-care of the ageing population in the northern part of Bangladesh.

Table 16.4 represents the association of demographic characteristics with usual activities and pain/discomfort of the ageing population in the northern part of Bangladesh. From Table 16.4, it is seen that place of residence, marital status, current occupation, previous occupation, family support and self-rated health status were the associated factors of usual activities of the ageing population in the northern part of Bangladesh. Religion, social benefits, family support and self-rated health status were the associated factors of pain/discomfort of the ageing population in the northern part of Bangladesh.

Table 16.1 Demographic characteristics of the ageing population in the northern part of Bangladesh

Variable	Group	Number (%)
Gender	Male	307 (56.90)
	Female	233 (43.10)
Place of residence	Rural	376 (69.60)
	Urban	164 (30.40)
Religion	Muslim	463 (65.70)
	Other (Hindu, Santal)	77 (14.30)
Age	60–70 years	347 (64.30)
	70–80 years	124 (23.00)
	80 years and above	69 (12.80)
BMI	Underweight	27 (5.00)
	Normal	319 (59.10)
	Overweight	194 (35.90)
Marital status	Married	413 (76.50)
	Other (unmarried, widow/widower, divorced, living separately)	127 (23.50)
Schooling years	Uneducated	121 (22.40)
	Primary	136 (25.20)
	High school	161 (29.80)
	College and above	122 (22.60)
Current occupation (after 60 years)	Working	257 (47.60)
	Not working	283 (52.40)
Previous occupation (before 60 years)	Farmer	135 (25.00)
	Service	114 (21.10)
	Self-employed	84 (15.60)
	Homemaker	207 (38.30)
Current family income (Tk.) (after 60 years)	20,000 and less	319 (59.10)
	20,001–40,000	129 (23.90)
	40,001 and above	92 (17.00)
Previous family income (Tk.) (before 60 years)	20,000 and less	289 (53.50)
	20,001–40,000	168 (31.10)
	40,001 and above	83 (15.40)
Social benefits	Receive pension	41 (7.60)
	Old age allowance	144 (26.70)
	No allowance	355 (65.70)
Family members	Less than 5	185 (34.30)
	5–10	320 (59.30)
	10 and above	35 (6.50)
Family support (caring)	Yes	445 (82.40)
	No	95 (17.60)
Self-rated health status	Healthy	178 (33.00)
	Fair	225 (41.70)
	Unhealthy	137 (25.40)

Table 16.2 Frequency of ageing population reporting levels 1–5 by dimension and by age group

Dimensions	Levels, N (%)	Age 60–70, N (%)	70–80, N (%)	≥80, N (%)	χ^2 value (*p*-value)
Mobility	No problems, 336 (62.22)	257 (47.59)	59 (10.93)	20 (3.70)	86.726 ($p<0.001$)
	Slight problems, 93 (17.22)	43 (7.96)	32 (5.93)	18 (3.33)	
	Moderate problems, 63 (11.67)	27 (5.00)	16 (2.96)	20 (3.70)	
	Severe problems, 32 (5.93)	17 (3.15)	12 (2.22)	3 (0.56)	
	Extreme problems, 16 (2.96)	3 (0.56)	5 (0.93)	8 (1.48)	
Self-care	No problems, 340 (62.96)	243 (45.00)	71 (13. 15)	26 (4.81)	41.598 ($p<0.001$)
	Slight problems, 94 (17.41)	55 (10.19)	24 (4.44)	15 (2.78)	
	Moderate problems, 65 (12.04)	36 (6.67)	15 (2.78)	14 (2.59)	
	Severe problems, 21 (3.89)	7 (1.30)	8 (1.48)	6 (1.11)	
	Extreme problems, 20 (3.70)	6 (1.11)	6 (1.11)	8 (1.48)	
Usual activities	No problems, 277 (51.30)	206 (38.15)	50 (9.26)	21 (3.89)	53.390 ($p<0.001$)
	Slight problems, 134 (24.82)	84 (15.56)	35 (6.48)	15 (2.78)	
	Moderate problems, 76 (14.07)	41(7.59)	21 (3.89)	14 (2.59)	
	Severe problems, 28 (5.19)	10 (1.85)	9 (1.67)	9 (1.67)	
	Extreme problems, 25 (4.63)	6 (1.11)	9 (1.67)	10 (1.85)	
Pain/ discomfort	No problem, 115 (21.30)	95 (17.59)	11 (2.04)	9 (1.67)	33.726 ($p<0.001$)
	Slight problems, 157 (29.07)	103 (19.07)	32 (5.93)	22 (4.07)	
	Moderate problems, 132 (24.44)	81 (15.00)	36 (6.67)	15 (2.78)	
	Severe problems, 70 (12.96)	39 (7.22)	20 (3.70)	11 (2.04)	
	Extreme problems, 66 (12.22)	29 (5.37)	25 (4.63)	12 (2.22)	
Anxiety/ depression	No problems, 161 (29.81)	105 (19.44)	32 (5.93)	24 (4.44)	3.733 (0.880)
	Slight problems, 158 (29.26)	98 (18.19)	38 (7.04)	22 (4.07)	
	Moderate problems, 118 (21.85)	79 (14.63)	28 (5.19)	11 (2.04)	
	Severe problems, 65 (12.04)	42 (7.78)	15 (2.78)	8 (1.48)	
	Extreme problems, 38 (7.04)	23 (4.26)	11(2.04)	4 (0.74)	

1 = No problems, 2 = slight problems, 3 = moderate problems, 4 = severe problems, 5 = extreme problems

Table 16.3 Associated factors of demographic characteristics with mobility and self-care of the ageing population in the northern part of Bangladesh

Variable	Group	Mobility AOR (95% CI), p	Self-care AOR (95% CI),p
Gender	Male vs female[R]	0.396 (0.168,0.935), 0.034[a]	0.641 (0.275,1.493), 0.303
Place of residence	Rural vs urban[R]	0.472 (0.283,0.788), 0.004[a]	0.317 (0.193,0.520), 0.000[a]
Religion	Muslim vs other[R]	0.895 (0.460,1.743), 0.744	0.636 (0.341,1.185), 0.154
Age	60–70 vs ≥80[R]	0.227 (0.112, 0.459), 0.000[a]	0.487 (0.250,0.946), 0.034[a]
	70–80 vs ≥80[R]	0.594 (0.278,1.268), 0.178	0.478 (0.231,0.989), 0.047[a]
BMI	Underweight vs overweight[R]	0.607 (0.221,1.668), 0.333	1.623 (0.596,4.117), 0.343
	Normal vs overweight[R]	0.922 (0.580,1.465), 0.731	0.800 (0.504,1.269), 0.343
Marital status	Married vs other[R]	0.493 (0.282,0.860), 0.013[a]	0.705 (0.400,1.240), 0.225
Schooling years	Uneducated vs college and above[R]	2.163 (0.990,4.728), 0.053	0.982 (0.448,2.148), 0.963
	Primary vs college and above[R]	1.042 (0.495,2.192), 0.914	1.378 (0.666,2.852), 0.387
	High school vs college and above[R]	0.892 (0.453,1.757), 0.741	1.032 (0.532,2.005), 0.925
Current occupation (after 60 years)	Working vs not working[R]	0.497 (0.304,0.811), 0.005[a]	0.353 (0.217,0.575), 0.000[a]

(continued)

Table 16.3 (continued)

Variable	Group	Mobility AOR (95% CI), p	Self-care AOR (95% CI),p
Previous occupation (before 60 years)	Farmer vs homemaker[R]	1.866 (0.685,5.084), 0.223	2.152 (0.797,5.808), 0.130
	Service vs homemaker[R]	1.570 (0.606,4.065), 0.353	2.025 (0.798,5.137), 0.137
	Self-employed vs homemaker[R]	2.494 (0.921,6.753), 0.072	1.634 (0.608,4.388), 0.330
Current family income (Tk.) (after 60 years)	Less than 20,000 vs greater than 40000[R]	0.668 (0.303,1.468), 0.315	1.062 (0.492,2.290), 0.878
	20,001–40,000 vs greater than 40000[R]	0.760 (0.364,1.587), 0.465	1.431 (0.703,2.912), 0.323
Previous family income (Tk.) (before 60 years)	Less than 20,000 vs greater than 40,000[R]	0.739 (0.317,1.724), 0.484	0.811 (0.356,1.846), 0.618
	20,001–40,000 vs greater than 40,000[R]	1.070 (0.507,2.257), 0.859	1.675 (0.814,3.445), 0.161
Social benefits	Receive pension vs no allowance[R]	1.800 (0.733,4.420), 0.200	1.945 (0.808,4.681), 0.138
	Old age allowance vs no allowance[R]	1.617 (0.958,2.730), 0.072	1.228 (0.739,2.040), 0.428
Family members	1–5 vs greater than 10[R]	2.689 (0.963,7.507), 0.059	0.212 (0.077,0.582), 0.003[a]
	5–10 vs greater than 10[R]	2.833 (1.091,7.356), 0.032[a]	0.342 (0.134,0.869), 0.024[a]
Family support	Yes vs no[R]	2.582 (1.379,4.835), 0.003[a]	0.784 (0.433,1.420), 0.421
Self-rated health status	Healthy vs unhealthy[R]	0.186 (0.100,0.346), 0.000[a]	0.194 (0.106,0.356), 0.000[a]
	Fair vs unhealthy[R]	0.515 (0.298,0.889), 0.017[a]	0.277 (0.161,0.477), 0.000[a]

[a]Significant at 5% level of significance; R = reference; AOR = adjusted odds ratio; CI = confidence interval

Table 16.4 Associated factors of demographic characteristics with usual activities and pain/discomfort of the ageing population in the northern part of Bangladesh

Variable	Group	Usual activities AOR (95% CI), p	Pain/discomfort AOR (95% CI), p
Gender	Male vs female[R]	0.687 (0.291,1.620), 0.391	0.448 (0.157,1.276), 0.133
Place of residence	Rural vs urban[R]	0.262 (0.158,0.434), 0.000[a]	0.766 (0.437,1.344), 0.353
Religion	Muslim vs other[R]	1.133 (0.596,2.152), 0.704	0.362 (0.143,919), 0.033[a]
Age	60–70 vs ≥80[R]	0.581 (0.287,1.175), 0.131	0.567 (0.235, 1.368), 0.207
	70–80 vs ≥80[R]	0.886 (0.415,1.893), 0.755	1.893 (0.671,5.341), 0.228
BMI	Underweight vs overweight[R]	0.911 (0.325,2.550), 0.859	1.398 (0.268,7.285), 0.691
	Normal vs overweight[R]	0.904 (0.577,1.416), 0.659	0.734 (0.436,1.237), 0.245
Marital status	Married vs other[R]	0.522 (0.298,0.915), 0.023[a]	0.803 (0.383,1.687), 0.563
Schooling years	Uneducated vs college and above[R]	1.307 (0.611,2.799), 0.490	0.940 (0.400,2.206), 0.886
	Primary vs college and above[R]	0.931 (0.454,1.911), 0.846	0.977 (0.436,2.186), 0.954
	High school vs college and above[R]	1.577 (0.816,3.046), 0.175	1.255 (0.621,2.536), 0.526
Current occupation (after 60 years)	Working vs not working[R]	0.455 (0.282,0.734), 0.001[a]	1.036 (0.598,1.795), 0.899

(continued)

Table 16.4 (continued)

Variable	Group	Usual activities AOR (95% CI), p	Pain/discomfort AOR (95% CI), p
Previous occupation (before 60 years)	Farmer vs homemaker[R]	2.753 (1.033,7.335), 0.043[a]	2.760 (0.876,8.697), 0.083
	Service vs homemaker[R]	1.656 (0.646,4.243), 0.293	1.619 (0.693,3.782), 0.395
	Self-employed vs homemaker[R]	1.396 (0.520,3.748), 0.508	2.410 (0.756,7.688), 0.137
Current family income (Tk.) (after 60 years)	Less than 20,000 vs greater than 40,000[R]	0.634 (0.296,1.358), 0.240	1.619 (0.693,3.782), 0.266
	20,001–40,000 vs greater than 40,000[R]	0.565 (0.275,1.161), 0.120	1.191 (0.554,2.563), 0.655
Previous family income (Tk.) (before 60 years)	Less than 20,000 vs greater than 40,000[R]	0.727 (0.321,1.643), 0.443	0.879 (0.347,2.228), 0.786
	20,001–40,000 vs greater than 40,000[R]	0.771 (0.373,1.591), 0.481	1.003 (0.453,2.224), 0.993
Social benefits	Receive pension vs no allowance[R]	1.761 (0.728,4.259), 0.209	1.572 (0.617,4.006), 0.343
	Old age allowance vs no allowance[R]	1.497 (0.897,2.497), 0.122	2.830 (1.455,5.501), 0.002[a]
Family members	1–5 vs greater than 10[R]	0.428 (0.154,1.191), 0.104	1.234 (0.404,3.766), 0.712
	5–10 vs greater than 10[R]	0.621 (0.238,1.618), 0.330	1.671 (0.596,4.689), 0.329
Family support	Yes vs no[R]	1.950 (1.066,3.567), 0.030[a]	2.107 (1.036,4.284), 0.040[a]
Self-rated health status	Healthy vs unhealthy[R]	0.107 (0.058,0.199), 0.000[a]	0.074 (0.028,0.197), 0.000[a]
	Fair vs unhealthy[R]	0.288 (0.165,0.503), 0.000[a]	0.214 (0.080,0.571), 0.002[a]

[a]Significant at 5% level of significance; R = reference; AOR = adjusted odds ratio; CI = confidence interval

Table 16.5 Associated factors of demographic characteristics with anxiety/depression and living arrangements of the ageing population in the northern part of Bangladesh

Variable	Group	Anxiety/depression AOR (95% CI), p	Living arrangements AOR (95% CI), p
Gender	Male vs female[R]	0.982 (0.402,2.401), 0.968	2.157 (0.851,5.465), 0.105
Place of residence	Rural vs urban[R]	0.265 (0.153,0.459), 0.000[a]	0.579 (0.344,0.975), 0.040[a]
Religion	Muslim vs other[R]	0.912 (0.462,1.799), 0.790	1.147 (0.576,2.286), 0.696
Age	60–70 vs ≥80[R]	1.044 (0.522,2.089), 0.902	1.240 (0.567,2.713), 0.589
	70–80 vs ≥80[R]	1.277 (0.605,2.692), 0.521	1.402 (0.593,3.311), 0.441
BMI	Underweight vs overweight[R]	3.430 (0.932,12.523), 0.064	0.933 (0.334,2.605), 0.895
	Normal vs overweight[R]	1.795 (1.145,2.815), 0.011[a]	2.592 (1.631,4.121), 0.000[a]
Marital status	Married vs other[R]	1.015 (0.556,1.853), 0.960	0.050 (0.020,0.121), 0.000[a]
Schooling years	Uneducated vs college and above[R]	0.760 (0.352,1.641), 0.485	2.987 (1.392,6.407), 0.005[a]
	Primary vs college and above[R]	0.619 (0.300,1.276), 0.194	2.072 (1.033,4.154), 0.040[a]
	High school vs college and above[R]	0.947 (0.482,1.863), 0.876	1.754 (0.952,3.232), 0.072

(continued)

Table 16.5 (continued)

Variable	Group	Anxiety/depression AOR (95% CI), p	Living arrangements AOR (95% CI), p
Current occupation (after 60 years)	Working vs not working[R]	0.997 (0.606,1.640), 0.990	0.935 (0.580,1.506), 0.781
Previous occupation (before 60 years)	Farmer vs homemaker[R]	1.357 (0.499,3.690), 0.550	0.723 (0.263,1.987), 0.529
	Service vs homemaker[R]	1.270 (0.469,3.436), 0.638	0.525 (0.195,1.412), 0.202
	Self-employed vs homemaker[R]	1.110 (0.398,3.095), 0.841	1.456 (0.488,4.347), 0.501
Current family income (Tk.) (after 60 years)	Less than 20,000 vs greater than 40,000[R]	2.656 (1.269,5.561), 0.010[a]	0.521 (0.232,1.170), 0.114
	20,001–40,000 vs greater than 40,000[R]	1.294 (0.668,2.508), 0.445	0.471 (0.220,1.007), 0.052
Previous family income (Tk.) (before 60 years)	Less than 20,000 vs greater than 40,000[R]	1.433 (0.652,3.150), 0.371	1.748 (0.744,4.108), 0.200
	20,001–40,000 vs greater than 40,000[R]	1.122(0.567,2.219), 0.741	1.320 (0.618,2.821), 0.474
Social benefits	Receive pension vs no allowance[R]	1.288 (0.517,3.211), 0.587	0.435 (0.183,1.035), 0.060
	Old age allowance vs no allowance[R]	1.393 (0.826,2.350), 0.213	0.825 (0.479,1.421), 0.488
Family members	1–5 vs greater than 10[R]	2.480 (0.945,6.503), 0.065	0.232 (0.069,0.782), 0.018[a]
	5–10 vs greater than 10[R]	1.849 (0.756,4.522), 0.178	0.424 (0.133,1.357), 0.148
Family support	Yes vs no[R]	0.602 (0.312,1.161), 0.130	2.542 (1.376,4.694), 0.003[a]
Self-rated health status	Healthy vs unhealthy[R]	0.313 (0.166,0.589), 0.000[a]	1.281 (0.697,2.357), 0.425
	Fair vs unhealthy[R]	0.680 (0.367,1.257), 0.219	1.341 (0.745,2.412), 0.328

[a]Significant at 5% level of significance; R = reference; AOR = Adjusted odds ratio; CI = confidence interval

Table 16.5 shows the association of demographic characteristics with pain/discomfort, anxiety/depression and living arrangements of the ageing population in the northern part of Bangladesh. Table 16.5 shows that place of residence, BMI, current family income and self-rated health status were the associated factors of anxiety/depression of the ageing population in the northern part of Bangladesh. Place of residence, BMI, marital status, schooling years, family members and family support were affecting the living arrangements of the ageing population in the northern part of Bangladesh.

16.4 Discussion

In the present study, we investigated the risk factors of HRQoL measured by EQ-5D-5L and the living arrangements of elderly people. Age, gender, educational level and marital status (Jafari et al. 2020; Lin et al. 2017; Avila-Funes et al. 2008) were significantly associated with mobility. We have found that gender, place of residence, age, marital status, current occupation, family members, family support and self-rated health status were the associated factors of mobility of the ageing population in the northern part of Bangladesh. Age, educational level and perceived health status (Kim and Lee 2019) were the associated factors of self-care in the ageing population. We observed that place of residence, age, current occupation; family members and self-rated health status were the associated factors of self-care of the ageing population in the northern part of Bangladesh. Age, family and social support factors (Chen et al. 2020) were the associated factors of the usual activities of the ageing population. We explored that place of residence marital status, current occupation, previous occupation, family support and self-rated health status were the associated factors of usual activities of the ageing population in the northern part of Bangladesh. Age (Shi et al. 2010; Elliott et al. 1999; Helme and Gibson 2001), gender (Shi et al. 2010) and educational level (Shi et al. 2010) were the associated factors of pain/discomfort of the ageing population. We observed that religion, social benefits, family support and self-rated health status were the associated factors of pain/discomfort of the ageing population in the northern part of Bangladesh. Family income (Siegel et al. 2004; Adams et al. 2004) and self-rated health status (Hybels et al. 2001; Biderman et al. 2002) were the associated factors of anxiety/depression in the ageing population. We found that place of residence, BMI, current family income and self-rated health status were the associated factors of anxiety/depression of the ageing population in the northern part of Bangladesh. Education (Panigrahi 2009; Prakash 1999), place of residence (Prakash 1999) and family size (Velkoff 2001) were affecting the living arrangements of the ageing population. We explored that place of residence, BMI, marital status, schooling years, family members and family support were affecting the living arrangements of the ageing population in the northern part of Bangladesh.

16.5 Limitations

There are some limitations to the current study. First, there might be respondent bias as the findings were self-reported. Second, this is a cross-sectional study; a longitudinal study might be helpful to reveal better results. Third, the assessment of chronic diseases was based on self-reporting, prescriptions and medications available to the individuals. Fourth, our study is limited to quantitative analysis, as we did not explore the qualitative aspects of older adults' HRQoL.

16.6 Conclusion

The results of this study provide an overview of important factors that influence HRQoL and living arrangements of older adults. In terms of self-rated health quality of life, mobility and usual activity were the two major problems for the elderly of the Northern part of Bangladesh. These factors, which were modifiable to some extent, could be potential targets for improving the health and quality of life among the oldest old adults.

References

Adams KB, Sanders S, Auth EA (2004) Loneliness and depression in independent living retirement communities: risk and resilience factors. Aging Ment Health 8(6):475–485
Anil R, Prasad K, Puttaswamy M (2016) The prevalence of loneliness and its determinants among geriatric population in Bengaluru City, Karnataka, India. Int J Commun Med Public Health 3(11):3246–3251
Avila-Funes JA, Gray-Donald K, Payette H (2008) Association of nutritional risk and depressive symptoms with physical performance in the elderly: the Quebec longitudinal study of nutrition as a determinant of successful aging (NuAge). J Am Coll Nutr 27(4):492–498
BBS (2011) Population and housing census 2011 (Zila Series and Community Series). Bangladesh Bureau of Statistics, Dhaka. Archived from the original on 2022-09-20. Accessed 23 July 2023
BBS (2022) Preliminary report on population and housing census 2022: Bangla version. Bangladesh Bureau of Statistics, Dhaka
Biderman A, Cwikel J, Fried AV, Galinsky D (2002) Depression and falls among community-dwelling elderly people: a search for common risk factors. J Epidemiol Community Health 56(8):631–636
Chen C, Liu GG, Shi QL, Sun Y, Zhang H, Wang MJ, Jia HP, Zhao YL, Yao Y (2020) Health-related quality of life and associated factors among oldest-old in China. J Nutr Health Aging 24:330–338
Cochran WG (1977) Sampling techniques. John Wiley and Sons Inc., New York
Cooper JK, Kohlmann T, Michael JA, Haffer SC, Stevic M (2001) Health outcomes. New quality measure for Medicare. Int J Qual Health Care 13(1):9–16
Elliott AM, Smith BH, Penny KI, Smith WC, Chambers WA (1999) The epidemiology of chronic pain in the community. Lancet 354(9186):1248–1252
Gold MR, Muennig P (2002) Measure-dependent variation in burden of disease estimates: implications for policy. Med Care 40:260–266
Guyatt G (1997) Insights and limitations from health-related quality-of-life research. J Gen Intern Med 12(11):720

Hahn EA, Cella D, Chassany O, Fairclough DL, Wong GY, Hays RD, Clinical Significance Consensus Meeting Group (2007) Precision of health-related quality-of-life data compared with other clinical measures. Mayo Clin Proc 82(10):1244–1254

Helme RD, Gibson SJ (2001) The epidemiology of pain in elderly people. Clin Geriatr Med 17(3):417–431

Hybels CF, Blazer DG, Pieper CF (2001) Toward a threshold for subthreshold depression: an analysis of correlates of depression by severity of symptoms using data from an elderly community sample. The Gerontologist 41(3):357–365

Jafari A, Aminisani N, Shamshirgaran SM, Rastgoo L, Gilani N (2020) Predictors of mobility limitation in older adults: a structural equation modelling analysis. Baltic J Health Phys Activity 12(1):3

Kim MY, Lee EJ (2019) Factors affecting self-care behaviour levels among elderly patients with type 2 diabetes: a quantile regression approach. Medicina 55(7):340

Lin SI, Lee HC, Chang KC, Yang YC, Tsauo JY (2017) Functional mobility and it's contributing factors for older adults in different cities in Taiwan. J Formos Med Assoc 116(2):72–79

Panigrahi AK (2009) Determinants of living arrangements of elderly in Orissa: an analysis. Institute for Social and Economic Change, Bangalore

Prakash IJ (1999) Ageing in India (No. WHO/HSC/AHE/99.2). World Health Organization, Geneva

Russell D, Peplau LA, Ferguson ML (1978) Developing a measure of loneliness. J Pers Assess 42(3):290–294

Santanasto AJ, Newman AB, Strotmeyer ES, Boudreau RM, Goodpaster BH, Glynn NW (2015) Effects of changes in regional body composition on physical function in older adults: a pilot randomized controlled trial. J Nutr Health Aging 19:913–921

Shi Y, Hooten WM, Roberts RO, Warner DO (2010) Modifiable risk factors for incidence of pain in older adults. Pain 151(2):366–371

Siegel MJ, Bradley EH, Gallo WT, Kasl SV (2004) The effect of spousal mental and physical health on husbands' and wives' depressive symptoms, among older adults: longitudinal evidence from the health and retirement survey. J Aging Health 16(3):398–425

Susanty S, Chung MH, Chiu HY, Chi MJ, Hu SH, Kuo CL, Chuang YH (2022) Prevalence of loneliness and associated factors among community-dwelling older adults in Indonesia: a cross-sectional study. Int J Environ Res Public Health 19(8):4911

Velkoff VA (2001) Living arrangements and Well-being of the older population: future research direction. Popul Bull United Nations 42(43):376–385

World Health Organization (2022) Ageing and Health. https://www.who.int/news-room/fact-sheets/detail/ageing-and-health

17 Prevalence of Loneliness and Its Associated Factors among Older Adults in the Northern Part of Bangladesh

Md. Abu Sayem, Md. Nurul Islam, and Md. Golam Hossain

17.1 Introduction

Loneliness is a prevalent mental health issue, particularly in older adults (Donovan and Blazer 2020), and is brought on by exposure to a number of aging-related issues. It is a subjective sensation of unhappiness (Russell et al. 1978), melancholy (Morlett Paredes et al. 2021), emptiness, distress, sorrow, loneliness, loss of purpose, non-belongingness, or loneliness (Perissinotto et al. 2012). According to some academics, persons who do not have enough or the right kind of social connections may experience loneliness as a result of their unfulfilled social needs (Hawkley and Cacioppo 2010).

The World Health Organization has estimated by 2030, one in six people in the world will be 60 years of age or older. The number of individuals over 60 will rise from 1 billion in 2020 to 1.4 billion by this time. By 2050, there will be 2.1 billion people in the globe who are 60 years of age or older, a doubling of the current figure. The number of adults 80 years of age or older is expected to triple, to 426 million, between 2020 and 2050 (WHO 2022).

In Bangladesh, as in other developing nations, the population is getting older (6.22% in 2001, 7.47% in 2011, and 9.25% in 2022). Bangladesh currently has 13 million people over the age of 60 years or over, which is 8% of the entire population (BBS 2022), and it is anticipated that this will rise in Bangladesh, reaching 11.5%

M. A. Sayem (✉)
EXIM Bank Agricultural University Bangladesh, Chapainawabganj, Bangladesh

Health Research Group, Department of Statistics, University of Rajshahi, Rajshahi, Bangladesh

M. N. Islam · M. G. Hossain
Health Research Group, Department of Statistics, University of Rajshahi, Rajshahi, Bangladesh

Department of Statistics, University of Rajshahi, Rajshahi, Bangladesh

M. Pal et al. (eds.), *Public Health and Nutrition*,
https://doi.org/10.1007/978-981-97-7890-4_17

(21.526 million) in 2030 and 21.5% (43.491 million) by 2050 (BBS 2022). The natural process of aging is influenced by a variety of biological and psychological variables (Anil et al. 2016). Older persons' mental, physical, and social well-being are all impacted by aging (Russell et al. 1978). In Europe, a significant proportion of the elderly population suffers from loneliness (Sandu et al. 2021). During the ongoing epidemic, the study found that elderly persons in Bangladesh had a decreased incidence of loneliness (Mistry et al. 2022). More than 54% of people who are older have experienced varying degrees of loneliness. Self-reported morbidities and socio-demographic characteristics were considered in order to identify the statistically significant risk factors for growing loneliness (Rahman et al. 2019). In older folks, loneliness is more common in some nations than others. The prevalence of loneliness varies from country to country. Loneliness, therefore, has become a major issue in a number of developed and developing countries, as well as developing countries such as Bangladesh.

Therefore, Bangladesh is not an exception to the global trend of an older population, and it is crucial for healthcare providers to comprehend the incidence of loneliness and its allied causes as loneliness has a negative effect on a person's mental and physical health. The incidence of loneliness among older persons in Bangladesh's northern region has, as far as we are aware, not been the subject of many studies conducted there. Therefore, this study set out to ascertain the prevalence of loneliness and the characteristics that are linked to it among the elderly population in the northern region of Bangladesh. The hypothesis of the study is to be a relationship between loneliness in older persons and their socio-demographic factors.

17.2 Materials and Methods

Study Area: The Rajshahi division (Rajshahi, Natore, Sirajganj, Bogura, Pabna, Naogaon, Chapainawabganj, Joypurhat) and the Rangpur division (Dinajpur, Kurigram, Gaibandha, Lalmonirhat, Nilphamari, Panchagarh, Rangpur, Thakurgaon) are included in the Northern part of Bangladesh. It generally refers to the region that is north of the Padma River and west of the Jamuna River, which includes the Barind Tract. According to the census conducted in 2022, the region has 37,964,075 residents. Islam is practiced by the majority of people (90.04%), followed by Hinduism (9.32%), the largest minority, and other religions (0.64%) (BBS 2022).

Study Population: The population of this study was all older adults 60 years of age and older living in the northern part of Bangladesh.

Sample Size Determination: The Cochran's (1977) sample size formula was used to get the required sample size for the study:

$$n = \frac{m}{M}$$

where p is the estimated percentage of a characteristic in the population which has been taken as 0.64 (Susanty et al. 2022), $q = 1—\mathrm{p} = 1–0.64 = 0.36$, Z is the Type I error at a 5% level of significance = 1.96, and d is the absolute error = 0.05. The formula estimated that 355 samples would be the minimum for our study. However, we collected data from 540 participants because larger sample sizes give more reliable results with greater precision and power.

Sampling Technique: We selected our sample from the population using multi-stage random sampling. Two Zilas (Chapainawabganj and Gaibandha) and two city corporations (Rajshahi and Rangpur) were randomly selected in the first stage from the two divisions (Rajshahi and Rangpur). In the second stage, two Upazilas (Shibganj Upazila and Chapainawabganj Sadar) were randomly selected out of the five Upazilas in the district of Chapainawabganj and two wards (11 and 18) were randomly selected from Rajshahi city corporation and two Upazilas (Gobindaganj and Sundarganj) were randomly selected from seven Upazilas of Gaibandha district and two wards (3 and 7) from Rangpur city corporation. In the third stage, four unions (Gobratola and Moharajpur from Chapainawabganj Sadar Upazila and Binodpur and Shahabajpur from Shibganj Upazila) were randomly selected and two mohallas (Malopara from 11 number ward and Shalbagan from 18 number ward) were randomly selected and four unions (Razahar and Mahimaganj from Gobindaganj Upazila and Haripur and Sreepur from Sundarganj Upazila) were randomly selected and two mohallas (Munsipara from 3 number ward and Babukhan from 7 number ward) were randomly selected. In the fourth stage, 376 (188 from Rajshahi division and 188 from Rangpur division) older women and men were chosen at random from each chosen Union (8X47 = 376) and 164 (82 from Rajshahi city corporation and 82 from Rangpur city corporation) older women and men were chosen at random from each chosen ward (4X41) =164). The necessary information for selecting the sample was obtained from the respective Union Parishad office and ward council office.

Data Collection: We discussed the objective of our current study with the selected subjects, and we obtained written consent from 540 older people. Data were gathered from 540 old individuals between June 5, 2022, and August 18, 2022, by 12 interviewers.

Outcome Variable: The outcome variable of the study was loneliness of older adults. Feelings of social isolation or loneliness were measured using the self-reported Three-Item Loneliness Scale, based on the Revised University of California, Los Angeles (UCLA) Loneliness Scale (Russell et al. 1978). The Three-Item Loneliness Scale is a questionnaire that is administered by interviewers, and there is a 3-point rating system for each question: 3 = frequently; 1 = hardly ever; 2 = sometimes. We classified our sample into two groups (1) not lonely (scores 3–5; code =0) and (2) lonely (scores 6–9, code = 1) (Steptoe et al. 2013).

Independent Variables: The survey questionnaire included age, marital status, family members, current occupation, current family income, social benefits, current dwelling, living arrangements, material deprivation, disability, family support, self-rated health status, and anxiety/depression as independent variables. All independent variables were categorical.

Statistical Analysis: The frequency distribution of categorical variables was computed using descriptive statistics. The chi-square test of association was used in bivariate analysis to identify the factors that are linked to loneliness. Afterward, using SPSS 23, the relevant components were added to a multiple binary logistic regression model in order to predict the risk factors for loneliness.

17.3 Results

Table 17.1 shows the general characteristics of aging people in the northern part of Bangladesh. From the table, it was observed that the majority (23.00%) of the older adults aged 60–70 years. Most (76.50%) of the older adults were married. The maximum (59.30%) of the older adults had less than five family members. The majority (52.40%) of the older adults were not working currently after 60 years. Currently, the family income of the maximum (59.10%) of the older adults was Tk. 20,000 and less. A lion's share (65.70%) of the older adults did not receive any allowance. Most (77.00%) of the older adults reported that they lived in their own house. Notably, 38.90% of the older adults lived with their spouse and 61.10% of the older adults were living with others (Alone, unmarried sons/daughters, married sons/daughters). The maximum (60.70%) of the older adults reported that they did not suffer any material deprivation. Notably, 72.60% of the older adults reported that they did not have any disability problems and 82.40% of the older adults said that they got formal family care. The majority (41.70%) of the older adults informed that their self-rated health status was fair and 72.20% of the older adults suffered from anxiety/depression.

Table 17.2 represents the prevalence of loneliness among aging people in the northern part of Bangladesh. From the table, we observed that the overall prevalence of self-reported loneliness was 61.85%. Prevalence of loneliness was higher among males than females (35.93% vs 25.92%).

Table 17.3 shows the association between the level of loneliness and socio-demographic characteristics of the older adults of the northern part of Bangladesh. From the table, it was obtained that marital status, disability, self-rated health status, and anxiety/depression were significantly associated with the level of loneliness of the older adults at a 5% level of significance.

Table 17.4 points out the binary logistic regression analysis to identify the associated factors of loneliness in older adults. From Table 17.5, it was seen that disabled elderly had a 2.032-fold higher chance of feeling loneliness compared to those who were not disabled. Elderly who had fair health had a 1.651-fold more chance of feeling loneliness than the healthy elderly. Unhealthy elderly had a 2.630-fold more chance of feeling loneliness than unhealthy elderly people. Elderly who suffered from anxiety/depression had a 1.621-fold higher chance of feeling loneliness compared to elderly who did not suffer from anxiety/depression.

Table 17.5 indicates the classification table for the level of loneliness of the older adults. From Table 17.4, it was observed that the model was correctly classified by 64.30% of cases. A cut point was identified that optimized sensitivity (85.60%) which was the percentage of correct prediction of category of interest and specificity (29.60%) which was the percentage of true negative.

Table 17.1 Different socio-demographic characteristics of the older adults

Variable	Group	Number (%)
Age	60–70	347 (64.30)
	70–80	124 (23.00)
	80 and above	69 (12.80)
Marital status	Married	413 (76.50)
	Other (unmarried, widow/widower, divorced, living separately)	127 (23.50)
Family members	Less than 5	185 (34.30)
	5–10	320 (59.30)
	10 and above	35 (6.50)
Current occupation	Working	257 (47.60)
	Not working	283 (52.40)
Current family income (Tk.)	20,000 and less	319 (59.10)
	20,001–40,000	129 (23.90)
	40,001 and above	92 (17.00)
Social benefits	Receive pension	41 (7.60)
	Old age allowance	144 (26.70)
	No allowance	355 (65.70)
Owns current dwelling	Yes	416 (77.00)
	No	124 (23.00)
Living arrangements	Living with spouse	210 (38.90)
	Other (alone, unmarried sons/daughters, married sons/daughters)	330 (61.10)
Material deprivation	Yes (at least one)	212 (39.30)
	No	328 (60.70)
Disability	Yes	148 (27.40)
	No	392 (72.60)
Family support (caring)	Yes	445 (82.40)
	No	95 (17.60)
Self-rated health status	Healthy	178 (33.00)
	Fair	225 (41.70)
	Unhealthy	137 (25.40)
Anxiety/depression	No problems	161 (29.80)
	Problems	379 (70.20)

Table 17.2 Prevalence of loneliness among older adults

Variable	Group	Male	Female	Total frequency (%)
Level of loneliness	Not lonely	113 (20.93)	93 (17.22)	206 (38.15)
	Lonely	194 (35.93)	140 (25.92)	334 (61.85)

Table 17.3 Association between level of loneliness and socio-demographic characteristics of the older adults

Variable	Group	χ^2 value (*p* value)
Age	60–70	1.939 (0.379)
	70–80	
	80 and above	
Marital status	Married	3.895 (0.048)*
	Other (unmarried, widow/widower, divorced, living separately)	
Family members	Less than 5	1.941 (0.379)
	5–10	
	10 and above	
Current occupation	Working	3.779 (0.052)
	Not working	
Current family income (Tk.)	20,000 and less	3.699 (0.157)
	20,001–40,000	
	40,001 and above	
Social benefits	Receive pension	0.389 (0.823)
	Old age allowance	
	No allowance	
Owns current dwelling	Yes	3.355 (0.067)
	No	
Living arrangements	Living with spouse	1.567 (0.211)
	Other (alone, unmarried sons/daughters, married sons/daughters)	
Material deprivation	Yes	3.375 (0.066)
	No	
Disability	Yes	6.204 (0.013)*
	No	
Family support (caring)	Yes	0.003 (0.955)
	No	
Self-rated health status	Healthy	19.711 (0.000)*
	Fair	
	Unhealthy	
Co-morbidities	Yes	0.992 (0.319)
	No	
Anxiety/depression	No problems	7.975 (0.005)*
	Problems	

*Significant at 5% level of significance

Table 17.4 Binary logistic regression analysis of loneliness of the older adults

Variables	B	S.E.	Wald	DF	P value	AOR	95% CI for AOR Lower	Upper
Marital status								
Other vs Married[R]	0.305	0.229	1.765	1	0.184	1.356	0.865	2.125
Disability								
Yes vs No[R]	0.709*	0.210	11.363	1	0.001	2.032	1.345	3.069
Self-rated health status								
Fair vs Healthy[R]	0.502*	0.212	5.594	1	0.018	1.651	1.090	2.502
Unhealthy vs Healthy[R]	0.967*	0.260	13.777	1	0.000	2.630	1.578	4.381
Anxiety/depression								
Problems vs no problems[R]	0.483*	0.203	5.661	1	0.017	1.621	1.089	2.414

N.B.: R: reference case; B: regression coefficient; SE: standard error; DF: degrees of freedom; AOR: adjusted odds ratio; CI: confidence interval
*Significant at 5% level of significance

Table 17.5 Classification table for the level of loneliness of the older adults

Observed		Predicted: Level of loneliness – Not lonely	Lonely	Percentage correct
Level of loneliness	Not lonely	61	145	29.60
	Lonely	48	286	85.60
Overall percentage				64.30

N.B.: The cut value is 0.50

17.4 Discussion

In this study, we investigated the loneliness experienced by senior citizens living in the northern region of Bangladesh. According to this study, loneliness affects 61.85% of older individuals in the part of Bangladesh. The results of the current study indicated a significant issue when compared to research done in Western and Eastern nations (Dahlberg et al. 2018; Tomstad et al. 2017; Perissinotto et al. 2012; Heikkinen and Kauppinen 2011). According to the findings from another study, older persons with physical limitations reported feeling more alone (Anil et al. 2016; Arslantaş et al. 2015; Aartsen and Jylhä 2011; Buchman et al. 2010; Wilson et al. 2007; Fried and Guralnik 1997; Ginn and Arber 1991). We found in the current study that older people with disabilities were more likely to experience loneliness. Previous studies found that poor self-reported health was significantly related to loneliness in older adults (Rouxel et al. 2017; Mansfield et al. 2016; Arslantaş et al. 2015; Burholt and Scharf 2014). In our study, self-reported health status (Fair and unhealthy) was notably connected to loneliness in older adults. We found that anxiety/depression was the most important predictor of loneliness among aging people, and the same findings had been found in different studies with different populations

(Igbokwe et al. 2020; Beutel et al. 2017; Chrostek et al. 2016; Muyan et al. 2016; Sündermann et al. 2014; Switaj et al. 2014; Aartsen and Jylhä 2011; Buchman et al. 2010; Ginn and Arber 1991).

17.5 Limitations

The major limitations of the current study were the following: (1) most of the information was gathered and self-reported by respondents, so respondent bias may exist, and (2) this was a cross-sectional study; we never looked at the change in behavior of the respondents the next time.

17.6 Conclusions

In the present study, we investigated the loneliness among aging people in the northern part of Bangladesh using suitable statistical techniques and model/s. A remarkable number of aging people reported that they were suffering from loneliness. Our selected statistical model provided that disability, health condition, and anxiety/depression were the most important predictors of loneliness among aging people. The results of this study can serve as a foundation for future studies on loneliness and well as provide the guidelines for improving the mental health policy of older adults for overcoming the problem.

References

Aartsen M, Jylhä M (2011) Onset of loneliness in older adults: results of a 28 year prospective study. Eur J Ageing 8:31–38

Anil R, Prasad K, Puttaswamy M (2016) The prevalence of loneliness and its determinants among geriatric population in Bengaluru City, Karnataka, India. Int J Commun Med Public Health 3(11):3246–3251. https://doi.org/10.18203/2394-6040.ijcmph20163944

Arslantaş H, Adana F, Ergin FA, Kayar D, Gülçin ACAR (2015) Loneliness in elderly people, associated factors and its correlation with quality of life: a field study from Western Turkey. Iran J Public Health 44(1):43

BBS (2022) Preliminary report on population and housing census 2022: Bangla version. Bangladesh Bureau of Statistics, Dhaka

Beutel ME, Klein EM, Brähler E, Reiner I, Jünger C, Michal M, Tibubos AN (2017) Loneliness in the general population: prevalence, determinants and relations to mental health. BMC Psychiatry 17(1):1–7. https://doi.org/10.1186/s12888-017-1262-x

Buchman AS, Boyle PA, Wilson RS, James BD, Leurgans SE, Arnold SE, Bennett DA (2010) Loneliness and the rate of motor decline in old age: the rush memory and aging project, a community-based cohort study. BMC Geriatr 10:1–8

Burholt V, Scharf T (2014) Poor health and loneliness in later life: the role of depressive symptoms, social resources, and rural environments. J Gerontol B Psychol Sci Soc Sci 69(2):311–324

Chrostek A, Grygiel P, Anczewska M, Wciórka J, Świtaj P (2016) The intensity and correlates of the feelings of loneliness in people with psychosis. Compr Psychiatry 70:190–199. https://doi.org/10.1016/j.comppsych.2016.07.015

Cochran WG (1977) Sampling techniques, 3rd edn. John Wiley & Sons, New York

Dahlberg L, Agahi N, Lennartsson C (2018) Lonelier than ever? Loneliness of older people over two decades. Arch Gerontol Geriatr 75:96–103. https://doi.org/10.1016/j.archger.2017.11.004

Donovan NJ, Blazer D (2020) Social isolation and loneliness in older adults: review and commentary of a national academies report. Am J Geriatr Psychiatry 28(12):1233–1244

Fried LP, Guralnik JM (1997) Disability in older adults: evidence regarding significance, etiology, and risk. J Am Geriatr Soc 45(1):92–100

Ginn J, Arber S (1991) Gender, class and income inequalities in later life. Br J Sociol 42(3):369–396

Hawkley LC, Cacioppo JT (2010) Loneliness matters: a theoretical and empirical review of consequences and mechanisms. Ann Behav Med 40(2):218–227

Heikkinen RL, Kauppinen M (2011) Mental Well-being: a 16-year follow-up among older residents in Jyväskylä. Arch Gerontol Geriatr 52(1):33–39

Igbokwe CC, Ejeh VJ, Agbaje OS, Umoke PIC, Iweama CN, Ozoemena EL (2020) Prevalence of loneliness and association with depressive and anxiety symptoms among retirees in north Central Nigeria: a cross-sectional study. BMC Geriatr 20:1–10

Mansfield J, Hazan H, Lerman Y, Shalom V (2016) Correlates and predictors of loneliness in older-adults: a review of quantitative results informed by qualitative insights. Int Psychogeriatr 28(4):557–576. https://doi.org/10.1017/S1041610215001532

Mistry SK, Ali AM, Yadav UN, Khanam F, Huda MN (2022) Changes in loneliness prevalence and its associated factors among Bangladeshi older adults during the COVID-19 pandemic. PLoS One 17(11):e0277247

Morlett Paredes A, Lee EE, Chik L, Gupta S, Palmer BW, Palinkas LA, Kim HC, Jeste DV (2021) Qualitative study of loneliness in a senior housing community: the importance of wisdom and other coping strategies. Aging Ment Health 25(3):559–566

Muyan M, Chang EC, Jilani Z, Yu T, Lin J, Hirsch JK (2016) Loneliness and negative affective conditions in adults: is there any room for hope in predicting anxiety and depressive symptoms? J Psychol 150(3):333–341

Perissinotto CM, Cenzer IS, Covinsky KE (2012) Loneliness in older persons: a predictor of functional decline and death. Arch Intern Med 172(14):1078–1084

Rahman MS, Rahman MA, Rahman MS (2019) Prevalence and determinants of loneliness among older adults in Bangladesh. Int J Emerg Trends Soc Sci 5(2):57–64

Rouxel P, Heilmann A, Demakakos P, Aida J, Tsakos G, Watt RG (2017) Oral health-related quality of life and loneliness among older adults. Eur J Ageing 14:101–109

Russell D, Peplau LA, Ferguson ML (1978) Developing a measure of loneliness. J Pers Assess 42(3):290–294

Sandu V, Zólyomi E, Leichsenring K (2021) Addressing loneliness and social isolation among older people in Europe. Policy Brief, pp 1–16

Steptoe A, Shankar A, Demakakos P, Wardle J (2013) Social isolation, loneliness, and all-cause mortality in older men and women. Proc Natl Acad Sci 110(15):5797–5801

Sündermann O, Onwumere J, Kane F, Morgan C, Kuipers E (2014) Social networks and support in first-episode psychosis: exploring the role of loneliness and anxiety. Soc Psychiatry Psychiatr Epidemiol 49(3):359–366

Susanty S, Chung MH, Chiu HY, Chi MJ, Hu SH, Kuo CL, Chuang YH (2022) Prevalence of loneliness and associated factors among community-dwelling older adults in Indonesia: a cross-sectional study. Int J Environ Res Public Health 19(8):4911

Tomstad S, Dale B, Sundsli K, Sævareid HI, Söderhamn U (2017) Who often feels lonely? A cross-sectional study about loneliness and its related factors among older home-dwelling people. Int J Older People Nursing 12(4):1–12

Wilson RS, Krueger KR, Arnold SE, Schneider JA, Kelly JF, Barnes LL, Tang Y, Bennett DA (2007) Loneliness and risk of Alzheimer disease. Arch Gen Psychiatry 64(2):234–240

Determinants of Neonatal and Infant Mortality in Bangladesh

18

Md. Kaderi Kibria, Susama Tanzim, Md. Mahmudul Alam, and Md. Monimul Huq

18.1 Introduction

Child mortality is a major public health concern across the world as it is frequently used to describe a country's overall social and economic well-being and progress (Roser et al. 2013). It is the most crucial indicator of a country's well-being and growth. Child mortality is a key measure of a country's standard of living and socio-economic progress; thus, social scientists and politicians throughout the world are keen to learn more about the variables that influence it (Gonzalez and Gilleskie 2017). The information on child and newborn mortality is a useful indication of qualifying demographic evaluation of a country's population. Children are most likely to die in the first month of life, with an average global rate of 17 fatalities per 1000 live births in 2020, down from 37 deaths per 1000 in 1990 (WHO 2022). In 2020, the risk of mortality after the first month and before reaching the age of 1 year was predicted to be 11 per 1000, while the risk of dying after reaching the age of 1 year and before reaching the age of 5 years was 9 per 1000 (You et al. 2018). In 2020, 2.4 million children perished in their first month of life worldwide almost 6500 neonatal fatalities each day with nearly a third of all neonatal deaths occurring during the first day after delivery and nearly three-quarters occurring within the first week (WHO 2022). Child mortality is divided into three categories based on the age of the child: neonatal, infant, and under-5. Neonatal mortality refers to deaths that occur within the first month of life, whereas infant mortality refers to deaths that occur within the first year of life (Alison 1959). Infant mortality was 38 per 1000

M. K. Kibria
Department of Statistics, Hajee Mohammad Danesh Science and Technology University, Dinajpur, Bangladesh

S. Tanzim · M. M. Alam · M. M. Huq (✉)
Department of Statistics, University of Rajshahi, Rajshahi, Bangladesh

M. Pal et al. (eds.), *Public Health and Nutrition*,
https://doi.org/10.1007/978-981-97-7890-4_18

live births, while child mortality was 7 per 1000 children (Darling 1911). The neonatal mortality rate was 30 fatalities per 1000 live births, accounting for 67% of all deaths in children under the age of 5 years. Over the previous two decades, the under-5 mortality rate has steadily decreased (Slabber 1989). However, the rate of decrease dropped substantially between 2014 and 2017–18. From 2014 to 2017–18, infant and neonatal death rates were steady. To identify children at higher risk of death and develop ways to lower this risk, such as increasing birth spacing, media exposure, prenatal care, and birthplace, among other things (Molitoris et al. 2019). A country's child mortality rate is an accepted and significant health measure (McGuire 2006). The rate of child mortality, which is also an important measure of the overall development of a country, is defined as the number of U5CM per 1000 live births (McGuire 2006). Reduce neonatal mortality to at least 12 deaths per 1000 live births and under-5 mortality to at least 25 deaths per 1000 live births, according to the third sustainable development goal (SDG-3.2.2). If we look at the geographical disparities, we can find that Sylhet has the greatest mortality rates for children under the age of 5 years (60 deaths per 1000 live births) and infants (52 deaths per 1000 live births), whereas Rangpur has the highest neonatal mortality rate (37 deaths per 1000 live births). All of the information comes from the "Bangladesh Demographic and Health Survey" (BDHS, 2017–18). Various research studies have been undertaken across the world to determine the factors that influence neonatal and infant mortality. An analytic approach to child endurance in developing countries focuses on a variety of biological, social, and environmental factors that determine neonatal and infant mortality (Mosley and Chen 1984). Chowdhury (2013) used Cox proportional hazard analysis to investigate the factors that influence under-5 mortality in Bangladesh (Chowdhury 2013). In his study, the location of residence, the area, and the mother's age were determined to be major factors influencing under-5 mortality. Another researchers investigated the factors that influence new born and child mortality in the Rajshahi area (Mondal et al. 2009). The outcomes of the review revealed that the mother's age at birth was the most important factor of neonatal, post-neonatal, and kid death. Residence, watching TV, kid's sex, and birth order were seen as enormous for child mortality, while mother's education and treatments were major markers for both neonatal and infant death. In Bangladesh, a researcher tried to explore at mother age, maternal education, and birth order as possible risk factors for newborn mortality (Kamal et al. 2012). Fatima et al. (2017) used a log-strategic parametric survival regression model to discover that the age of the mother at birth, maternal education, the sex of the child, the size of the child at birth, the location of transportation, and NGO membership all had a significant influence on infant mortality (Fatima-Tuz-Zahura et al. 2017). Financial ability, mother's education, clinical check-ups during pregnancy, and watching TV are all important factors in newborn, toddler, and under-5 mortality (Islam and Biswas 2021). Rahman et al. (2021) conducted a study of BDHS data using the Cox proportional hazard model and discovered that the site of birth, mother's education, source of drinking water, availability of power, and wealth index all played a significant role in lowering the child mortality rate (Rahman et al. 2021). Despite the fact that Bangladesh achieved Millennium Development Goal—4 with a 65% reduction rate from 1993 to 2014, a substantial number of children in Bangladesh are still dying every year owing to a lack of suitable awareness and actions. As a result, proper efforts are still necessary to improve the situation and boost the survival rates of children.

18.2 Methods

18.2.1 Study Sampling and Setting

The entire study has been carried out through the use of secondary data from BDHS 2017. It is the national demographic and health survey that aims to provide information on social progress, childhood mortality and causes of death, and nutritional status of mothers and children.

BDHS promises its national representatives and hence covers the entire population residing noninstitutional dwelling units in the country. The enumeration areas (EAs) prepared for the 2017–18 population and housing census comprised a sampling frame collected from BBS (Bangladesh Bureau of Statistics). The sampling methodology utilized in this study is outlined in Fig. 18.1.

18.2.2 Outcome Variables

According to the objectives of the study, we used neonatal and infant mortality as the dependent variable. On the contrary, based on the study purpose, we consider the independent variables at individual and community levels, while mother's age at birth, mother's education level, husband's education level, wealth index, sex of the

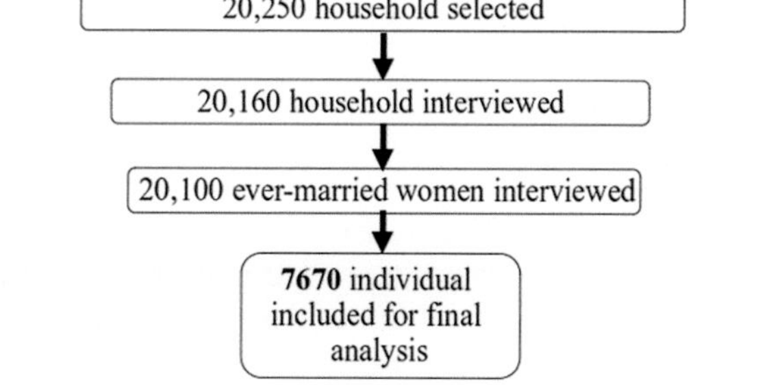

Fig. 18.1 Sampling design of this study

child, number of antenatal visits, delivery by C-section, size of the child at birth, birth order, delivery assistance, place of delivery, breastfeeding, postnatal care (PNC) by a qualified person, media exposure, source of water, and type of toilet facility are considered as individual-level factors. Under the community level, we considered the type of residential area, region, electricity availability, telephone availability, NGO activity, availability of field workers, presence of pharmacy, and contraceptive use.

18.2.3 Statistical Analysis

To analyze the data, we used IBM SPSS (Version 26.0), and visualization was performed using the R software (Version 4.2). The chi-square test analysis was used to check the association between neonatal and infant mortality with the individual and community level factors. Also to explore the significant factors in the case of neonatal and infant mortality, we used binary logistic regression analysis.

18.3 Results

18.3.1 Demographic and Socio-Economic Characteristics of the Respondents

The main aim of this study is to observe the factors that influence neonatal and infant mortality from the perspective of Bangladesh. The sample for this study consists of ever-married women aged 15–49 years who have had at least one child in the last 3 years. Table 18.1 represents the demographic and socioeconomic characteristics at the individual level of the respondents. It is observed that the rate of newborn mortality is 30 per 1000 births, while the infant mortality rate is 38 per 1000 live births. Almost 46% of mothers had a secondary education and their spouses (51%) are uneducated or partially educated. Notably, 67% of women reported having a normal birth, while 33% reported having a cesarean section. However, 39.7% of women said they nursed their kids right after birth or within an hour, which is a highly beneficial practice. A smaller percentage of mothers (31.6%) said that they attended postnatal checks in the first 2 days, while the remainder did not. According to the birth order, most of the children (53%) appear to be their mother's second to fourth child. Notably, 34% of mothers stated that their birth gap was between 2 and 4 years, which is essential for healthy kids. A greater proportion of women (57.7%) reported getting their PNC from a qualified individual. More than half of the mothers did not take any vitamin-A and drank tubewell water, while 67.3% of them used a pit latrine.

Distributions of the covariates at the community level are shown in Table 18.2. Electricity availability is a basic determinant of Bangladesh's socioeconomic standing. It is shown that 80.6% of families live in communities with electricity. According to the study, 72.5% of ever-married women aged 15–49 years are members of at least one NGO. Notably, 38% of women live in a community where health services are

Table 18.1 Percentage distribution of the selected demographic and socioeconomic characteristics at individual level of the respondents

Variable name	Category	Frequency (%)	Variable name	Category	Frequency (%)
Neonatal mortality	Yes	229 (2.9)	**Birth order**	First order	2798 (36.5)
	No	7441 (97.1)		Second to fourth order	4428 (57.7)
Infant mortality	Yes	295 (3.8)		>Fourth order	444 (5.8)
	No	7375 (96.2)	**Delivery assistance**	Unqualified	2225 (46.9)
Mother age	<15 years	22 (0.3)		Qualified	2516 (53.1)
	15–24 years	3422 (44.6)	**Place of delivery**	Hospital/ clinic	2292 (49.1)
	>24 years	4226 (55.1)		Home/others	2370 (50.9)
Mother's education level	≤ Primary	2990 (39)	**Breastfeeding**	Exclusive	3203 (60.3)
	Secondary	3514 (45.8)		Initiative	2108 (39.7)
	Higher	1166 (15.2)	**Postnatal visit**	Within 2 days	3107 (68.3)
Father's education level	≤ Primary	3828 (49.9)		Others	1443 (31.7)
	Secondary	2354 (30.7)	**Postnatal care by qualified person**	No	2751 (42.3)
	Higher	1328 (17.3)		Yes	3760 (57.7)
Wealth Index	Rich	3059 (39.9)	**Media exposure**	Not at all	2811 (36.6)
	Middle/ poor	4611 (60.1)		Sometimes	4859 (63.4)
Gender	Female	4150 (47.8)	**Mother received Vit-A**	No	2520 (58.3)
	Male	4526 (52.2)		Yes	1802 (41.7)
Sex of deceased child	Female	155 (55.8)	**Multiple gestation**	No	7524 (98.1)
	Male	240 (44.2)		Yes	146 (1.9)
No. of neonatal visits	No Visit	364 (8.4)	**Source of water**	Piped water	543 (7.2)
	1–3 times	1895 (43.8)		Tubewell	6906 (91.4)
	> = 4 times	2063 (47.7)		Dugwell	57 (0.8)
Delivery by C-section	No	3060 (67)		Others	51 (0.7)
	Yes	1508 (33)	**Type of toilet**	Flush	2364 (30.8)
Size of child	Not small	1705 (84.2)		Pit latrine	5159 (67.3)
	Small	320 (15.8)		Others	147 (1.9)

provided by field workers belonging to government, non-governmental, private, businesses, religious organizations, and so on. The remaining 62% receive health care facilities without fieldworkers. The results suggest that 69.5% of respondents live in a neighborhood where family planning methods are offered. According to the findings, 63.7% of women reside in a neighborhood where a pharmacy is available and almost 70% of them use contraceptives to prevent pregnancy-related health risks.

18.3.2 Association

Table 18.3 represents the association of child neonatal and infant mortality with respect to individual-level covariates. The neonatal mortality and infant mortality rate are significantly related to wealth index, whereas child from both wealthy

Table 18.2 Percentage distribution of the selected covariates at the community level

Variable name	Category	Frequency	Percentage
Place of resident	Dhaka	1170	15.3
	Rajshahi	786	10.2
	Rangpur	864	11.3
	Sylhet	1134	14.8
	Mymensingh	906	11.8
	Khulna	809	10.5
	Chittagong	1213	15.8
	Barishal	788	10.3
Region	Urban	2728	35.6
	Rural	4942	64.4
Electricity	No	1487	19.4
	Yes	6183	80.6
Telephone	Using telephone services	4727	61.6
	Deprived of telephone services	2943	38.4
NGO activity	No	3150	72.5
	Yes	1193	27.5
Availability of field worker	No	3117	62.4
	Yes	1876	37.6
Presence of pharmacy	Yes	3122	63.7
	No	1782	36.3
Use contraceptive	Not using	2338	30.5
	Use	5332	69.5

(98.2%) and middle/poor (96.2%) family died before the age of 28 days. Similarly, in the case of neonatal mortality, most of the rich (97.7%) and middle/poor (95.1%) family children died before 12 months from their birth. Sex of deceased child is significantly associated with both neonatal and infant mortality rate, while many male and female children were deceased after 28 days in neonatal cases and more than 1 month in case of infant mortality. Delivery by C-section is also significantly associated with neonatal mortality, whereas almost 98% of the child died before 28 days and the death rate after 28 days is very low. On the contrary, size of child is another covariate significantly associated with both neonatal and infant mortality and both sizes of the child died before 28 days for neonatal cases and before 12 months for infant mortality cases. However, birth order of the child is a significant factor of infant mortality. Delivery assistance is also an important factor significantly associated with both neonatal and infant mortality. Almost 95% child died by unqualified assistance and almost 93% of the infants died by unqualified assistance before 12 months of age. Also, the factors of breastfeeding and postnatal visits were significantly associated with both neonatal and infant mortality. Vitamin A is also an important factor related to a healthy baby. Mothers receiving vitamin A are highly significant with neonatal mortality.

Table 18.4 represents the association of child neonatal and infant mortality with respect to the community level covariates. Among the covariates, telephone use was highly associated with neonatal and infant mortality, while almost 68% of the

Table 18.3 Association of child neonatal and infant mortality with respect to individual level

Variable	Category	Neonatal mortality			Infant mortality		
		>28 days	≤28 days	P-value	>12 months	≤12 months	*P*-value
Mother Age	<15 years	20 (90.9)	2 (9.1)	0.202	20 (90.9)	2 (9.1)	0.395
	15–24 years	3287 (96.9)	135 (3.1)		3287 (96.1)	135 (3.9)	
	>24 years	4105 (97.1)	121 (2.9)		4068 (96.3)	158 (3.7)	
Mother's education level	> = Primary	2890 (96.7)	100 (3.3)	0.240	2859 (95.6)	131 (4.4)	0.088
	Secondary	3413 (97.1)	101 (2.9)		3385 (96.3)	129 (3.7)	
	Higher	1138 (97.6)	28 (2.4)		1131 (15.3)	35 (3.0)	
Father's education Level	> = Primary	3729 (97.4)	100 (2.6)	0.134	3698 (96.6)	131 (3.4)	0.132
	Secondary	2271 (96.5)	82 (3.5)		2249 (95.6)	104 (4.4)	
	Higher	1286 (96.8)	42 (3.2)		1275 (96.0)	53 (4.0)	
Wealth index	Rich	3004 (98.2)	55 (1.8)	**0.000**	2990 (97.7)	69 (2.3)	**0.000**
	Middle/poor	4437 (96.2)	174 (3.8)		4385 (95.1)	226 (4.9)	
Gender	Female	3899 (97.2)	113 (2.8)	0.362	3867 (96.4)	145 (3.6)	0.269
	Male	3542 (96.8)	116 (3.2)		3508 (95.9)	150 (4.1)	
Sex of deceased child	Female	27 (22.3)	94 (77.7)	**0.000**	1 (0.8)	120 (99.2)	**0.000**
	Male	38 (22.0)	135 (78)		0 (0)	173 (100)	
No. of neonatal visits	No Visit	358 (98.4)	6 (1.6)	0.893	356 (97.80)	8 (2.2)	0.154
	1–3 times	1858 (98)	37 (2.0)		1833 (96.7)	62 (3.3)	
	> = 4 times	2026 (98.2)	37 (1.8)		2015 (97.7)	48 (2.3)	
Delivery by C-section	No	2959 (96.7)	101 (3.3)	**0.026**	2929 (95.7)	131 (4.3)	0.108
	Yes	1476 (97.9)	32 (2.1)		1465 (97.1)	43 (2.9)	
Size of child	Not small	1671 (98.0)	34 (2.0)	**0.001**	1658 (97.2)	47 (2.8)	**0.000**
	Small	303 (94.7)	17 (5.3)		296 (92.5)	24 (7.5)	

(continued)

Table 18.3 (continued)

Variable	Category	Neonatal mortality			Infant mortality		
		>28 days	≤28 days	P-value	>12 months	≤12 months	*P*-value
Birth order	First order	2698 (96.4)	100 (3.6)	0.072	2669 (95.4)	129 (4.6)	**0.023**
	Second to fourth order	4311 (97.4)	117 (2.6)		4280 (96.7)	148 (3.3)	
	>Fourth order	432 (97.3)	12 (2.7)		426 (95.9)	18 (4.1)	
Delivery assistance	Unqualified	2106 (94.7)	119 (5.3)	**0.041**	2074 (93.2)	151 (6.8)	**0.022**
	Qualified	2413 (95.9)	103 (4.1)		2385 (94.8)	131 (5.2)	
Place of delivery	Hospital/Clinic	2212 (96.5)	80 (3.5)	**0.002**	2191 (95.6)	101 (4.4)	**0.000**
	Home/others	2248 (94.6)	128 (5.4)		2213 (93.1)	163 (6.9)	
Breastfeeding	Exclusive	3093 (96.6)	110 (3.4)	**0.021**	3061 (95.6)	142 (4.4)	**0.010**
	Initiative	2009 (95.3)	99 (4.7)		1981 (94.0)	127 (6.0)	
Postnatal visit	Within 2 days	3005 (96.7)	102 (3.3)	**0.034**	2975 (95.8)	132 (4.2)	**0.021**
	Others	1412 (97.9)	31 (2.1)		1402 (97.2)	41 (2.8)	
Postnatal care by qualified person	No	2681 (97.5)	70 (2.5)	0.294	2657 (96.6)	94 (3.4)	0.443
	Yes	3648 (97.0)	112 (3.0)		3618 (96.2)	142 (3.8)	
Media exposure	Not at all	2733 (97.2)	78 (2.8)	0.409	2706 (96.3)	105 (3.7)	0.701
	Sometimes	4708 (96.9)	151 (3.1)		4669 (96.1)	190 (3.9)	
Mother received vit-a	No	2460 (97.6)	60 (2.4)	**0.002**	2442 (96.9)	79 (3.1)	0.054
	Yes	1782 (98.9)	20 (1.1)		1763 (97.8)	39 (2.2)	
Source of water	Piped water	529 (97.4)	14 (2.6)	0.552	524 (96.5)	19 (3.5)	0.693
	Tubewell	6698 (97.0)	208 (3.0)		6637 (96.1)	269 (3.9)	
	Dugwell	56 (98.2)	1 (1.8)		56 (98.2)	1 (1.8)	
	Others	48 (94.1)	3 (5.9)		48 (94.1)	3 (5.9)	
Type of toilet	Flush	2294 (97.0)	70 (3.0)	0.955	2274 (96.2)	90 (3.8)	0.842
	Pit latrine	5005 (97.0)	154 (3.0)		4961 (96.2)	198 (67.1)	
	Others	142 (96.6)	5 (3.4)		140 (95.2)	7 (4.8)	

Table 18.4 Association of child neonatal and infant mortality with respect to the community level covariates

		Neonatal mortality			Infant mortality		
Variable	Category	>28 days	≤28 days	*P*-value	>12 month	≤12 month	*P*-value
Place of resident	Dhaka	1134 (96.9)	36 (3.1)	0.382	1124 (96.2)	46 (3.9)	0.278
	Rajshahi	765 (97.3)	21 (2.7)		756 (96.2)	30 (3.8)	
	Rangpur	834 (96.5)	30 (3.5)		830 (96.1)	34 (3.9)	
	Sylhet	1096 (96.6)	38 (3.4)		1086 (95.8)	48 (4.2)	
	Mymensingh	887 (97.9)	19 (2.1)		880 (97.1)	26 (2.9)	
	Khulna	783 (96.8)	26 (3.2)		780 (96.4)	29 (3.6)	
	Chittagong	1184 (97.6)	29 (2.4)		1173 (96.7)	40 (3.3)	
	Barishal	758 (96.2)	30 (3.8)		746 (94.7)	42 (5.3)	
Region	Urban	2641 (96.8)	87 (3.2)	0.437	2622 (96.1)	106 (3.9)	0.894
	Rural	4800 (97.1)	142 (2.9)		4753 (96.2)	189 (3.8)	
Electricity	No	1443 (97.0)	44 (3.0)	0.946	1425 (95.8)	62 (4.2)	0.470
	Yes	5998 (97.0)	185 (3.0)		5950 (96.2)	233 (3.8)	
Telephone	Using telephone services	1428 (97.9)	31 (2.1)	**0.026**	1417 (97.1)	42 (2.9)	**0.018**
	Deprived of telephone services	2998 (96.7)	103 (3.3)		2967 (95.7)	134 (4.3)	
NGO activity	No	3078 (97.7)	72 (2.3)	0.125	3046 (96.7)	104 (3.3)	0.531
	Yes	1156 (96.9)	37 (3.1)		1149 (96.3)	44 (3.7)	
Availability of field worker	No	2627 (98.1)	52 (1.9)	0.575	2601 (97.1)	78 (2.9)	0.350
	Yes	1615 (98.3)	28 (1.7)		1603 (97.6)	40 (2.4)	
Availability of qualified doctor	No	2681 (97.5)	70 (2.5)	**0.029**	2657 (96.6)	94 (3.4)	**0.043**
	Yes	3648 (97.0)	112 (3.0)		6275 (96.4)	236 (3.6)	
Presence of pharmacy	Yes	20 (95.2)	1 (4.8)	0.511	20 (95.2)	1 (4.8)	0.736
	No	3850 (97.5)	99 (2.5)		3814 (96.6)	135 (3.4)	
Use contraceptive	Not using	2234 (95.6)	104 (4.4)	**0.000**	2208 (94.4)	130 (5.6)	**0.000**
	Use	5207 (97.7)	125 (2.3)		5167 (96.9)	165 (3.1)	

neonatal mortality occurred due to unavailability of telephone service. Availability of qualified doctors is another factor that is significantly related to neonatal and infant mortality in this study. Use of contraceptive is another important factor that is significantly related to both neonatal and infant mortality.

18.3.3 Binary Logistic Regression

The logistic regression analysis identifies the individual's level factors are significantly associated with the neonatal and infant mortality (Fig. 18.2). Wealth index indicates that the rich people are 54% (OR: 0.467%, 95% CI: 0.17–0.76, $p < 0.05$) and 55% (OR: 0.448%, 95% CI: 0.20–0.86, $p < 0.05$) less likely of dying of neonatal and infant death, respectively, than those people, belonging to the poor or middle class. Gender of the child result showed that female children are almost 38% (OR: 0.62%, 95% CI: 0.24–0.87, $p < 0.05$) and 58% (OR: 0.42%, 95% CI: 0.12–0.81, $p < 0.05$) less likely to occur neonatal and infant mortality, respectively than the male children. Also size of child at birth is another significant factor, while not small size child are 64% (OR: 0.36%, 95% CI: 0.21–0.67, $p < 0.05$) and 65% (OR: 0.35%, 95% CI: 0.09–0.77, $p < 0.05$) less likely to occur neonatal and infant mortality, respectively, than those child who were small of size at birth. Delivery assistance is

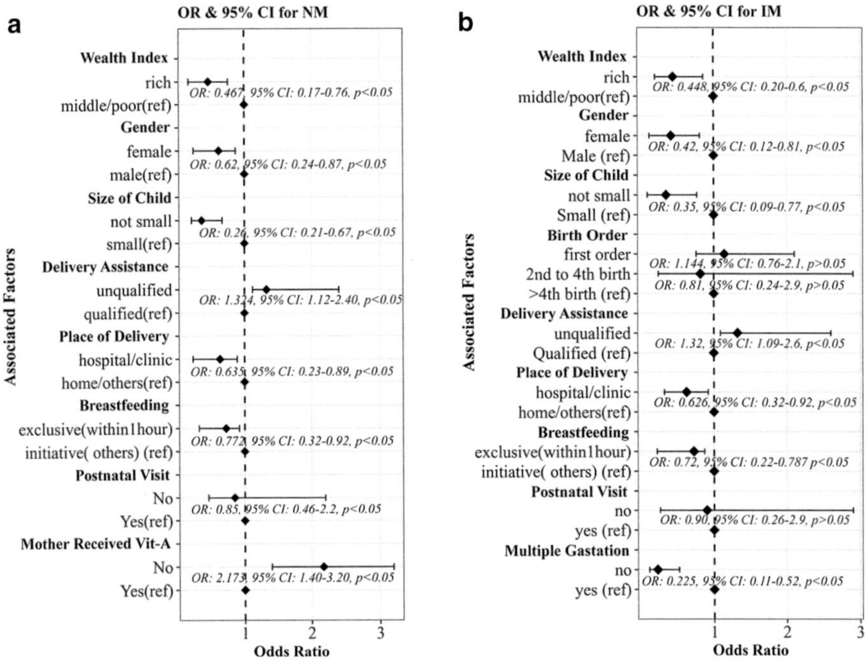

Fig. 18.2 Estimated binary logistic regression adjusting for individual level characteristics of (**a**) NM and (**b**) IM

also another important factor related to neonatal and infant mortality death. It is observed that, in unqualified birth attendance, almost 32% (OR: 1.324, 95% CI: 1.12–2.40, $p < 0.05$) and 32.6% (OR: 1.326, 95% CI: 1.09–2.60, $p < 0.05$) more likely to occur the neonatal and infant death, respectively, than the deliveries with the qualified birth attendance. Place of delivery result showed that deliveries in hospitals/clinics have 36% (OR: 0.635, 95% CI: 0.23–0.89, $p < 0.05$) and 37% (OR: 0.626, 95% CI: 0.32–0.92, $p < 0.05$) less likely to occur the neonatal and infant mortality, respectively, than the place of delivery at home/others. Breastfeeding is another significant factor, while breastfeeding within 1 h has 22.8% (OR: 0.772, 95% CI: 0.32–0.92, $p < 0.05$) and 27.6% (OR: 0.724, 95% CI: 0.22–0.87, $p < 0.05$) less likely to occur neonatal and infant mortality, respectively, than those who were breastfeeding more than 1 h. Also, vitamin A is a significant factor, while the mother who did not receive vitamin A (OR: 2.173, 95% CI: 1.40–3.20, $p < 0.05$) is almost two times more likely to occur neonatal death than the mothers who received vitamin A. Finally, multiple gestation showed that not multiple gestation has (OR: 0.225, 95% CI: 0.11–0.52, $p < 0.05$) less likely to occur the infant death than the child with multiple gestation.

In Fig. 18.3, binary logistic regression analysis identifies the community level factors that are significantly associated with neonatal and infant mortality. Among the community level, telephone indicates that the respondents having telephone availability has almost 58% (OR: 1.58, 95% CI: 1.12–1.98, $p < 0.05$) and 51% (OR:1.512, 95% CI: 1.22–2.80, $p < 0.05$) more likely to neonatal and infant death, respectively, than the respondents who did not use telephone service. Also use of contraceptive is another important factor; while the mother who used contraceptive, the child had almost two times (OR:1.939, 95% CI: 1.33–3.40, $p < 0.05$) and 84% (OR:1.844, 95% CI: 1.43–2.80, $p < 0.05$) more likely to occur neonatal and infant mortality, respectively, than the mother who used it.

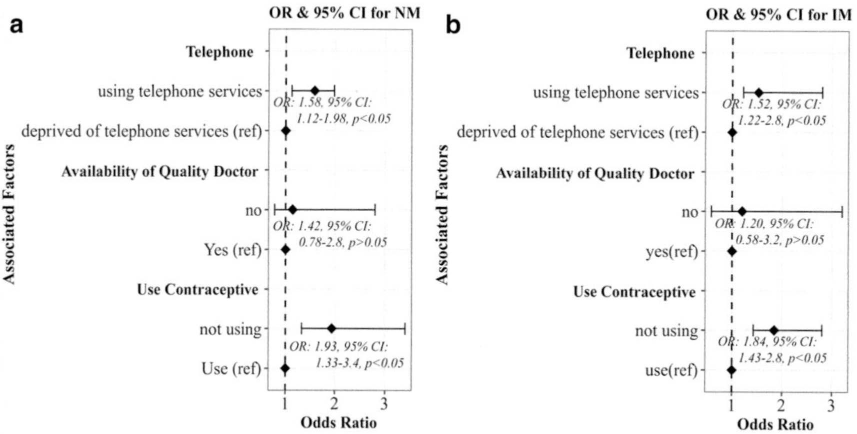

Fig. 18.3 Estimated binary logistic regression adjusting for community level characteristics: (**a**) NM and (**b**) IM

18.4 Discussion

Neonatal and infant mortality are crucial measures of a healthy population. External environment in which an infant lives has the greatest impact on the infant's survival after 1 month (Nair et al. 2011). The factors that contribute to neonatal and infant mortality are critical in reducing under-5 child mortality (Murad et al. 2023). The research looked at two layers of parameters, one is individual level, and another is community level factors. In bivariate analysis, individual level factors such as wealth index, sex of deceased child, delivery assistance, cesarean section delivery, size of the child, place of delivery, breastfeeding, and postnatal care (PNC) are found to be significant in both neonatal and infant mortality. The wealth index is used to describe a household's financial situation of the respondents. According to the findings, unwealthy households have a greater death rate than wealthier households. Similar results were found in Sudan and Pakistan (Bashir et al. 2013; Nisar and Dibley 2014). Furthermore, logistic analysis reveals that it has a significant impact on delivery factors according to BDHS (2017–18). Skilled delivery assistance can help to reduce the chance of death. The study discovered that it had a significant impact on both neonatal and infant mortality. Place of delivery was significantly associated with neonatal mortality in case of Ethiopia population (Wake et al. 2022; Ahmed et al. 2023) that is similar to our findings but not significantly associated with early neonatal mortality in Bangladesh (Ijdi et al. 2022). It is assumed that the death rate for home deliveries would be higher than for deliveries in a hospital or other reputable facility which is like our results. Cesarean section has been a widespread practice in recent years, particularly in more developed areas in Bangladesh (Ahmmed et al. 2021). According to the findings of the study, the rate of newborn and infant death is low among mothers who deliver by C-section (Sarker et al. 2016; Abdulla et al. 2023). In both bivariate analyses, the results demonstrate substantial outcomes for both neonatal and newborn children. Breast milk is a newborn's only source of nutrition. According to the study, children who receive breast milk within an hour have a better chance of living to their first birthday than children who do not (Alison 2009). As both the mother and the child may encounter a variety of problems following delivery, it is critical that they receive competent advice and guidance within the first two days of delivery. PNC has been identified as a key factor in both neonatal and newborn death (Singh et al. 2014, 2017). Furthermore, any qualified person should provide PNC. This was also discovered to be a relevant predictor for PNC in both the bivariate levels of this study. Community level factors such as telephone, availability of qualified doctors, and use of contraceptive have a significant impact on neonatal and infant mortality (Shukla et al. 2020; Bradshaw et al. 2023). As a result, these were investigated in a univariate analysis excluding the location of residence because clusters coincide with districts, which could lead to a misinterpretation of the overall conclusion. The availability of a telephone service has been identified as a critical issue in both sectors' analyses. It has been discovered that neonatal and newborn mortality rates are low in communities with telephone service which is similar to sub-Saharan African study (Flückiger and Ludwig 2023). The presence of a pharmacy is a sign of a thriving community, particularly in rural areas where medication is rarely available. In bivariate analysis, this indicator reveals almost the same outcome for neonatal and infant death (Khan et al. 2022). The presence of a doctor in any community lowers the risk of death. The neonatal and newborn mortality rates do not differ significantly among them. When there is a trained doctor in a community, however, the death rate is substantially lower than in communities where there is none (Harvey and Trudgill 2021). In comparison to metropolitan areas, rural areas have a greater prevalence of neonatal and infant mortality. This could be due to a lack of resources in rural areas compared with urban areas. The presence of an electricity infrastructure is another evidence of a developed town. In communities where electricity is available, the rate of neonatal and infant mortality is low (Mohammed and Akuoko 2022). Again, mothers who participated in NGO activities had a low rate of neonatal and infant mortality. We discovered a community level impact in both neonatal and newborn death from a null model in multivariate analysis.

18.5 Conclusion

In our study, we found that wealth index, sex of deceased child, assistance in delivery, C-section delivery, child size, place of delivery, breastfeeding, and PNC are the important factors for individual-level those were associated with both neonatal and infant mortality. In addition, telephone facilities, availability of a qualified doctor, and use of contraceptives were significant community-level factors associated with a child's neonatal and infant mortality. The strength of the study is that it was able to achieve its objectives and provide various factors at individual and community levels that will contribute to reducing neonatal and infant mortality, followed by child mortality among children under 5 years of age, thus achieving its achievement to contribute to the goal of SDG 3.

References

Abdulla F, Hossain MM, Rahman MM, Rahman MS, Rahman A (2023) Risk factors of caesarean deliveries in Urban–rural areas of Bangladesh. Front Reprod Heal 5:1101400. https://doi.org/10.3389/frph.2023.1101400

Ahmed KT, Karimuzzaman M, Mahmud S, Rahman L, Hossain MM, Rahman A (2023) Influencing factors associated with maternal delivery at home in Urban areas: a cross-sectional analysis of the Bangladesh demographic and health survey 2017–2018 data. J Health Popul Nutr 42:83. https://doi.org/10.1186/s41043-023-00428-9

Ahmmed F, Manik MMR, Jamal Hossain M (2021) Caesarian section (CS) delivery in Bangladesh: a Nationally representative cross-sectional study. PLoS One 16:e0254777. https://doi.org/10.1371/journal.pone.0254777

Alison F (1959) Neonatal mortality. Rev Med Moyen Orient 16:159–162

Alison S (2009) The risks of not breastfeeding for mothers and infants. Rev Obstet Gynecol 2:222

Bashir AO, Ibrahim GH, Bashier IA, Adam I (2013) Neonatal mortality in Sudan: analysis of The Sudan Household Survey, 2010. BMC Public Health 13:1. https://doi.org/10.1186/1471-2458-13-287

Bradshaw CJA, Perry C, Judge MA, Saraswati CM, Heyworth J, Le Souëf PN (2023) Lower infant mortality, higher household size, and more access to contraception reduce fertility in low-and middle-income Nations. PLoS One 18:e0280260. https://doi.org/10.1371/journal.pone.0280260

Chowdhury AH (2013) Determinants of under-five mortality in Bangladesh, vol 03. Open J, Stat, p 213. https://doi.org/10.4236/ojs.2013.33024

Darling R (1911) Infant and child mortality. J R Stat Soc 74:207–208. https://doi.org/10.2307/2339837

Fatima-Tuz-Zahura M, Mohammad KA, Bari W (2017) Log-logistic proportional odds model for analyzing infant mortality in Bangladesh. Asia-Pacific J Public Heal 29:60–69. https://doi.org/10.1177/1010539516680023

Flückiger M, Ludwig M (2023) Mobile phone coverage and infant mortality in Sub-Saharan Africa. J Econ Behav Organ 211:462–485. https://doi.org/10.1016/j.jebo.2023.05.013

Gonzalez RM, Gilleskie D (2017) Infant mortality rate as a measure of a Country's health: a robust method to improve reliability and comparability. Demography 54:701–720. https://doi.org/10.1007/s13524-017-0553-7

Harvey PR, Trudgill NJ (2021) The Association between physician staff numbers and mortality in English Hospitals. EClinicalMedicine 32:100709. https://doi.org/10.1016/j.eclinm.2020.100709

Ijdi RE, Tumlinson K, Curtis SL (2022) Exploring association between place of delivery and newborn care with earlyneonatal mortality in Bangladesh. PLoS One 17:e0262408. https://doi.org/10.1371/journal.pone.0262408

Islam MA, Biswas B (2021) Socio-economic factors associated with increased neonatal mortality: a mixed-method study of Bangladesh and 20 other developing Countries based on demographic and health survey Data. Clin Epidemiol Glob Heal 11:100801. https://doi.org/10.1016/j.cegh.2021.100801

Kamal SMM, Ashrafuzzaman M, Narreen SA (2012) Risk factors of neonatal mortality in Bangladesh. J Nepal Paediatr Soc 32:37–46. https://doi.org/10.3126/jnps.v32i1.4845

Khan N, Trisha NI, Rashid M (2022) Availability and readiness of health care facilities and their effects on under-five mortality in Bangladesh: analysis of linked data. J Glob Health 12:04081. https://doi.org/10.7189/jogh.12.04081

McGuire JW (2006) Basic health care provision and under-5 mortality: a cross-National study of developing Countries. World Dev 34:405–425. https://doi.org/10.1016/j.worlddev.2005.08.004

Mohammed M, Akuoko M (2022) Subnational variations in electricity access and infant mortality: evidence from Ghana. Heal Policy Open 3:100057. https://doi.org/10.1016/j.hpopen.2021.100057

Molitoris J, Barclay K, Kolk M (2019) When and where birth spacing matters for child survival: an International comparison using the DHS. Demography 56:1349–1370. https://doi.org/10.1007/s13524-019-00798-y

Mondal MNI, Hossain MK, Ali MK (2009) Factors influencing infant and child mortality: a case study of Rajshahi District, Bangladesh. J Hum Ecol 26:31–39

Mosley WH, Chen LC (1984) An analytical framework for the study of child survival in developing Countries. Child Surviv Strateg Res 10:25–45. https://doi.org/10.2307/2807954

Murad MW, Abdullah ABM, Islam MM, Alam MM, Reaiche C, Boyle S (2023) Determinants of neonatal, infant and under-five mortalities: evidence from a developing country, Bangladesh. J Public Health Policy 44:230–241. https://doi.org/10.1057/s41271-023-00413-w

Nair M, Webster P, Arianaa P (2011) Impact of non-health policies on infant mortality through the social determinants pathway. Bull World Health Organ 89:778

Nisar Y, Bin, Dibley MJ (2014) Determinants of neonatal mortality in Pakistan: secondary analysis of Pakistan demographic and health survey 2006-07. BMC Public Health 14:663. https://doi.org/10.1186/1471-2458-14-663

Rahman MM, Ara T, Mahmud S, Samad N (2021) Revisit the correlates of infant mortality in Bangladesh: findings from two Nationwide cross-sectional studies. BMJ Open 11:e045506. https://doi.org/10.1136/bmjopen-2020-045506

Roser M, Ritchie H, Dadonaite B (2013) Child and infant mortality. Publ online OurWorldInDataorg. "https://ourworldindata.org/child-mortality"

Sarker BK, Rahman M, Rahman T, Hossain J, Reichenbach L, Mitra DK (2016) Reasons for preference of home delivery with traditional birth attendants (TBAs) in Rural Bangladesh: a qualitative exploration. PLoS One 11:e0146161. https://doi.org/10.1371/journal.pone.0146161

Shukla A, Kumar A, Mozumdar A, Aruldas K, Acharya R, Ram F, Saggurti N (2020) Association between modern contraceptive use and child mortality in India: a calendar data analysis of the national family health survey (2015-16). SSM Popul Heal 11:100588. https://doi.org/10.1016/j.ssmph.2020.100588

Singh K, Brodish P, Haney E (2014) Postnatal care by provider type and neonatal death in Sub-Saharan Africa: a multilevel analysis. BMC Public Health 14:941. https://doi.org/10.1186/1471-2458-14-941

Singh K, Brodish P, Chowdhury ME, Biswas TK, Kim ET, Godwin C, Moran A (2017) Postnatal care for newborns in Bangladesh: the importance of health-related factors and location. J Glob Health 7:020507. https://doi.org/10.7189/jogh.07.020507

Slabber CF (1989) Under-five mortality. South Afr Med J 75:501. https://doi.org/10.1007/springerreference_84984

Wake GE, Chernet K, Aklilu A, Yenealem F, Wogie Fitie G, Amera Tizazu M, Mittiku YM, Sisay Chekole M, Behulu GK (2022) Determinants of neonatal mortality among neonates admitted to neonatal intensive care unit of dessie comprehensive and specialized hospital, Northeast Ethiopia; an unmatched case-control study. Front Public Heal 10:979402. https://doi.org/10.3389/fpubh.2022.979402

World Health Organization Dashboard WHO Coronavirus (COVID-19) Dashboard With Vaccination Data (2022). Https://Covid19.Who.Int/. 1

You D, Hug L, Hill K (2018) Child mortality. In: Routledge handbook of Asian demography. Routledge, London, pp 168–189. https://doi.org/10.4324/9781315148458-10

Infant, Neonatal and Maternal Mortality in ASEAN Countries: A Panel Data Analysis

19

Shrabani Das, Raju Maiti, Premananda Bharati, and Manoranjan Pal

19.1 Introduction

As the title suggests, this chapter intends to see the mortality situations in ASEAN countries. The term ASEAN should not be confused with "Asian," which means the Asian continent. ASEAN means the "Association of South-east Asian Nations." It is mainly composed of ten countries, namely, Brunei, Burma (Myanmar), Cambodia, Indonesia, Laos, Malaysia, Philippines, Singapore, Thailand, and Vietnam. Later, East Timor (Timor-Leste) and Papua New Guinea joined the Association as observer States[1] (see Fig. 19.1). SEAP has a population of about 700 million at present, which is more than 8% of the world's population. The association was founded on 8 August 1967. The main purpose is to promote economic development through economic exchanges and socio-cultural development through social and economic interactions. Besides, the member nations have signed a treaty to make their zone free of nuclear weapons, which became effective on 21 June 2001. Public health is also a major concern of ASEAN. To fight against severe acute respiratory syndrome (SARS) outbreak pandemic, the ten member countries in ASEAN worked together with three other nations China, Japan, and South Korea (ASEAN+3) and successfully coordinated to stop the pandemic. They realized that, to achieve their goal, it is necessary to maintain regional peace, treat each other with mutual respect and

[1] https://en.wikipedia.org/wiki/ASEAN.

S. Das (✉) · R. Maiti
Economic Research Unit, Indian Statistical Institute, Kolkata, West Bengal, India

P. Bharati
Biological Anthropology Unit, Indian Statistical Institute (ISI), Kolkata, West Bengal, India

M. Pal
Economic Research Unit, Indian Statistical Institute (ISI), Kolkata, West Bengal, India

M. Pal et al. (eds.), *Public Health and Nutrition*,
https://doi.org/10.1007/978-981-97-7890-4_19

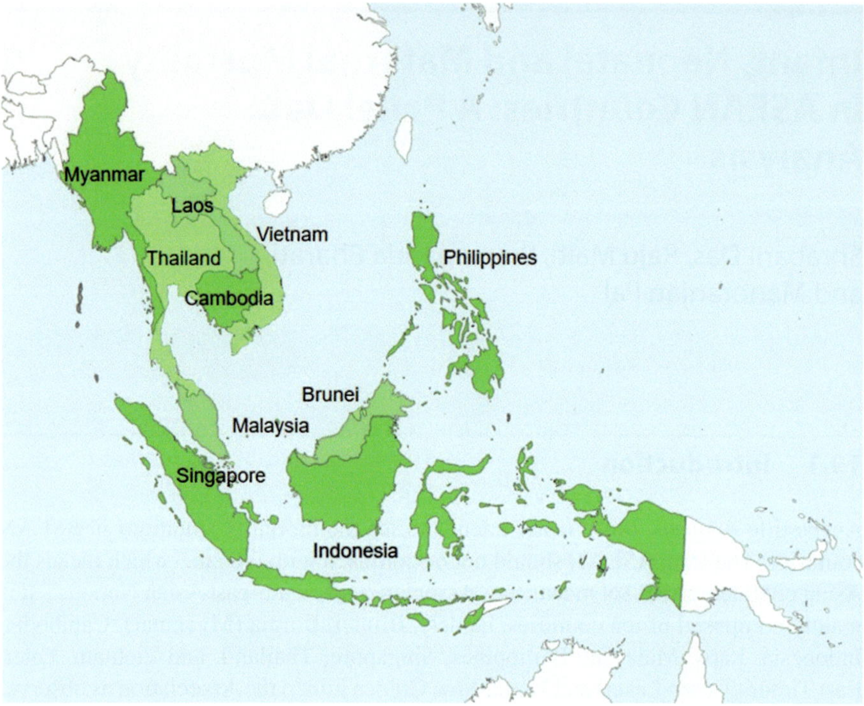

Fig. 19.1 Member States of ASEAN (Source: https://en.wikipedia.org/wiki/ASEAN)

reverence, and adhere to the principles of the United Nations Charter. They also wanted to strengthen their joint security in the style of NATO.

Education and poverty alleviation are the two most important factors for the socioeconomic development of the World. One of the objectives of the new Millennium Development Goals (MDGs) in 2000 was to improve the Human Development Index within the next 15 years, which mainly targets health improvement, education attainment, and poverty reduction. At the end of 2015, the UN General Assembly further redefined these goals as 17 Sustainable Development Goals (SDGs). The target period of these goals was the next 15 years. Despite all these efforts, we see that almost 2.6 million children cannot reach 1 month of their age. The sad reality is that about 40% of them do not survive their first day. UNICEF's report also highlights the causes of stillbirths, complications during early pregnancy, and insufficient nutrition for women. Mortality rates tend to differ based on the specific conditions in each country. For example, infant mortality rate (IMR) in Japan is only 1 infant death per 1000 births, whereas it is 46 in Pakistan which is the worst among the ASEAN countries. Proper initiatives should be taken in order to improve the socioeconomic situation in developing countries as they are lagging compared with developed countries.

"Health Outcome" refers to the indicators of healthcare that affect a country's population. Health outcome is better if there are reductions in chronic diseases, morbidity, mortality, healthcare costs, and improvements in longevity, quality of life, physical functionality, satisfaction with care, and mental well-being. According to the New South Wales Health Department in Australia, a health outcome is defined as the "change in the health of an individual, group, or population due to an intervention or series of interventions." This encompasses all health-related aspects, including the cost of providing proper healthcare, effective patient supervision, and the duration of treatments. Researchers utilize these parameters to assess situations and enhance the quality of life and care for patients. In terms of mortality, the widely recognized and easily understood health outcome indicators are the IMR,[2] Neonatal Mortality Rate (NMR)[3], and Maternal Mortality Ratio (MMR).[4]

It is true that life expectancy has been gradually increasing, but mortality rates do not decrease over time at the same pace in many developing countries. It is crucial to focus on improving the quality of life for vulnerable infants to reduce the IMR . Recent estimates show that IMR, along with NMR and MMR , have decreased significantly, with infant deaths dropping from 12 million in 1990 to 2.6 million in 2017 (Sari et al. 2021). Despite this decline, it is important to analyze the actual patterns of this decrease and understand the factors contributing to it, as well as their significance, particularly in ASEAN countries. Therefore, the aim of this study is to use fixed and random effects models to examine how various socioeconomic conditions in ASEAN countries affect IMR, NMR, and MMRs. The paper is organized as follows: Section 19.2 provides a literature review, Section 19.3 describes the data used for the analysis, Section 19.4 presents the model and estimates the parameters, and the final section concludes with remarks on the strengths and weaknesses of the study.

---

[2] IMR: Number of resident newborns in a specified geographic area (country, state, county, etc.) dying under 1 year of age divided by the number of resident live births for the same geographic area (for a specified time period, usually a calendar year) and multiplied by 1000, that is

$$IMR = \frac{\text{Number of Infant Deaths in less than 1 Year}}{Number\ of\ Live\ Births} \times 100.$$

[3] NMR: Number of resident newborns in a specified geographic area (country, state, county, etc.) dying at less than 28 days of age divided by the number of resident live births for the same geographic area (for a specified time period, usually a calendar year) and multiplied by 1000, that is

$$NMR = \frac{\text{Number of Infant Deaths in 0–28 days}}{Number\ of\ Liver\ Births} \times 1000.$$

[4] MMR: Number of maternal deaths from pregnancy-related causes in a specific geographic area within 42 days of pregnancy termination, divided by the total number of live births in the same area during a specific time period, that is

$$MMR = \frac{\text{Number of Maternal Deaths in 42 Days of pregnancy termination}}{Number\ of\ Live\ Births} \times 100{,}000.$$

19.2 Literature Review

According to Hanmer et al. (2003) the overall development of a Nation is not only measured by per capita income but also by child mortality rate and other social pointers including socio-profitable conditions of the Nation. Rollen (2016) emphasize that the child mortality rate is a pivotal index of a nation's public health. Enhancing the quality of mortal life is of prime importance, and this is one of the basic aspects of development. This should begin from the antenatal stage to postnatal stages, nonage education, and continue into adulthood.

Motherly fertility rates, nutritive status in gestation, smoking, and environmental pollution are set up to have a strong influence on child mortality rates according to numerous experimenters. It has been seen that the educational level of mothers has a strong influence on the status of health of children. According to Bhatia et al. (2018), Dallolio et al. (2012), Hay et al. (2019), and Ullah et al. (2017), women who are not duly educated have a tendency to marry beforehand, and lack knowledge of the importance of gestational period and its care and usually have an advanced threat of mortality during parturition. As health expenditure increases, health programs expand, and access to healthcare becomes easier, the growth of newborns becomes facile. Motherly and child healthcare is generally better in developed countries than in poor countries (Ullah et al. 2017). Erdoğan et al. (2013) found a long-run empirical negative relationship between infant mortality and GDP. Ollo (2019) in his paper explained that child mortality may be caused by inheritable factors and uterine complaints. According to Mohammed and Wunnava (1999), the significant influence of socioeconomic factors, such as motherly fertility rate, womanish labor force, educational status of the mothers, and GDP per capita on child mortality rate in several countries. Shobande and Abdul (2020) linked the negative influence of energy consumption and pollution on the child mortality rate in Africa. The child mortality rate is therefore useful for measuring the trend of future population over time. The knowledge of child mortality rate is also necessary to make strategies to ameliorate motherly and child health programs in developing nations. Houweling and Kunst (2010) observed that the difference in socioeconomic conditions in developed and developing countries is a cause of child mortality, in addition to other health factors such as motherly health, nutrition, and complaint. Dallolio et al. (2012) stated that the Gini Index and the severance rate had a positive influence on the child mortality rate, while the education position of the mama had a negative influence. Iram and Butt linked social factors videlicet neighborhood of living area, education position of the mother, exclusive breastfeeding, and income had a significant influence on the child mortality rate in Pakistan. According to Rezaei et al. (2015), the child mortality rate in Iran was explained by numerous socio-profitable factors such as GDP per capita, the rate of croakers per 1000 total population, womanish labor force participation, neighborhood, and education position. On the contrary, Oloo and Alan (2005) conducted a study in developing countries and set up that the health expenditure per capita and immunization programs had no significant influence on child mortality rate, but per capita income and motherly fertility had a significant influence on child mortality rate. Rezaei et al. (2015)

in their paper examined and analyzed in detail the influence of per capita GDP, the number of health workers, fertility rate, and many other factors on the child mortality rate in Iran. They found a positive relationship between fertility and child mortality rates. Sarkar et al. (2018) also studied the impacting socioeconomic factors of child mortality rates in several ASEAN countries and found that educational status and the population had a significant influence on child mortality rate. Even social inequality was seen to have an influence on the child mortality rate in Brazil (Goldani et al. 2002) and other countries (Hosseinpoor et al. 2006; Bhatia et al. 2018). In fact, Hosseinpoor et al. (2006) showed that socioeconomic inequality had an influence on the child mortality rate between different businesses in Iran. According to Bhatia et al. (2018), in India, programs reducing socioeconomic inequality also reduced child mortality rates, which emphasizes the need for enforcing proper socio-profitable programs. Energy consumption causes pollution, and it has been seen to have a negative and significant influence on the child mortality rate in Africa (Shobande and Abdul 2020). ASEAN nations frequently defy the challenge of dwindling child and motherly mortality rates. High child mortality is nearly associated with shy motherly and child health services. Government enterprises bear community backing to foster preventative care for expectant matters, maintain a healthy living terrain, and promote healthy cultures. Therefore, a thorough health policy is pivotal to ameliorating the quality of motherly and infant care services.

19.3 Data Description

The data for this work have been taken from the World Bank website.[5] It is panel data consisting of mortality rates for different stages of growth after birth like infant, neonatal, and maternal mortality and the associated variables from the year 2000 to the year 2020. The summary statistics of all the variables are given in Table 19.1. However, in the panel data regression, some of the variables are dropped due to multicollinearity.

Similarly, from Figs. 19.2, 19.3 and 19.4, IMR, NMR, and MMR in ASEAN countries are also found to be decreasing during 2000–2020. Timor-Leste is found to have the highest NMR and MMR compared with other ASEAN countries. The rates are decreasing over time showing the possible developments in socioeconomic conditions, whereas Singapore is found to have the lowest mortality rates among the 12 ASEAN countries.

Using the dataset, it is also possible to check the heterogeneity of mortality rates across countries and over time under consideration from Figs. 19.5 and 19.6, respectively. It is clearly visualized that mortality rates are falling over time in ASEAN Countries.

Before fitting any model for the panel dataset under consideration, it is important to check the correlation between variables, particularly here the correlation between IMR, NMR, and MMR with other explanatory variables is important. From Tables

[5] https://databank.worldbank.org/source/world-development-indicators.

Table 19.1 Summary statistics for selected variables

Variable	Mean	Minimum	Median	Maximum
Infant mortality rate	29.50	1.80	24.85	87.00
Neonatal mortality rate	16.49	0.80	15.05	39.10
Maternal mortality ratio	181.10	6.00	135.00	750.00
Population growth	1.53	1.47	1.46	5.32
SRB	1.07	1.05	1.07	1.12
Male population	10.19	3.88	10.12	16.62
Female population	9.83	4.00	9.77	16.22
Fertility rate	2.65	1.10	2.43	6.02
LEB	70.07	56.51	70.26	84.47
CBR	20.94	8.50	20.16	39.12
Undernourishment	12.72	0.00	9.75	47.00
Domestic health	245.93	3.97	117.31	2773.32
Domestic Pvt. health Exp.	46.65	4.86	52.73	85.90
Out-of-pocket health Exp.	37.52	4.86	37.41	85.90
Domestic Govt. health Exp.	322.17	2.55	75.67	3054.24
Current health Exp.	579.15	19.36	226.44	5827.57
Open defecation (%)	15.05	0.00	9.090	87.45
Low birth weight (%)	13.84	6.31	12.68	21.18
Sanitation facility (%)	67.07	10.19	70.11	100.00
Anemia	37.35	16.80	36.70	100.20

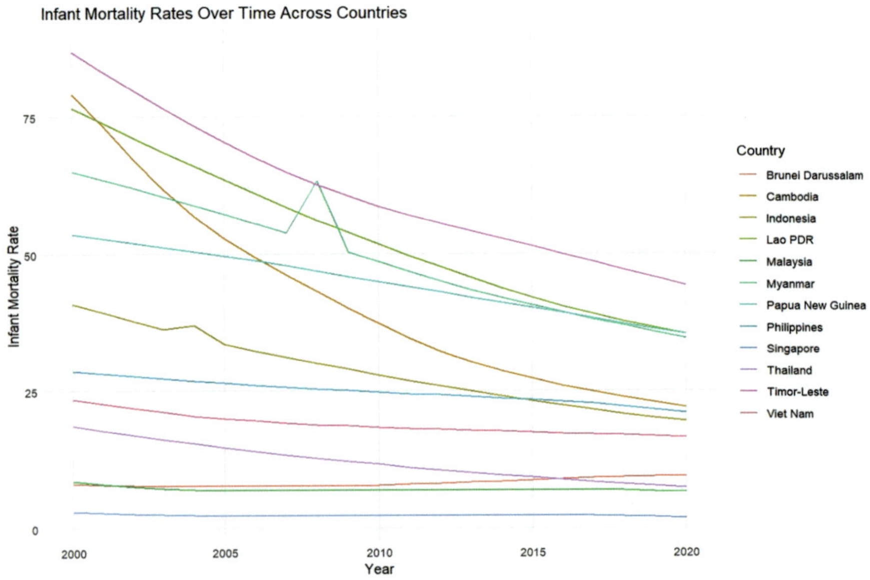

Fig. 19.2 Infant mortality rate in ASEAN 2000–2020

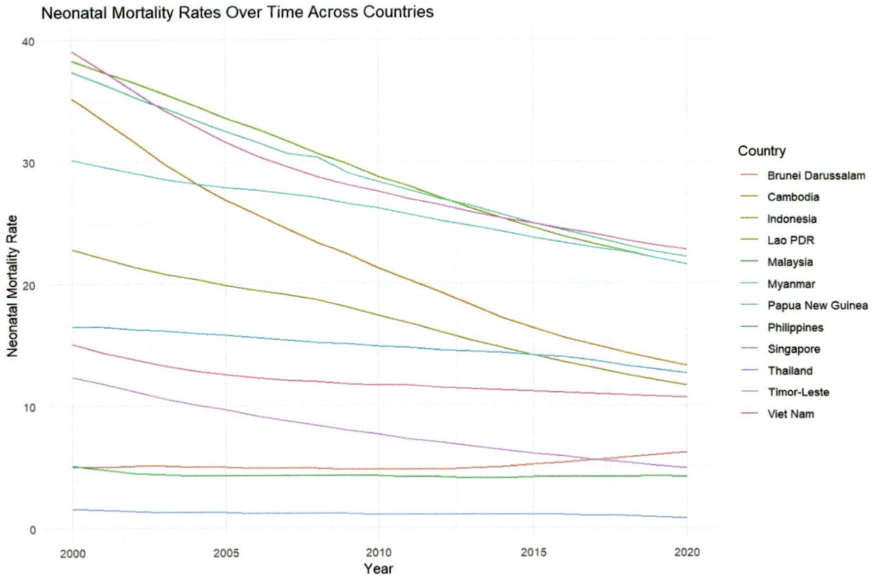

Fig. 19.3 Neonatal mortality rate in ASEAN 2000–2020

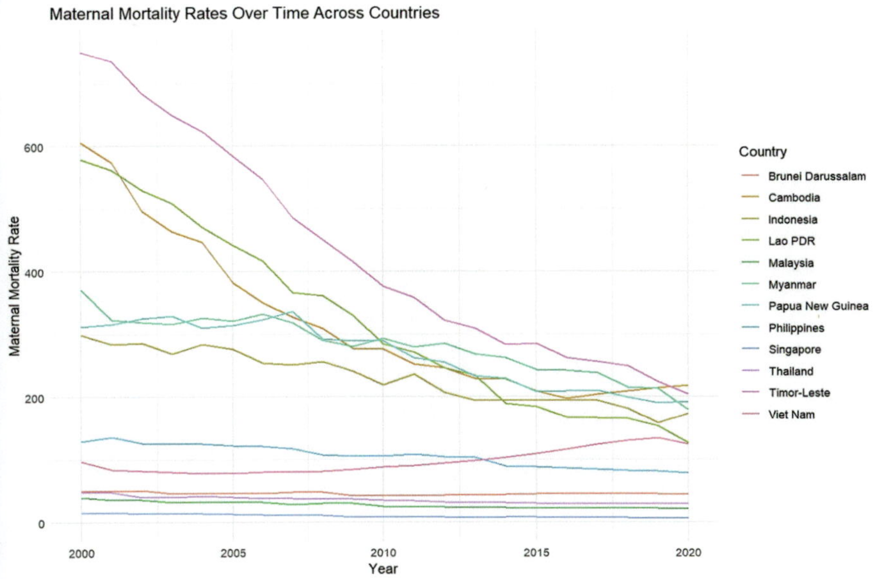

Fig. 19.4 Maternal mortality rate in ASEAN 2000–2020

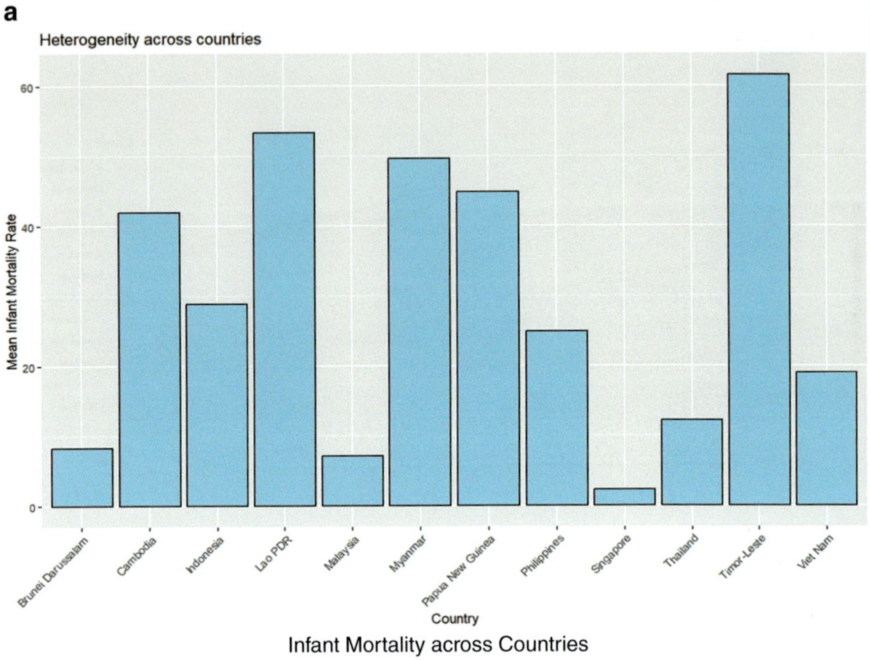

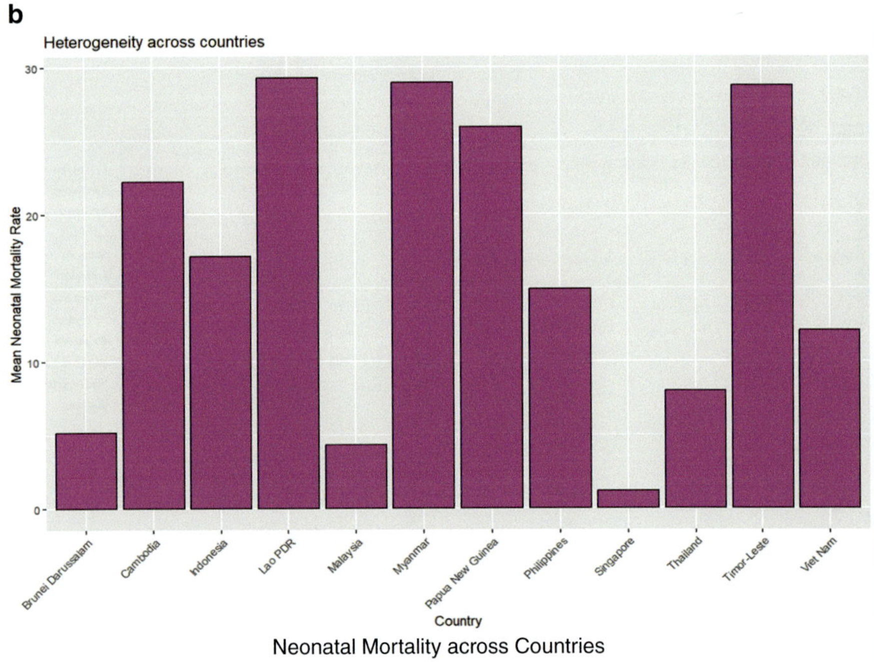

Fig. 19.5 Heterogeneity across countries. (**a**) Infant Mortality across Countries. (**b**) Neonatal Mortality across Countries. (**c**) Maternal Mortality across Countries

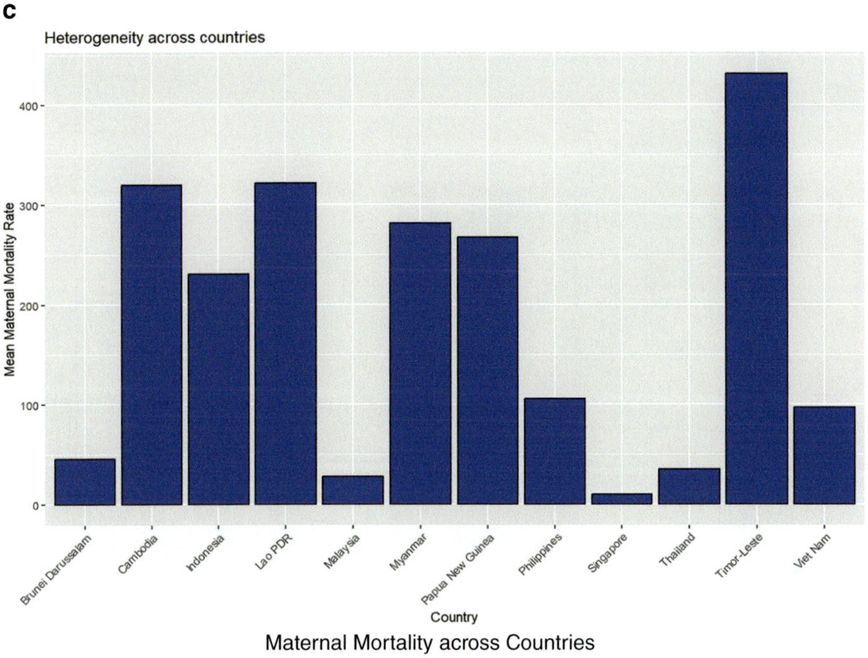

Fig. 19.5 (continued)

19.2, 19.3 and 19.4, it can be concluded that dependent variables like IMR, NMR, and MMR are highly positively correlated with other socioeconomic variables both across countries as well as overall. The correlations are also statistically significant at a 1% or 5% level of significance.

a

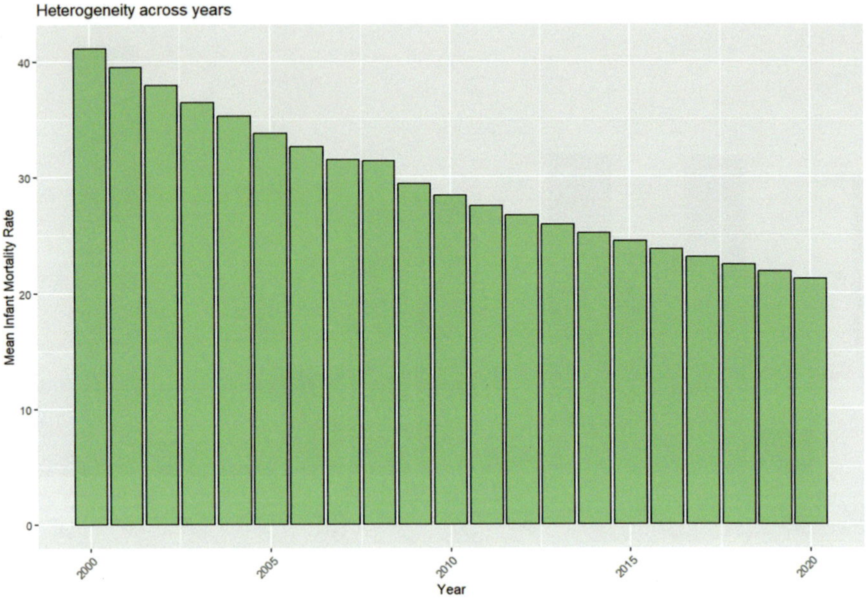

Infant Mortality over Countries

b

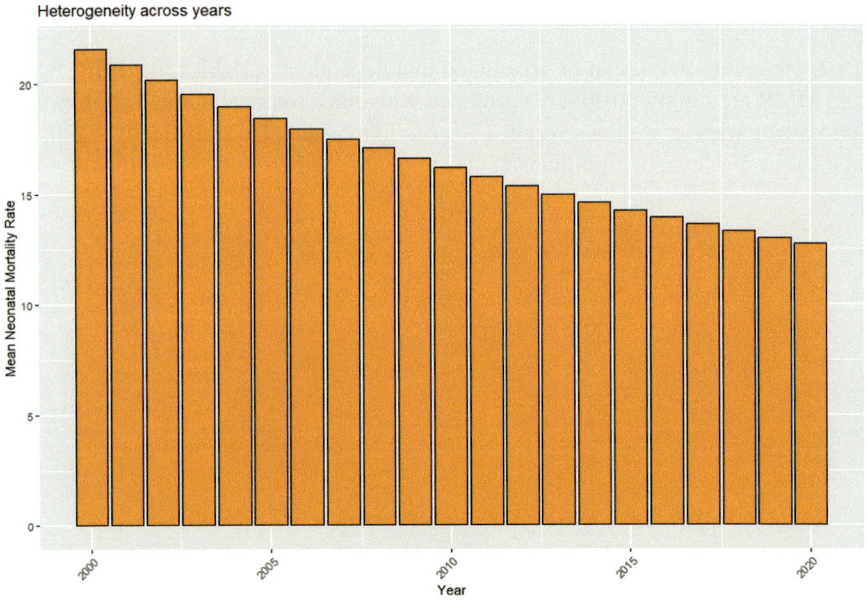

Neonatal Mortality over Time

Fig. 19.6 Heterogeneity over time. (**a**) Infant Mortality over Countries. (**b**) Neonatal Mortality over Time. (**c**) Maternal Mortality over time

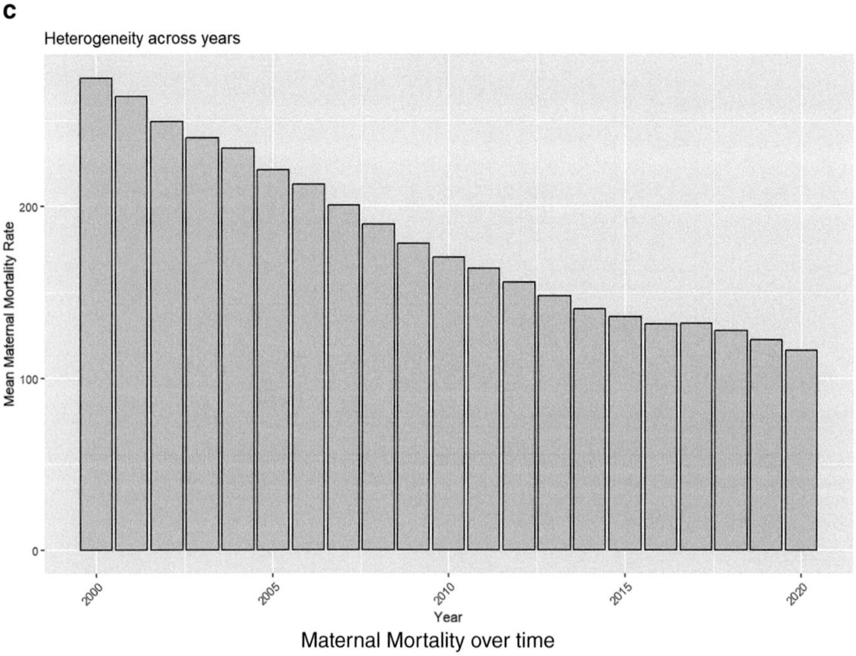

Fig. 19.6 (continued)

Table 19.2 Correlation with infant mortality rate

	Population Growth	Population Ages 00_04 (Female)	Life Expectancy at Birth	Undernourishment	Dom. Gen. Gov. Health Exp	Open Defecation	LBW Babies	Anemia Pregnant Women
Indonesia	0.894[a]	0.925[a]	−0.937[a]	0.936[a]	−0.862[a]	0.995[a]	0.930[a]	−0.214
Cambodia	0.922[a]	0.968[a]	−0.999[a]	0.992[a]	−0.816[a]	0.966[a]	0.974[a]	0.994[a]
Lao PDR	0.454[b]	0.996[a]	−0.997[a]	0.996[a]	−0.744[a]	0.998[a]	0.971[a]	0.951[a]
Myanmar	0.469[b]	0.966[a]	−0.954[a]	0.932[a]	−0.855[a]	0.970[a]	−0.622[a]	0.742[a]
Malaysia	0.707[a]	0.814[a]	−0.809[a]	−0.534[b]	−0.720[a]	0.823[a]	−0.695[a]	0.814[a]
Philippines	0.934[a]	0.992[a]	−0.997[a]	0.979[a]	−0.914[a]	0.993[a]	−0.828[a]	0.969[a]
Papua New Guinea	0.993[a]	0.998[a]	−0.982[a]	0.841[a]	−0.881[a]	−0.993[a]	−0.990[a]	0.986[a]
Singapore	0.156	0.868[a]	−0.909[a]	0.060	−0.767[a]	0.405	−0.831[a]	0.677[a]
Thailand	0.956[a]	0.981[a]	−0.993[a]	0.982[a]	−0.991[a]	0.999[a]	0.994[a]	−0.838[a]
Timor Leste	0.167	0.929[a]	−1.000[a]	0.938[a]	−0.903[a]	0.985[a]	0.488[b]	−0.013
Vietnam	0.432	0.981[a]	−0.890[a]	0.978[a]	−0.877[a]	0.959[a]	0.957[a]	0.980[a]
Brunei Darussalam	−0.831[a]	−0.693[a]	0.115	−0.156	−0.664[a]	−0.983[a]	0.832[a]	−0.603[a]
Overall	**0.191**[a]	**0.780**[a]	**−0.941**[a]	**0.855**[a]	**−0.586**[a]	**0.742**[a]	**0.499**[a]	**0.714**[a]

[a]Correlation is significant at the 0.01 level (two-tailed)
[b]Correlation is significant at the 0.05 level (two-tailed)

Table 19.3 Correlation with neonatal mortality

	Population Growth	Population Ages 00_04 (Female)	Life Expectancy at Birth	Undernourishment	Dom. Gen. Gov. Health Exp	Open Defecation	LBW Babies	Anemia Pregnant Women
Indonesia	0.942[a]	0.952[a]	−0.908[a]	0.960[a]	−0.908[a]	0.996[a]	0.973[a]	−0.353
Cambodia	0.953[a]	0.985[a]	−0.990[a]	0.994[a]	−0.869[a]	0.989[a]	0.993[a]	0.987[a]
Lao PDR	0.439[b]	0.992[a]	−0.999[a]	0.994[a]	−0.765[a]	0.999[a]	0.975[a]	0.939[a]
Myanmar	0.628[a]	0.993[a]	−0.852[a]	0.974[a]	−0.832[a]	0.996[a]	−0.710[a]	0.831[a]
Malaysia	0.683[a]	0.804[a]	−0.776[a]	−0.682[a]	−0.684[a]	0.827[a]	−0.654[a]	0.813[a]
Philippines	0.896[a]	0.989[a]	−0.993[a]	0.974[a]	−0.945[a]	0.992[a]	−0.764[a]	0.980[a]
Papua New Guinea	0.995[a]	0.996[a]	−0.980[a]	0.830[a]	−0.881[a]	−0.988[a]	−0.986[a]	0.984[a]
Singapore	0.254	0.879[a]	−0.958[a]	0.125	−0.852[a]	0.357	−0.909[a]	0.628[a]
Thailand	0.954[a]	0.982[a]	−0.991[a]	0.984[a]	−0.989[a]	0.998[a]	0.995[a]	−0.831[a]
Timor Leste	0.100	0.901[a]	−0.997[a]	0.946[a]	−0.879[a]	0.970[a]	0.529[b]	0.047
Vietnam	0.449[b]	0.973[a]	−0.879[a]	0.965[a]	−0.849[a]	0.941[a]	0.939[a]	0.976[a]
Brunei Darussalam	−0.644[a]	−0.493[b]	0.015	−0.298	−0.448[b]	−0.868[a]	0.608[a]	−0.362
Overall	**0.164**[a]	**0.761**[a]	**−0.963**[a]	**0.831**[a]	**−0.636**[a]	**0.697**[a]	**0.488**[a]	**0.783**[a]

[a]Correlation is significant at the 0.01 level (two-tailed)
[b]Correlation is significant at the 0.05 level (two-tailed)

Table 19.4 Correlation with maternal mortality ratio

	Population Growth	Population Ages 00_04 (Female)	Life expectancy at birth	Undernourishment	Dom. Gen. Gov. Health Exp	Open Defecation	LBW Babies	Anemia Pregnant Women
Indonesia	0.883[a]	0.906[a]	−0.927[a]	0.954[a]	−0.857[a]	0.976[a]	0.937[a]	−0.299
Cambodia	0.865[a]	0.926[a]	−0.991[a]	0.968[a]	−0.728[a]	0.920[a]	0.934[a]	0.985[a]
Lao PDR	0.470[b]	0.995[a]	−0.993[a]	0.996[a]	−0.708[a]	0.991[a]	0.953[a]	0.964[a]
Myanmar	0.547[b]	0.928[a]	−0.803[a]	0.866[a]	−0.835[a]	0.954[a]	−0.503[b]	0.655[a]
Malaysia	0.962[a]	0.981[a]	−0.959[a]	−0.795[a]	−0.938[a]	0.973[a]	−0.935[a]	0.970[a]
Philippines	0.894[a]	0.982[a]	−0.975[a]	0.960[a]	−0.903[a]	0.983[a]	−0.765[a]	0.972[a]
Papua New Guinea	0.965[a]	0.961[a]	−0.985[a]	0.907[a]	−0.898[a]	−0.970[a]	−0.929[a]	0.965[a]
Singapore	0.149	0.943[a]	−0.951[a]	0.042	−0.765[a]	0.213	−0.822[a]	0.739[a]
Thailand	0.913[a]	0.948[a]	−0.958[a]	0.957[a]	−0.958[a]	0.972[a]	0.955[a]	−0.785[a]
Timor Leste	0.187	0.944[a]	−0.997[a]	0.905[a]	−0.910[a]	0.980[a]	0.513[b]	0.003
Vietnam	−0.456[b]	−0.701[a]	0.697[a]	−0.740[a]	0.917[a]	−0.837[a]	−0.841[a]	−0.572[a]
Brunei Darussalam	0.630[a]	0.739[a]	−0.758[a]	0.105	0.164	0.361	−0.647[a]	0.775[a]
Overall	**0.193**[a]	**0.748**[a]	**−0.882**[a]	**0.802**[a]	**−0.510**[a]	**0.802**[a]	**0.396**[a]	**0.656**[a]

[a]Correlation is significant at the 0.01 level (two-tailed)
[b]Correlation is significant at the 0.05 level (two-tailed)

19.4 Methods and Model Estimation

This paper uses simple fixed & random effect models for Panel data analysis using the given dataset to understand the effects of the explanatory variables on different mortality rates to understand the patterns of the change. As there are two models, it calls for the suitability and superiority of one model to the other model, which is done by the Hausman Specification test. The following are some basic details of the overall models used.

Pooled Panel Data Model: The pooled panel data model is the simplest and the basic form of panel data models, though it does not incorporate the characteristics of panel data. It assumes that all individual units have the same intercept and slope coefficients. The model is

$$y_{it} = \beta_0 + \beta_1 x_{it} + u_{it},$$

where x_{it} is a vector of explanatory variables and u_{it}'s are independent of each other. Also,

$$u_{it} \sim N\left(0, \sigma^2\right).$$

Fixed Effects Model: The fixed effects model includes individual-specific effects, allowing for different intercepts for different individual units and time points. The basic model is the same as above.

Random Effects Model: The random effects model treats the individual-specific effects as random variables assuming they are uncorrelated with the regressors. The basic model remains the same.

It is important to note that Fixed Effect Model is also called least square dummy variable (LSDV) model where we can introduce the Cross-section (N) specific and time (T) specific dummies. But here the problem arises when N is very large, since then it causes huge loss in Degrees of freedom

Hausman Specification Test: The Hausman test is used to choose between the fixed effects (FE) and random effects (RE) models by testing whether the individual-specific effects are correlated with the regressors. The null hypothesis is H_0: RE is consistent versus alternative hypothesis H_1: FE is consistent. The test statistic is given by

$$\mathrm{H} = \left(\hat{\beta}_{\mathrm{RE}} - \hat{\beta}_{\mathrm{FE}}\right)' \left[\mathrm{Var}\left(\hat{\beta}_{\mathrm{RE}}\right) - \mathrm{Var}\left(\hat{\beta}_{\mathrm{FE}}\right)\right]^{-1} \left(\hat{\beta}_{\mathrm{RE}} - \hat{\beta}_{\mathrm{FE}}\right),$$

where $\hat{\beta}_{\mathrm{FE}}$ is the coefficient estimate from the fixed effects model, $\hat{\beta}_{\mathrm{RE}}$ is the coefficient estimate from the random effects model, $\mathrm{Var}\left(\hat{\beta}_{\mathrm{FE}}\right)$ is the variance-covariance matrix of $\hat{\beta}_{\mathrm{FE}}$, and $\mathrm{Var}\left(\hat{\beta}_{\mathrm{RE}}\right)$ is the variance-covariance matrix of $\hat{\beta}_{\mathrm{RE}}$. The test statistic H follows a chi-squared distribution with degrees of freedom equal to the difference in the number of parameters estimated in the two models. In fact, we estimate both the fixed effects and random effects models, compute the value of the test statistic H, and compare the computed H value with the critical value of the chi-squared distribution at a chosen significance level. If H is greater than the critical value, reject the null hypothesis that the random effects model is consistent and choose the fixed effects model.

The results of the regression analysis of the pooled panel data model are given in Tables 19.5, 19.6 and 19.7. From these regression results, it is found that overall models are significant when pooled regression is performed to see the effects of other variables on the mortality rates. To maintain the value of VIF to ≤ 10 for the explanatory variables, we have taken only a few explanatory variables, which means that there is no multicollinearity. Population Growth, Life Expectancy at Birth, and Percentage of Anemic Pregnant Women have negative effects on all three mortality rates. Percentages of Open Defecation and LBW Babies have a positive effect on the mortality rates. Other variables have mixed effects, having positive effects for one/some of the mortality rates and negative effects on other(s). The interpretations of these results are not very clear. Hopefully, the situation will improve in the FE and RE models.

In the FE model, the problem of multicollinearity arises when dummy variables are introduced for countries and years. In order to avoid this problem, variables are taken one by one in the models so as to eliminate the problem of multicollinearity. Thus, we are finally left with four explanatory variables, namely, Population Growth Rate, Undernourishment, Domestic General Government Health Expenditure, and Percentage of Open Defecation. The results of FE Panel Data Regression of IMR,

Table 19.5 Regression: Infant mortality rate

Variable	Coefficient	t	Sig.	Tolerance	VIF
(constant)	243.083	19.793	0.000		
Population growth	−1.290	−2.870	0.004	0.600	1.667
Population ages 00–04 female	−1.290	−5.136	0.000	0.122	8.215
Life expectancy at birth	−2.909	−21.199	0.000	0.100	9.984
Undernutrition	0.514	11.140	0.000	0.283	3.533
Dom. Gen. Gov. health Exp.	0.001	0.862	0.389	0.442	2.264
Open defecation	0.306	14.476	0.000	0.477	2.094
LBW babies	0.556	4.850	0.000	0.360	2.781
Anemia of pregnant women	−0.382	−6.576	0.000	0.191	5.243

Table 19.6 Regression: Neonatal mortality rate

Variable	B	t	Sig.	Tolerance	VIF
(constant)	124.137	20.446	0.000		
Population growth	−0.575	−2.589	0.010	0.600	1.667
Population ages 00–04 female	−0.888	−7.149	0.000	0.122	8.215
Life expectancy at birth	−1.513	−22.299	0.000	0.100	9.984
Undernutrition	0.223	9.789	0.000	0.283	3.533
Dom. Gen. Gov. health Exp	7.531E-5	0.199	0.843	0.442	2.264
Open defecation	0.077	7.388	0.000	0.477	2.094
LBW babies	0.334	5.900	0.000	0.360	2.781
Anemia of pregnant women	−0.018	−0.644	0.520	0.191	5.243

Table 19.7 Regression: Maternal mortality ratio

Variable	Coefficient	t	Sig.	Tolerance	VIF
(constant)	1687.382	12.848	0.000		
Population growth	−7.230	−1.505	0.134	0.600	1.667
Population ages 00–04 female	2.780	1.035	0.302	0.122	8.215
Life expectancy at birth	−19.771	−13.472	0.000	0.100	9.984
Undernutrition	2.721	5.515	0.000	0.283	3.533
Dom. Gen. Gov. health Exp.	0.015	1.855	0.065	0.442	2.264
Open defecation	3.729	16.483	0.000	0.477	2.094
LBW babies	−4.703	−3.836	0.000	0.360	2.781
Anemia of pregnant women	−4.532	−7.303	0.000	0.191	5.243

NMR, and MMR on the four regressors stated above with Country Dummies are given in Table 19.8. We have also run the Panel Data FE regression model taking both country and time dummies and this is given in Appendix A. This improves the goodness of fit of the model but very little.

It can be seen from Table 19.9 that many of the Country Dummies are very significant implying significant country variations. Surprisingly, the effect of all four regressors is positive on all three mortality rates. Why Government Health Expenditure has positive effect on mortalities is not clear.

Even after the introduction of time dummies in Table 19.9, the overall model does not statistically improve much as most of the time dummies are statistically insignificant; it is not worthwhile to keep the time dummies in the model which requires here degrees of freedom due to introduction of one variable corresponding to each year avoiding one in order to avoid falling into Dummy variable Trap or Perfect Multicollinearity. Both fixed and random effects models are estimated and then selected out of two models. Hausman specification tests are performed with the results summarized in Table 19.10. For IMR , NMR null hypothesis, i.e., the RE model is consistent is rejected at a 5% significance level, whereas for MMR, the RE model is found to be consistent.

The results of the RE model for the same set of variables are given in Table 19.10, 19.11, 19.12.

Table 19.13 shows the result of the Hausman Specification Test. It shows that we should take the FE model for IMR and NMR and the RE model for MMR.

From the above results of regression through origin population growth, Domestic General Government Health expenditure is found to be insignificant, whereas undernutrition and percentage of open defecation are found to be statistically significant at 5% level of significance. Mortality rates are positively affected by undernutrition and open defecation as it is supposed to be. Improvement of Domestic Government health through an increase in health expenditure has a mitigating impact on mortality rates though the results are insignificant.

Table 19.8 Result of fixed effect panel data regression of IMR, NMR and MMR with Country Dummy Only

	IMR	NMR	MMR
Population growth	0.500 (0.225)	0.266 (0.075)	3.350 (0.597)
Undernutrition	0.623 (0.000)	0.317 (0.000)	3.390 (0.000)
Dom. Gen. Gov. health Exp.	0.000 (0.957)	0.000 (0.427)	0.002 (0.876)
Open defecation	0.558 (0.000)	0.195 (0.000)	6.056 (0.000)
Dummy_Indonesia	9.626 (0.000)	9.079 (0.000)	68.284 (0.000)
Dummy_Cambodia	3.891 (0.010)	7.492 (0.000)	−47.909 (0.039)
Dummy_Lao PDR	21.918 (0.000)	16.559 (0.000)	37.393 (0.037)
Dummy_Myanmar	34.283 (0.000)	21.866 (0.000)	171.605 (0.000)
Dummy_Malaysia	3.240 (0.006)	2.482 (0.000)	2.163 (0.904)
Dummy_Philippines	12.299 (0.000)	9.147 (0.000)	12.802 (0.432)
Dummy_Papua	19.749 (0.000)	14.410 (0.000)	86.421 (0.000)
Dummy_Singapore	1.484 (0.369)	1.017 (0.089)	1.442 (0.955)
Dummy_Thailand	5.182 (0.000)	4.579 (0.000)	−5.408 (0.695)
Dummy_Timur Leste	24.415 (0.000)	12.447 (0.000)	139.012 (0.000)
Dummy_Vietnam	6.662 (0.000)	6.586 (0.000)	2.721 (0.834)
Dummy Brunei	6.391 (0.001)	4.724 (0.000)	23.353 (0.414)
R-square	0.994	0.997	0.968

The values in parentheses represent *p*-values

Table 19.9 Regression with Country and Time (Year) Dummy

	IMR	NMR	MMR
Population growth	0.379 (0.416)	0.124 (0.452)	2.653(0.715)
Undernourishment	0.551 (0.000)	0.275 (0.000)	2.618(0.001)'
Dom.Gen.Gov health Exp.	0.001 (0.565)	0.000 (0.533)	0.008(0.615)
Open defecation	0.546 (0.000)	0.185 (0.000)	5.967(0.000)
Dummy_Indonesia	10.176 (0.000)	9.249 (0.000)	78.276(0.000)
Dummy_Cambodia	4.888 (0.006)	8.067 (0.000)	−34.598(0.212)
Dummy_LaoPDR	22.967 (0.000)	17.113 (0.000)	51.872(0.026)
Dummy_Myanmar	34.951 (0.000)	22.054 (0.000)	183.422(0.000)
Dummy_Malaysia	2.842 (0.055)	2.041 (0.000)	2.497(0.914)
Dummy_Philippines	12.725 (0.000)	9.252 (0.000)	21.484(0.310)
Dummy_Papua	21.354 (0.000)	15.317 (0.000)	106.927(0.001)
Dummy_Singapore	0.261 (0.898)	−0.017 (0.981)	−6.121(0.847)
Dummy_Thailand	5.096 (0.000)	4.243 (0.000)	−0.988(0.960)
Dummy_TimurLeste	26.528 (0.000)	13.638 (0.000)	165.041(0.000)
Dummy_Vietnam	6.928 (0.000)	6.538 (0.000)	10.180(0.581)
Dummy_Brunei	4.934 (0.031)	3.498 (0.000)	13.750(0.698)
Dummy_Y2000	2.936 (0.059)	1.870 (0.001)	22.243(0.357)
Dummy_Y2001	2.340 (0.128)	1.597 (0.004)	18.745(0.433)
Dummy_Y2002	1.979 (0.181)	1.413 (0.008)	13.353(0.562)
Dummy_Y2003	1.700 (0.232)	1.278 (0.012)	12.455(0.574)
Dummy_Y2004	1.292 (0.364)	1.040 (0.040)	13.021(0.557)

(continued)

Table 19.9 (continued)

	IMR	NMR	MMR
Dummy_Y2005	0.752 (0.596)	0.897 (0.075)	7.749(0.726)
Dummy_Y2006	0.475 (0.735)	0.779 (0.119)	6.604(0.763)
Dummy_Y2007	0.210 (0.880)	0.684 (0.167)	1.305(0.952)
Dummy_Y2008	0.863 (0.532)	0.618 (0.208)	−3.375(0.875)
Dummy_Y2009	−0.058 (0.965)	0.565 (0.231)	−6.739(0.745)
Dummy_Y2010	0.071 (0.957)	0.601 (0.195)	−6.710(0.741)
Dummy_Y2011	0.175 (0.892)	0.647 (0.159)	−5.141(0.798)
Dummy_Y2012	0.116 (0.928)	0.556 (0.220)	−6.810(0.732)
Dummy_Y2013	0.143 (0.910)	0.497 (0.266)	−7.896(0.687)
Dummy_Y2014	0.179 (0.886)	0.417 (0.345)	−8.963(0.643)
Dummy_Y2015	0.233 (0.850)	0.373 (0.394)	−7.518(0.695)
Dummy_Y2016	0.216 (0.860)	0.307 (0.481)	−5.708(0.765)
Dummy_Y2017	0.279 (0.819)	0.283 (0.513)	0.807(0.966)
Dummy_Y2018	0.303 (0.803)	0.230 (0.592)	2.758(0.884)
Dummy_Y2019	0.251 (0.836)	0.146 (0.733)	2.651(0.888)
R-square	0.994	0.998	0.969

Figures in parentheses represent the level of significance

Table 19.10 Random effect model of infant mortality rate

Variable	Estimate	*z*-value	Significance
Intercept	12.514 (2.618)	4.779	<0.001***
Population	0.437 (0.412)	1.060	0.2891
Domestic GG health	−0.00034 (0.00093)	−0.368	0.713
Undernourishment	0.635 (0.041)	15.507	<0.001***
Defecation	0.555 (0.029)	18.879	<0.001***
R-squared		0.88019	
Adjusted R-squared		0.87825	
Chi-sq		1814.65	
P-value		<2.22e-16	

Standard errors are in parentheses. Significance codes: ***$p<0.001$, **$p<0.01$, and *$p<0.05$

Table 19.11 Random effect model of neonatal mortality rate

Variable	Estimate	*z*-value	Significance
Intercept	9.228 (1.576)	5.856	<0.001***
Population	0.248 (0.149)	1.660	0.0970 .
Domestic GG health	−0.00034 (0.00034)	−1.019	0.3082
Undernourishment	0.319 (0.015)	21.474	<0.001***
Defecation	0.195 (0.011)	18.232	<0.001***
R-squared		0.9085	
Adjusted R-squared		0.90702	
Chisq		2452.56	
P-value		< 2.22e−16	

Standard errors are in parentheses. Significance codes: ***$p < 0.001$, **$p < 0.01$, and *$p < 0.05$

Table 19.12 Random effect model of maternal mortality ratio

Variable	Estimate	Std. error	Significance
(intercept)	41.1607 (19.2097)	2.1427	0.0321*
Population	2.3143 (6.1069)	0.3790	0.7047
Domestic GG health	−0.0032 (0.0132)	−0.2450	0.8065
Undernourishment	3.9953 (0.6012)	6.6455	< 0.001***
Defecation	5.7551 (0.4200)	13.7016	< 2.2e-16***
Total sum of squares		1,760,400	
Residual sum of squares		502,940	
R-squared		0.7143	
Adj. R-squared		0.7096	

Standard errors are in parentheses. Significance codes: ***$p<0.001$, **$p<0.01$, and *$p<0.05$

Table 19.13 Hausman specification test

	Model 1	Model 2	Model 3
Dependent variable	IMR	NMR	MMR
P-value	0.001525	$8.375e^{-11}$	0.2222
Result	FE is consistent	FE is consistent	RE is consistent

19.5 Conclusion

The policymakers and governments of the ASEAN member countries should concentrate on balanced socioeconomic development of the nations to promote the health status of the respective countries. One of the most important objects should be to take enterprise to ameliorate the mortality rates. This present study examined and analyzed in detail the socio-profitable determinants of child mortality rate, NMR, and MMR in ASEAN member countries. Socioeconomic variables such as population growth, health expenditure, low birth weight babies, life expectation at birth, undernourishment, open defecation, and anemia in pregnant women have preliminarily been anatomized in other studies and unambiguously found their significant influence on child mortality rate, NMR, and MMR in their respective countries. High Domestic Government health expenditure was found to reduce child, neonatal, and maternal mortality. The present study estimated the influence of socioeconomic factors on child mortality rate, NMR, and MMR in ASEAN. Stationary balanced panel data model was used. The fixed effect model was seen to have a better fit for IMR and NMR. For MMR, any of the FE and ME models can be taken. There was a significant influence of undernourishment and chance of open defecation on child mortality rate, NMR, and MMR in ASEAN countries. Health expenditure had no significant influence on child mortality rate but has a positive influence.

Ultramodern health services are more accessible for mothers and children, but this must also be balanced with income equalization and enhancement in health structure so that services are fluently accessible by all groups. Continued social and profitable inequality causes high child mortality rates to be concentrated on poor families. Child mortality rate counts are demanded for development programs, especially in the health and social fields. Also, empowering women has both direct and circular impacts on mindfulness of motherly and child health. Thus, it is necessary to formulate effective health programs to reduce child mortality rates, because the mother's and child's well-being determines the health of the coming generation.

Therefore, the recommendations of this study are as follows. (1) Strategies are demanded to give accessible and affordable health installations to all groups. (2) Increase mindfulness of women's commissions through educational programs on motherly and child health. (3) Ameliorate social conditions in society, and income equalization to ameliorate citizen weal. This study was limited by banning other socio-profitable variables that may impact child mortality rate, NMR, and MMR in ASEAN. This study could also be extended by the selection of variables in Panel data frame as suggested by Smith, Timmerman (2019).

References

Bhatia B, Kailash P et al (2018) Consensus statement on the classification of tremors. From the task force on tremor of the International Parkinson and Movement Disorder Society. Mov Disord 33(1):75–87

Dallolio D, Di Laura V, Gregori JL, Franchino G, Calugi S, Domenighetti G, Fantini MP (2012) Socio-economic factors associated with infant mortality in Italy: an ecological study. Int J Equity Health 11:1–5

Elizabeth BB et al (2011) Dimensions of perceived racism and self-reported health: examination of racial/ethnic differences and potential mediators. Ann Behav Med 42(1):14–28

Erdoğan E, Engin ME, Arıca F (2013) The strategic role of infant mortality in the process of economic growth: an application for high income OECD countries. Procedia Soc Behav Sci 99:19–25

Goldani G, Zubaran M et al (2002) Narrowing inequalities in infant mortality in Southern Brazil. Rev Saude Publica 36:478–483

Hanmer H, Lucia RL, White H (2003) Infant and child mortality in developing countries: analysing the data for robust determinants. J Dev Stud 40(1):101–118

Hay H, Katherine LMD, Percival V, Henry S, Klugman J, Wurie H, Raven J et al (2019) Disrupting gender norms in health systems: making the case for change. Lancet 393(10190):2535–2549

Hosseinpoor ARH, Van Doorslaer E, Speybroeck N, Naghavi M, Mohammad K, Majdzadeh R, Vega J (2006) Decomposing socioeconomic inequality in infant mortality in Iran. Int J Epidemiol 35(5):1211–1219

Houweling TA, Kunst AE (2010) Socio-economic inequalities in childhood mortality in low-and middle-income countries: a review of the international evidence. Br Med Bull 93(1):7–26

Mohammed ZZ, Wunnava PV (1999) Factors affecting infant mortality rates: evidence from cross–sectional data. Appl Econ Lett 6(5):271–227

Ollo GG (2019) Predictors of preterm birth among women of pastoralist communities in Marsabit county, Kenya, Diss. Kenyatta University, Nairobi

Oloo O, Alan J (2005) Child mortality in developing countries: challenges and policy options. East Afr Soc Sci Res Rev 21(2):1–17

Rezaei S, Matin BK, Rad EH (2015) Socioeconomic determinants of infant mortality in Iranian children: a longitudinal econometrics analysis. Int J Pediatr 3.1.1:375–380

Rollen SS, Tubayan EJC (2016) The relationship of health-related factors to labor productivity of the ASEAN-5. Rev Integr Bus Econ Res 5(4):138

Sari S, Kartika V, Prasetyani D (2021) Socioeconomic determinants of infant mortality rate in Asean: a panel data analysis. J ASEAN Stud 9(1):1

Sarkar S, Dhar B, Rouhoma H (2018) Socio-economic determinants of infant mortality in the south Asian region—A cross sectional analysis. Int J Business Soc 2(2):1–6

Shobande S, Abdul O (2020) The effects of energy use on infant mortality rates in Africa. Environ Sustain Indicators 5:100015

Ullah U, Anzar M, Husseni AM, Mahmood SU (2017) Consanguineous marriages and their detrimental outcomes in Pakistan: an urgent need for appropriate measures. Int J Community Med Public Health 5(1):1–3

Part IV

Miscellaneous

Role of Mass Media on Health Awareness Among Rural Mothers: A Qualitative Study

20

Md. Belal Hossain and Md. Golam Hossain

20.1 Introduction

Health is a complex phenomenon that involves many factors, including an individual's physical and mental well-being as well as the quality of their social environment. The condition of women during their pregnancies, deliveries, and postpartum periods is referred to as maternal health. To ensure that women and their infants achieve their optimum potential for good health and happiness, every stage should be enjoyable (WHO 2022). A healthy lifestyle and high-quality medical care are crucial for society's effective setup. Social inequalities characterize health and healthcare quality (Kruk et al. 2018).

Mass media is one of the best communication methods for disseminating information and raising awareness. To stop the spread of various diseases, the mass media makes health information available to raise public awareness. Mass media has many forms, including television, the Internet, newspapers, magazines, traditional media, and folk media (Anwar et al. 2020). Due to its accessibility in distant places and affordability, radio, like in other developing nations, is Bangladesh's primary source of information and entertainment. News, commentary, analysis, and commercials are all included in broadcasts. The general people are becoming less interested in this media nowadays (Azad 2023).

Television is one of the most significant communication tools for inspiring individuals to contribute to a better society. It can significantly affect people, increase

M. B. Hossain (✉)
Department of Mass Communication and Journalism, University of Rajshahi, Rajshahi, Bangladesh

Department of Mass Communication and Journalism, Comilla University, Cumilla, Bangladesh

M. G. Hossain
Department of Statistics, University of Rajshahi, Rajshahi, Bangladesh

M. Pal et al. (eds.), *Public Health and Nutrition*,
https://doi.org/10.1007/978-981-97-7890-4_20

knowledge, shape public opinion, and introduce new lifestyles. The newest development in electronic communication is the Internet. It is quickly bringing about a momentous shift in the world of communication. The medium offers immediate access to the world's most extensive databases and information repositories (Alam 2014).

Many academics have used content analysis to look into health-related study subjects. According to Bonnie and George (1975), they thought about how radio and television would affect public service messages for family planning (Bonnie and George 1975). Dubey and Bardhan (1981) developed a module on content analysis of messages and programs in health and population communication to assist medium and lower-level field workers in becoming more familiar with and comprehending communication research (Dubey and Bardhan 1981). Singh Archana (2007) examined the role of mass communication in avoiding behaviors and managing AIDS using content analysis of Indian newspapers and mass media. The public health community widely relies on the media for support, attention, and endorsement because it is recognized as a primary source of information about science and health, even among health professionals (Archana 2007). Bryant and Finklea (2022) found that this aligns with the agenda-setting idea regarding the quantity of commercial, graphic, and other timeslots offered. Content analysis is a useful method to understand how the media spreads health messages and how the public obtains this health information (Bryant and Finklea 2022). Chandra Shekhar Ghanta (2012) emphasizes that one of the fundamental tenets of the media is to disseminate information to raise public awareness of the state's welfare. The mass media are widely acknowledged as a crucial social institution in today's societies. The study focused on the health-related advertisements that may be found on radio and television, which are forms of mass media. The analysis uses two communicative instruments that were chosen at random (Ghanta 2012). Achala Gupta and A. K. Sinha (2010) found that mass media are widely acknowledged as a crucial social institution in today's societies. The study looked at the health-related messages broadcast on television, radio, and in print (newspapers and magazines) and electronic (magazines and newspapers). The newspapers, magazines, radio and television stations, and other sources used for the analysis were randomly picked. However, print and mass media primarily covered political, social, criminal, and sporting news, according to a thorough content study of numerous communication mediums (Gupta and Sinha 2010). Mashreky et al. (2015) found that the results of a community trial in rural Bangladesh show that inadequate IYCF (Infant and Young Children Feeding) practices contribute to the undernutrition of newborns and young children in developing nations like Bangladesh (Mashreky et al. 2015). Paula Bylaska-Davies (2011) noted that breastfeeding has long been recognized as the best and most complete form of nutrition for newborns because it supports growth and promotes good health. It has been proposed that the mass media is a potent, global communication tool that can change societal norms (Bylaska-Davies 2011).

However, mass media disseminates information among the general public to foster acceptance of any notion intended to spark interest. Interactive user feedback and creative engagement in a meaningful and valuable way for national development in any country is also encouraged by those media, either directly or indirectly (Naveena 2015). As a result, mass media interact with people so much that even people with limited literacy skills can understand information about social, political, and developmental issues. Mass media can focus public attention on specific problems while drawing attention to various concerns that must be addressed to address them. Therefore, the present study investigates the role of mass media like television, radio, and the Internet in creating awareness among rural mothers about their health and their breastfeeding children.

20.2 Study Methods

A qualitative study has been conducted by applying the survey method. The primary data were collected from 100 mothers having breastfeeding children from July 2017 to June 2018. The respondents aged 18–59 years residing in the study areas have been surveyed through a structured questionnaire following a purposive sampling technique. This study was conducted at Adda Union of Barura Upazila under the Comilla district of Bangladesh. This Upazila is a typical rural area of Bangladesh. Five villages have been selected purposively based on proximity and cooperation from Adda Union. Twenty respondents were selected from each village, like Adda, Kandirpar, Osshodia, Khatla, and Chotopotia. The demographic variables and patterns are presented through the frequency tables. The different relationships and associations are studied by using descriptive statistics.

20.3 Results and Analysis

Table 20.1 represents the socio-demographic profile of the respondents. The study findings show that a maximum of 74% of respondents are 18–29 years of age, and 18% of respondents are between 30 and 39 years of age. Notably, 2% of respondents are between 40 and 49 years old, and 3% of respondents are between 50 and 59 years of age, which is a low percentage of the entry. Therefore, the study found that most of the respondents are young and middle-aged. Young women are playing a dominating role in the rural areas of Bangladesh (Anam 2021). It is known to all that no nation can prosper without education. The present study represents the educational condition of the respondents also. Notably, 2% are entirely uneducated; 2% of respondents could sign and have had primary education; about 18% of respondents have attained a lower-secondary level of education; 48% of respondents have had a secondary level of education; about 27% of the respondents have attained a higher secondary level of education. However, only 1% of respondents have an undergraduate level. The study indicates that many respondents were at a secondary level of education. Therefore, the educational achievement of the respondents creates more opportunities for getting social, economic, and other facilities. It is also found that in some cases, the educational gap thrashes respondents in underprivileged situations in their practical lives.

Table 20.1 Socio-demographic profile of the respondents

SL	Background characteristics ($N = 100$)	Number	%
1.	Age (years)		
	18–29	74	74
	30–39	18	18
	40–49	5	5
	50–59	3	3
2	Educational qualification		
	Illiterate	2	2
	Class 5	4	4
	Class 8	18	18
	SSC	48	48
	HSC	27	27
	Undergraduate	1	1
3.	Occupation		
	Housewife	99	99
	Service	1	1
4.	Religious status		
	Islam	100	100
5.	Number of children		
	0–1	40	40
	2–3	52	52
	4–5	8	8

It is essential to analyze the occupational position to know the present situation of the respondents. The study disclosed that there are only two types of occupation of the respondents in the study area. Almost 99% of respondents a housewife, and only 1% are engaged in service. Therefore, the study revealed that most of the respondents are involved in household maintenance activities in the rural areas of Bangladesh. On the contrary, all the respondents belong to Islam, and nobody belongs to other religious status in the study areas. So, the Muslim peoples dominate the Adda Union under the Barura Upazila of the Comilla district of Bangladesh. Finally, the study also represents the number of children of the respondents who live in the study areas. Notably, 40% of respondents have zero to one child, 55% of respondents have two to three children, and only 8% of respondents have four to five children. So, the study confirmed that most respondents have two to three children in rural areas of Bangladesh.

Table 20.2 represents that the central exciting area of this study is understanding the mass people's awareness, perceptions, and knowledge about mass media—particularly the role of mass media in creating mother and child health awareness in rural areas of Bangladesh. The study shows that all (100%) respondents give positive opinions about the role of mass media concerning mother and child health awareness. So, all women have an idea about mass media in the rural areas of Bangladesh. Most of the respondents (47%) are watching television; 6% use radio and the Internet as mass media. About 4% of respondents used mobile phones and

Table 20.2 Awareness, perceptions, and knowledge about mass media

SL	Background characteristics (*N* = 100)	Number	%
1.	Opinion of respondents about mass media		
	Yes	100	100
2.	Perception about different mass media		
	Television	47	47
	Radio	6	6
	Mobile	4	4
	Internet	6	6
	Above all	37	37
4.	Health-related messages from mass media		
	About taking physical care of the mother	14	14
	To know how to preserve the nutrition of the children	13	13
	About taking proper care of the children	8	8
	About the necessity of breastfeeding	7	7
	To achieve knowledge for taking proper care of the children	6	6
	Above all	52	52
5.	Interest in watching mass media		
	No interest at all	4	4
	Not so much interest	57	57
	Keep neutral	2	2
	Interested	31	31
	Much interested	6	6
6.	Essential programs of mass media		
	Drama	74	74
	Cinema	4	4
	Amusing show	8	8
	Health-related show	6	6
	News	2	2
	Others	6	6
7.	Mass media used for getting health-related messages		
	Television	87	87
	Mobile	5	5
	Internet	7	7
	Others	1	1

37% directly used all the media to get different health-related messages for their children's health awareness. So, most rural mothers use television for health-related messages regarding mother and child health issues. On the contrary, 14% of respondents get messages from mass media about taking physical care of rural mothers, 13% of respondents for knowing how to preserve the nutrition of their children, about 8% about taking proper care of the children, 7% about the necessity of the breastfeeding of the children, 6% respondents for achieving knowledge for taking proper care of the children, and most respondents (52%) are getting health-related messages from above all through mass media. The study also discussed the respondent's level of interest in mass media. From the respondents, 57% of rural mothers are not interested in watching mass media, 31% are interested, 6% are interested, 6% have no interest, and another 2% are neutral about watching mass media. This study also discussed what mass media broadcasts important programs. Almost 74% of respondents answered about the different types of drama broadcast on a television channel, 8% of respondents replied about the amusing show, 6% about the health-related show, 4% about the cinema, but only 2% of respondents said the news is broadcasted in mass media, and another 6% replied different programs are broadcasting in mass media beyond that responded. To educate rural mothers about health-related issues, it is essential to know how they prefer to learn about them. Understanding the rural mothers' preferred method for learning is just as important as understanding how they currently learn about it. All the respondents asked about the mother and child health information news source. The study found that 87% of respondents replied that television is the primary source for getting health-related messages in mass media. About 7% used the Internet as mass media, and 5% of respondents replied about mobile phones as mass media. Only 1% replied about other sources (i.e., public lectures, discovery channels, cultural events, etc.) used for getting health-related messages. However, surprisingly, nobody responded about radio as a mass media where radio was a significant and available source of mass media once upon a time.

The study shows the effects of mass media on the personal lives of rural mothers through watching mass media. Table 20.3 shows that among the total respondents, 100% gave positive responses to the role of mass media in their personal lives. That means they can gather information concerning mother and child health awareness through mass media, which creates positive signs in their personal lives. It should be mentioned here that rural mothers have an idea about mass media and get the opportunity to gather information about mother and child health awareness through it, which ultimately plays a vital role in their everyday lives. About 62% gave a positive answer, 35% said very good, and only 3% said moderate answers about mother and child health awareness. So, the figure shows that most rural mothers said that mass media plays a vital role in mother and child health awareness. All the respondents were asked about the respondents' opinions concerning the present effect of mass media on accruing knowledge about mother and child health issues. The majority of the respondents (74%) replied that it is essential, and about 25% said it is crucial. However, only 1% said they have no idea about the effect of mass media on mother and child health awareness. They said they did not know about that. It was found that 98% of respondents answered positively about the necessity of giving extra foods side by side with breastfeeding through mass media, and only 2% did not answer concerning giving extra foods side by side with breastfeeding. Of the respondents, 70% respondents said vegetable mixed hospose is taken as extra foods by the babies, 20% said other liquid food, 3% respondents said rice and halua as a portion of extra food for the babies, and 4% respondents did not comment on the extra food of their babies.

The findings also show the information on the health-related advertisements that respondents can watch regarding mother and child health awareness issues through mass media. It was found that 99% of respondents gave their opinion about the

Table 20.3 Effects of mass media on mother and child health awareness

SL	Background characteristics (N = 100)	Number	%
1.	Role of mass media in personal life		
	Yes	100	100
2.	Effect of mass media on mother and child health awareness		
	Good	62	62
	Very good	35	35
	Not so good	3	3
3.	The implication of mass media for mother and child health-related knowledge		
	Important	25	25
	Very important	74	74
4.	Programs related to the importance of breastfeeding through mass media		
	Yes	98	98
	No	2	2
5.	We are giving extra foods side by side with breastfeeding through mass media		
	Yes	98	98
	No	2	2
6.	Extra foods should be taken by the babies		
	Vegetable mixed hospose	70	70
	Other liquid food	20	20
	Rice	3	3
	Halua	3	3
	No comment	4	4
7.	Health-related advertisements from mass media		
	Yes	99	99
	No	1	1
8.	Other sources for getting health messages beyond mass media		
	Health-related posters	16	16
	Leaflet	8	8
	Wall writing	4	4
	Audiovisual media	35	35
	Other sources	37	37

advertisement they can watch regarding mother and child health awareness through mass media, and only 1% of respondents gave their negative opinion about the advertisement. So, the study confirmed that almost all rural mothers get health-related messages from mass media advertisements. This study discussed with all respondents the types of sources other than mass media from which they can get information regarding mother and child health issues. It was found that 16% of respondents replied for health-related posters, about 4% said for leaflets, about 4% replied wall writing, 35% answered audiovisual media, and 37% replied about other sources for getting health-related messages beyond mass media.

20.4 Discussion

The mass media has a crucial role in advancing health literacy, modifying health-related behaviors, and providing public health information. Unfortunately, the majority of public health interventions in the media's coverage are determined externally and do not adequately involve the local population. Because of this, relatively little is understood about the consequences of mass media promotion that is prompted locally (Zamawe et al. 2016). Rural mothers and essential health information are largely connected to the mass media. The radio and television are examples of mass media that can be used to effectively remind people of important information or influence target audiences to adopt new behaviors. They can also provide updates to the public in addition to telling them about newly discovered ailments and where to get assistance (Naveena 2015). Television is one of the most significant forms of mass media used to inspire people to create a better society. It has the power to greatly affect individuals, introducing new ideas, expanding knowledge, and influencing public opinion. It is already a strong advocate for healthy lifestyles in the health sector and in both rural and urban communities (Ghanta 2012). The present study shows that the programs through mass media related to the importance of breastfeeding. Among the total respondents, 98% answered positively about the importance of breastfeeding, and only 2% did not answer concerning the importance of breastfeeding. The findings show that most rural mothers admit they can benefit from watching mass media as it gives different messages, especially about mother and child health issues. It should be mentioned here that rural mothers benefit from mass media regarding mother and child health awareness. The study also shows information from the respondents regarding giving extra foods side by side with breastfeeding through mass media. It is mentionable here that the present role of mass media for accruing knowledge about mother and child health issues is remarkable in the rural areas of Bangladesh concerning mother and child health issues. Moreover, radio and television are the primary mass media platforms that provide information to both urban and rural populations in many countries. It is interesting to see that even uneducated people can benefit from these two mass media instruments. Geographic variations in media exposure are notable. However, compared to their rural counterparts, urban women and men have had better access to all three media sources regardless of where they live. Additionally, comparing exposure along gender lines revealed that the distribution favors men over women. Mass media can provide different tasks such as education, information, making public opinion, and entertainment to the people of the country. They also play a vital role in creating various health-related awareness to the mass people like mothers with their breastfeeding children across the rural areas of the country.

20.5 Conclusion

The present study investigates the role of mass media on rural mothers' knowledge of health awareness for their children. The focus of this study is the investigative description of the role of mass media on rural mothers and children about their health awareness issues. As a result, this study provides an overall idea for understanding the respondents' socioeconomic position. One hundred rural women with breastfeeding children were polled to gather information about these concerns and to see their thoughts on overall livelihood patterns and health awareness through mass media. As a powerful audiovisual medium, television touches a sizable portion of the population. Additionally, it is a crucial communication tool for spreading the word about healthcare services through commercials and other programs with a health focus. This study has furnished empirical information regarding women's access to mass media and illuminated the significant correlation between it and their knowledge of maternal health. The study's overall summary presents the mass media as an effective means of educating women about maternal health issues and raising their awareness of such information. Mass media also plays an important role in creating health-related awareness among rural mothers and their breastfeeding children throughout the country. Finally, this study suggested the curiosity of researchers for additional information and offered fresh ideas for future studies regarding the health awareness of rural mothers and their children.

20.6 Limitations

As a researcher in the field of mass communication, it is an opportunity for the researcher to know the mass media activities concerning the health awareness of rural women. Some constraints were appended which are as follows:

1. The limitation of time, resources, grants, and other facilities caused problems for the researchers in conducting an in-depth study.
2. This study describes the role of mass media on rural women concerning health awareness.
3. This study is included with a smaller sample size due to the shortage of time, resources, grants, and other facilities.
4. The study is designed to target rural mothers having breastfeeding children. Ideally, the research team should have interviewed every mother in the study areas, which is not possible due to funding constraints.

Acknowledgments The researcher(s) is grateful to the Comilla University Research Grant (Fiscal Year: 2017–2018) for granting funds to conduct this study.

References

Alam S (2014) The role of Media in Bangladesh. MSS thesis, Department of Political Science, University of Dhaka

Anam S (2021) Let our rural women rise and claim their rights. https://www.thedailystar.net/views/opinion/news/let-our-rural-women-rise-and-claim-their-rights-2199111

Anwar A, Malik M, Raees V, Anwar A (2020) Role of mass media and public health communications in the COVID-19 pandemic. Cureus 12(9):e10453

Archana SR (2007) Mass communication in prevention and control of AIDS: content analysis of Indian newspapers. Development communication. Publication Bureau Punjabi University, Patiala, pp 115–144

Azad A Kalam (2023). Media Landscapes, Expert Analyses of the State of Media. https://medialandscapes.org/country/bangladesh/traditional-communication/overview

Bonnie R, George D (1975) Radio television spot announcement for family Planning. World Wide, University of Chicago, Chicago

Bryant J, Finklea BW (2022) Fundamentals of media effects. Waveland Press

Bylaska-Davies P (2011) The role of the mass Media in Women's infant feeding decisions: a dissertation

Dubey DC, Bardhan A (1981) Content analysis of messages and Programmes: modules on health and population communication research. National Institute of Health and Family Welfare, New Delhi

Ghanta CS (2012) In his study on coverage of health information in mass media: a study. J Arts, Sci Commerce 2(1):1

Gupta A, Sinha A (2010) Health coverage in mass media: a content analysis. J Commun 1:19. https://doi.org/10.1080/0976691X.2010.11884766

Kruk ME, Gage AD, Arsenault C, Jordan K, Leslie HH, Roder-DeWan S, Pate M (2018) High-quality health systems in the sustainable development goals era: time for a revolution. Lancet Glob Health 6(11):e1196–e1252

Mashreky SR, Rahman F, Rahman A, Talab A, Rahman Z (2015) Role of mass media in increasing mothers' knowledge and practices on IYCF: findings from a community trial in rural Bangladesh. South East Asia J Public Health 5(1):18–24

Naveena N (2015) Importance of mass media in communicating health messages: an analysis. IOSR-JHSS 20:36–41

WHO (2022) Mental Health. https://www.who.int/news-room/fact-sheets/detail/mental-health-strengthening-our-response

Zamawe CO, Banda M, Dube AN (2016) The impact of a community-driven mass media campaign on the utilization of maternal health care services in rural Malawi. BMC Pregnancy Childbirth 16:1–8

Psychometric Properties of Walsh Family Resilience Questionnaire (WFRQ) in the Malaysian Context

21

Bee Seok Chua, Suzanna Awang Bono, Geetha Vithilingam, Ching Sin Siau, Mimi Fitriana Zaini, Noran Naqiah Hairi, Hairil Fadzly Md Akir, and Wah Yun Low

21.1 Introduction

In recent years, many parties, including scientists, policymakers, and others, have shown significant interest in the study of resilience, particularly in the context of family resilience (Luthar and Cicchetti 2000). Focusing on resilience is essential as it emphasizes the well-being of individuals, families, and society (Armitage et al. 2012). This focus will be able to improve lives and reduce the possible social costs that are associated with stresses endured by individuals and communities (Armitage et al. 2012). However, research in this area in Malaysia is still very much lacking. Furthermore, there is a definite need to assess the theoretical and empirical

B. S. Chua
Faculty of Psychology and Social Work, Universiti Sabah Malaysia, Sabah, Malaysia
e-mail: chuabs@ums.edu.my

S. A. Bono (✉)
School of Social Sciences, Universiti Sains Malaysia, Penang, Malaysia
e-mail: suzanna.bono@usm.my

G. Vithilingam · N. N. Hairi · W. Y. Low
Faculty of Medicine, Universiti Malaya, Kuala Lumpur, Malaysia
e-mail: geethav@tarc.edu.my; noran@um.edu.my; lowwy@um.edu.my

C. S. Siau
Centre for Community Health Studies, Faculty of Health Sciences, Universiti Kebangsaan Malaysia, Kuala Lumpur, Malaysia
e-mail: chingsin.siau@ukm.edu.my

M. F. Zaini
Faculty of Behavioural Sciences, Help University Malaysia, Kuala Lumpur, Malaysia

H. F. M. Akir
National Population and Family Development Board, Kuala Lumpur, Malaysia
e-mail: hairil@lppkn.gov.my

M. Pal et al. (eds.), *Public Health and Nutrition*,
https://doi.org/10.1007/978-981-97-7890-4_21

foundation of family resilience study in Malaysia. This study, hence, was designed to assess the Walsh Family Resilience Questionnaire (WFRQ) in the Malaysian context. According to Walsh (2015), resilience is the ability to rebound from disruptive and stressful happenings and to be able to endure the happenings of an individual or a family. Nieto and his colleagues (2023) studied 439 adults and found a positive association between resilience and personality traits. Furthermore, using social resources aptly has also been indicated as a form of resilience (Yıldırım and Celik 2020).

Thus, in this study, we have studied the interplay between family characteristics and social factors during the COVID-19 pandemic, in relation to resilience. Family is the most essential unit that fosters resilience, as this is where closeness, intimacy, and emotional bonding of familial relationships are formed (Carr and Kellas 2018). Moreover, family is where resilience is hindered or fostered since this is also where each family member perceives and responds to adversity and adapts to it (Carr and Kellas 2018). As discussed by Procentese and colleagues in their 2019 study involving 227 Italian parents, a family is an interconnected system, in which each member of the family shares relationships and makes both positive and negative memories together (Procentese et al. 2019). These shared relationships and memories formed are noted by Walsh (2021) to impact a family's ability to operate as a functional system that utilizes coping and adaptations. In this study, we explored this interconnected system in relation to the adversity and adaptability created by the COVID-19 pandemic.

The WFRQ (2015) has three essential domains: Belief System, Organizational Pattern, and Communication and Problem-Solving. Each of these encompasses three components that are characteristically dynamic, synergistic, and interactive, within and across, each of the above domains. In this study, the questions of the three domains of the WFRQ were forward and backward-translated and were administered in a bi-lingual format to Malaysian families. It is imperative to quantitatively assess the psychometric properties of WFRQ in the Malaysian context. Hence, this study looks at the factor structure, reliability, and validity of WFRQ in the Malaysian context.

21.2 Methods

21.2.1 Participants

The demographic profile of the respondents who took part in the study was described in this section. Data collection began in March 2023 and finished early in April 2023. A total of 215 data were collected from parents of children between the ages of 21 and 65 years (mean = 43.96, SD = 9.42). In the study, 143 (66.2%) mothers and 70 (or 32.4%) fathers participated. Malay respondents comprised 71.2% of the sample, with Indians (19.5%) and Chinese (9.3%) following closely behind. Muslims comprised 73% of the respondents, Hindus made up 15.3%, Buddhists made up 7.4%, and Christians made up 2.8%. The majority just completed secondary school, and 43.1% had a meager monthly salary of less than RM2,000. The summary of the demographic characteristics of the respondents is presented in Table 21.1.

Table 21.1 Demographic characteristics of the respondents ($N = 215$)

Variables	Frequency	Percent (%)
Gender		
Male	70	32.6
Female	143	66.5
Race		
Malay	153	71.2
Chinese	20	9.3
Indian	42	19.5
Religion		
Islam	73.0	73.0
Buddhism	7.4	7.4
Hinduism	15.3	15.3
Christianity	2.8	2.8
Others	1.4	1.4
Number of children		
One child	18	8.4
Two children	40	18.6
Three children	76	35.3
Four children	45	20.9
More than 4 children	36	16.7
Income per month		
Below RM2,000	93	43.3
RM2,000–RM3,000	68	31.6
RM3,001–RM4,000	39	18.1
RM4,001–RM5,000	9	4.2
RM5,000 and above	6	2.8
Employment		
Not working	4	1.9
Agriculture/farming	5	2.3
Daily worker	35	16.3
Private company	142	66.0
Government employee	13	6.0
Business owner	16	7.4
Education level		
Primary school	20	9.3
Secondary school	158	73.5
Tertiary education	35	16.3

Percentages of variables do not add up to 100% due to missing values
US$1 = 4.3 RM (Malaysian Ringgits)

21.2.2 Instruments

The Perceived Relationship Quality Component (PRQC) Inventory and the WFRQ were given to the respondents to complete as self-reported assessments. Walsh (2003) invented the WFRQ. The 32 items in the WFRQ measure three primary scales: communication processes (10 items), organizational processes (9 items), and belief systems (13 items). The processes that foster resilience, such as finding meaning in adversity, having an optimistic outlook, and transcending into spirituality, were measured by the family beliefs. The organizational process scale assessed how well a family used its social and financial resources, how flexible its structure was, and how attached its members were to one another. The third component is the communication process, which entails clear methods, honest emotional expression, and cooperative problem-solving. The items assess the degree to which individual claims about how their family is handling crises and ongoing issues are true. The ratings range from 1 (rarely/never) to 5 (nearly often). Item 32 of the WFRQ was an open-ended question concerning practices and beliefs that are particularly useful for helping the family deal with trying and stressful times.

The PRQC Inventory (Fletcher et al. 2000) was used to assess relationship quality. Six categories were created from the 18 PRQC measures: intimacy (items 7–9), trust (items 10–12), relationship satisfaction (items 1–3), passion (items 13–15), commitment (items 4–6), and love (items 16–18). Each component evaluation of three items, each of which had a 7-point Likert-type scale with 1 representing not at all and 7 representing excessively.

21.2.3 Data Analysis

The IBM SPSS Statistics Version 21.0 was used to analyze the data. Principal axis factoring was used in an exploratory factor analysis (EFA) to determine the WFRQ's factor structure in the Malaysian context. The data were examined for suitability for factor analysis using Bartlett's test of sphericity and Kaiser–Meyer–Olkin's (KMO's) measure of sample adequacy before an EFA was carried out. The number of components to be preserved was determined using scree plots, Kaiser's criterion (eigenvalues $\geq$1.0), and the proportion of variation accounted by the number of factors (Costello and Osborne 2005). The number of factors that should be generated from the EFA is identified by the slope that clearly levels off the curve of scree plot (the "elbow"; Thompson 2004). If an item's factor loading on a single factor was greater than 0.4 and differed by at least 0.2 from other factors, it was kept.

The method of internal consistency Cronbach's alpha was used to test the reliability of the scales; a criterion of 0.70 was used to indicate good reliability (Ursachi et al. 2015). The convergent validity of the scale was evaluated to determine the instrument's validity. The WFRQ would significantly and positively correlate with scores on the PRQC Inventory, based on the evidence that the scale captures important aspects of family functioning. The significant positive correlation between the WFRQ total score and the PRQC Inventory is expected to support the convergent validity of the scale. This aligns with Walsh's (2017) and Fletcher et al.'s (2000) findings that revealed the interconnectedness between family resilience and the quality of relationships within the family. The observed relationships between specific dimensions of family resilience, such as transcendence and spirituality, clear information and resources, and connectedness among family members, with corresponding aspects of relationship quality, including satisfaction, commitment, intimacy, trust, and passion, provide additional evidence for the construct validity of the WFRQ in the Malaysian context. These findings underscore the utility of the WFRQ as a comprehensive measure that not only assesses family resilience but also aligns with key components of positive relationship dynamics within families.

21.2.4 Results

21.2.4.1 Factor Structure of Walsh Family Resilience Questionnaire (WFRQ)

The results of the first two initial analyses, which included Bartlett's test of sphericity and the KMO test, indicated that the scale's coefficient was 0.806 and that the Bartlett result was significant ($\chi^2 = 2852.96$, $p < 0.001$). The dataset's factorability was confirmed by the outcomes of these two analyses.

Promax Oblique with Kappa 4 Rotation primary axis factoring was used in EFA to determine the first factor structure of the WFRQ in the Malaysian context. The factors were examined for each of the 31 WFRQ items. The scale comprised eight factors with eigenvalues greater than 1, according to the results. However, the scree plot revealed a five- or six-factor solution (refer to Fig. 21.1) instead of the WFRQ original nine-factor structure. Following up on these plot results, factor analyses using Promax Oblique Rotation were carried out once more, this time with the number of components fixed at six.

The six-factor solution's factor analysis accounted for 57.78% of the variance. Items 19, 30, and 31 were eliminated due to their insufficient factor loading of 0.40. Table 21.3 displays the six factors together with the corresponding items, factor loadings, eigenvalues, and percentage of variance.

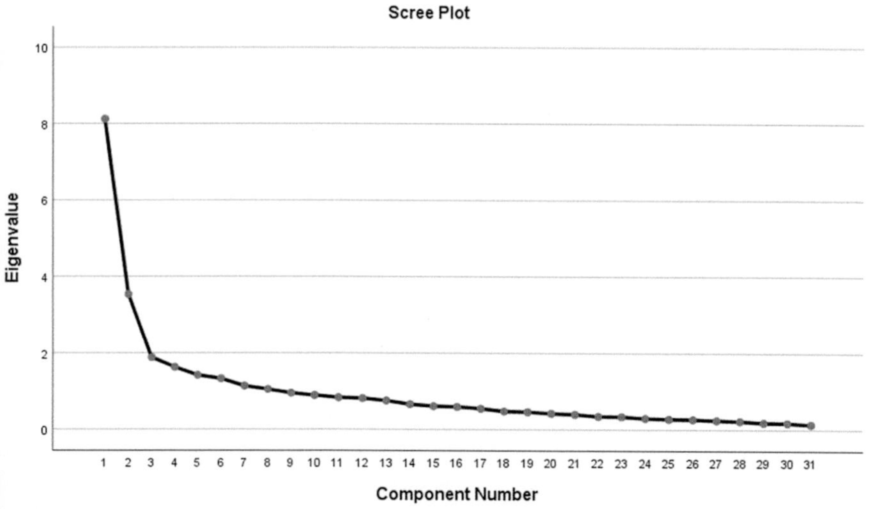

Fig. 21.1 Scree plot for the Walsh Family Resilience Questionnaire (WFRQ)

Table 21.3 Factor structure, items, factor loadings, eigenvalues, and percentage of variance of the Walsh Family Resilience Questionnaire (WFRQ)

	Factor loading					
Item	1 Eigenvalue= 8.12% variance = 26.20	2 Eigenvalue = 3.54% variance = 11.41	3 Eigenvalue = 1.88% variance = 6.07	4 Eigenvalue = 1.63% variance = 5.25	5 Eigenvalue = 1.42% variance = 4.57	6 Eigenvalue = 1.33% variance = 4.28
11	0.855					
10	0.761					
12	0.595					
15	0.577					
14	0.565					
13	0.520					
9	0.406					
19						
30						
23		0.828				
24		0.683				
22		0.636				
21		0.457				
31						
17			0.900			
16			0.733			
18			0.610			
20			0.600			
8				0.766		
7				0.687		

Item	Factor loading					
	1 Eigenvalue= 8.12% variance = 26.20	2 Eigenvalue = 3.54% variance = 11.41	3 Eigenvalue = 1.88% variance = 6.07	4 Eigenvalue = 1.63% variance = 5.25	5 Eigenvalue = 1.42% variance = 4.57	6 Eigenvalue = 1.33% variance = 4.28
6				0.675		
5				0.611		
26					0.845	
27					0.728	
25					0.583	
29					0.422	
28					0.409	
2						0.778
1						0.761
4						0.701
3						0.648

Walsh (2003) states that the promotion of family resilience is facilitated by nine critical processes that fall into three categories of family functioning. Making sense of adversity, having a positive attitude, transcendence, and spirituality are among the activities that foster resilience in the first domain of family functioning or family beliefs. The use of social and financial resources, connectivity among family members, and structural flexibility are all processes that promote resilience in the second domain of family functioning or organizational patterns. According to Walsh (2003), communication is the third component of family functioning. It entails clear processes, honest emotional expression, and cooperative problem-solving. The EFA in our study produced a six-factor solution that reflected the aspects of family resilience proposed by Walsh's conceptual framework. The six components were identified as follows: (1) transcendence and spirituality; (2) clear knowledge and resources; (3) family member connectedness; (4) creating the meaning of adversity; (5) open emotional expression; and (6) good perspective.

21.2.4.2 Reliability and Validity of WFRQ

With a Cronbach's alpha value of 0.87, the overall WFRQ scale demonstrated a high level of internal consistency. WFRQ subscales were formed by adding the 27 items in accordance with their corresponding factors since all of them had factor loadings greater than 0.40. Table 21.4 presents the subscales' Cronbach's alpha coefficients, which ranged between 0.73 and 0.80. The WFRQ total score, which measures family resilience, and the PRQS total scale score, which measures perceived relationship quality, showed a significant positive relationship ($r = 0.34$, $p < 0.001$), as predicted. Referring to Table 21.5, the correlation between the WFRQ total scale score and the PRQS subscale revealed a positive relationship with a range of 0.26–0.34 ($p < 0.001$). The findings showed that people with greater family resilience scores also had higher levels of relationship quality (Table 21.5).

Table 21.4 Internal consistencies Cronbach's alphas for the Walsh Family Resilience Questionnaire (WFRQ)

Scale	Number of items	Items	Cronbach's Alpha Coefficients
WFRQ total scale			0.866
Transcendence and spirituality (factor 1)	7	9, 10, 11, 12, 13, 14, 15	0.767
Clear information and resources (factor 2),	4	21, 22, 23, 24	0.734
Connectedness among family members (factor 3)	4	16, 17,18, 20	0.773
Making meaning of adversity (factor 4)	4	5, 6, 7, 8	0.804
Open emotional expression (factor 5)	4	25, 26, 27, 28, 29	0.789
Positive outlook (factor 6)	4	1, 2, 3, 4	0.762

Table 21.5 Intercorrelation between the Walsh Family Resilience Questionnaire (WFRQ) Score and the Perceived Relationship Quality Component (PRQC) Inventory Score

Scale/Subscale	WFRQ_ Total Score	PRQS_ Total Score	Relationship Satisfaction	Commitment	Intimacy	Trust
WFRQ_Total						
PRQS_Total	0.342**					
Relationship satisfaction	0.335**	0.881**				
Commitment	0.285**	0.902**	0.844**			
Intimacy	0.312**	0.912**	0.739**	0.773**		
Trust	0.311**	0.876**	0.663**	0.713**	0.787**	
Passion	0.265**	0.842**	0.640**	0.662**	0.716**	0.703**

**$p < 0.01$

21.3 Discussion

The findings of this study contribute valuable insights into the psychometric properties of the WFRQ in the Malaysian context. The examination of factor structure, reliability, and validity of the WFRQ in the Malaysian population offers a foundation for understanding family resilience in this cultural context.

The EFA revealed a six-factor solution for the WFRQ in Malaysia, accounting for 57.78% of the total variance. These factors were identified as transcendence and spirituality, clear information and resources, connectedness among family members, making meaning of adversity, open emotional expression, and a positive outlook. This structure aligns with Walsh's conceptual framework, emphasizing the significance of family beliefs, organizational patterns, and communication processes in promoting family resilience.

The emergence of these factors suggests that Malaysian families draw on spiritual resources, maintain flexibility in facing challenges, and emphasize familial connectedness. Additionally, the importance of clear information, economic security, and open emotional expression in fostering resilience was highlighted. The identified factors provide a nuanced understanding of how families in Malaysia navigate adversities, especially during the challenging period of the COVID-19 pandemic.

The internal consistency of the WFRQ was found to be high ($\alpha = 0.92$), indicating strong reliability. The individual subscales also demonstrated good internal consistency, with Cronbach's alpha coefficients ranging from 0.73 to 0.80. This suggests that the WFRQ is a reliable instrument for measuring family resilience in the Malaysian context, with each subscale contributing consistently to the overall reliability of the questionnaire. Validation studies in varied cultural contexts, such as Duncan et al. (2021) in the United States, echo our findings. They confirmed the WFRQ's reliability and its three-factor structure: belief systems, organization patterns, and communication/problem-solving. These results underscore the instrument's reliability across cultures. Additionally, Li and Li (2021) translated the WFRQ-R into Chinese and assessed its reliability among stroke survivors and caregivers. Their findings revealed strong internal consistency ($\alpha = 0.83$) and supported its validity through factor analysis. This highlights its reliability and validity in assessing family resilience in different cultural contexts.

The validity of the WFRQ was supported by its positive correlation with the PRQC Inventory, reinforcing its concurrent validity. Additionally, the subscale analysis revealed positive relationships between specific dimensions of family resilience and relationship quality (e.g., satisfaction, commitment, intimacy, trust, passion), providing evidence for convergent validity. These findings align with research by Feinberg et al. (2022), demonstrating that intervention families in the Family Foundations program exhibited higher levels of positive family relationship quality, further emphasizing the WFRQ's utility in capturing various aspects of family resilience and its positive relationship dynamics. Similarly, research by Zarei et al. (2013) found that family communication patterns, such as conversation and conformity orientation, were significant predictors of quality of life among female high school students, with resilience emerging as a key predictor of positive relationship dynamics. These findings collectively underscore the validity of the WFRQ in assessing family resilience and its relationship with positive relationship experiences.

These findings hold implications for both research and practice. The identified factors offer a comprehensive understanding of the components that contribute to family resilience in the Malaysian context. Researchers can use this validated instrument to further explore the dynamics of family resilience in diverse populations within Malaysia. Practitioners can leverage this knowledge to develop targeted interventions and support systems that enhance family resilience, especially during challenging circumstances like the COVID-19 pandemic.

It is important to acknowledge some limitations of the study, such as the specific demographic characteristics of the sample, which may limit the generalizability of the findings. Future research could include more diverse samples to ensure broader applicability. Additionally, longitudinal studies could provide a deeper understanding of how family resilience evolves over time.

21.4 Conclusion

This study provides evidence supporting the psychometric properties of the WFRQ in the Malaysian context. The identified factors, high reliability, and positive correlations with relationship quality suggest that the WFRQ is a valuable tool for assessing family resilience in Malaysia. Further research and application of the WFRQ can enhance our understanding of family resilience dynamics and contribute to the development of targeted interventions to support families in times of a health crisis.

Acknowledgments Thanks to the National Population and Family Development Board (LPPKN), Ministry of Women, Family and Community Development Malaysia for the research funding.

References

Armitage D, Béné C, Charles AT, Johnson D, Allison EH (2012) The interplay of Well-being and resilience in applying a social-ecological perspective. Ecol Soc 17(4):17

Carr KR, Kellas JK (2018) The role of family and marital communication in developing resilience to family-of-origin adversity. J Fam Commun 18:68–84

Costello AB, Osborne JW (2005) Best practices in exploratory factor analysis: four recommendations for getting the most from your analysis. Pract Assess Res Eval 10(7):1–9

Duncan JM, Garrison ME, Killian TS (2021) Measuring family resilience: evaluating the Walsh family resilience questionnaire. Fam J 29(1):80–85. https://doi.org/10.1177/1066480720956641

Feinberg ME, Gedaly L, Mogle J, Hostetler ML, Cifelli JA, Tornello SL, Jones DE (2022) Building long-term family resilience through universal prevention: 10-year parent and child outcomes during the covid-19 pandemic. Fam Process 61(1):76–90

Fletcher GJO, Simpson JA, Thomas G (2000) The measurement of perceived relationship quality components: a confirmatory factor analytic approach. Personal Soc Psychol Bull 26(3):340–354. https://doi.org/10.1177/0146167200265007

Li X, Li H (2021) Reliability and validity of the Chinese version of the revised Walsh family resilience questionnaire. Ann Palliat Med 10:8709–8717

Luthar SS, Cicchetti D (2000) The construct of resilience: implications for interventions and social policies. Dev Psychopathol 12(4):857–885

Nieto M, Visier ME, Silvestre IN, Navarro B, Serrano JP, Martínez-Vizcaíno V (2023) Relation between resilience and personality traits: the role of hopelessness and age. Scand J Psychol 64(1):53–59

Procentese F, Gatti F, Napoli I (2019) Families and social media use: the role of parents' perceptions about social media impact on family Systems in the Relationship between family collective efficacy and open communication. Int J Environ Res Public Health 16:5006. https://doi.org/10.3390/ijerph16245006

Thompson B (2004) Exploratory and confirmatory factor analysis: understanding concepts and applications. American Psychological Association, Washington, DC

Ursachi G, Horodnic IA, Zait A (2015) How reliable are measurement scales? External factors with indirect influence on reliability estimators. Procedia Econ Finance 20:679–686. https://doi.org/10.1016/S2212-5671(15)00123-9

Walsh F (2003) Family resilience: a framework for clinical practice. Fam Process 42:1

Walsh F (2015) Strengthening family resilience, 3rd edn. New York, Guilford Press

Walsh F (2017) Strengthening family resilience, 3rd edn. New York, Guilford Press

Walsh F (2021) Family resilience: a dynamic systemic framework. In: Ungar M (ed) Multisystemic resilience: adaptation and transformation in contexts of change. Oxford Academic, New York. https://doi.org/10.1093/oso/9780190095888.003.0015

Yıldırım M, Celik F (2020) Social support, resilience and subjective Well-being in college students. J Posit School Psychol 5:127–135. https://doi.org/10.47602/jpsp.v5i2.229

Zarei E, Fallahchai SR, Vahedi Sarrigani N (2013) The study of relationship between family communications patterns with resilience and quality of life the high school girl's students. J Life Sci 3(4):289–293

References

Socioeconomic and Demographic Factors: Scenario of Fertility Differentials in Bangladesh

22

Md. Nasim Mahmud and K. M. Abdul Mumin

22.1 Introduction

Every animal increases family. Human beings are not an exception to it. To give birth to a child is a general characteristic of a woman. However, the capacity to give birth is not the same for all women. At a time, the variation that is seen in different regions and within the same region is called differential fertility.

The fertility of humans is influenced by various factors such as socioeconomic, socio-cultural, biological, and demographic conditions. Socioeconomic and socio-cultural elements indirectly impact fertility by affecting the proximate determinants. Additionally, the socioeconomic status and variations within it have an impact on fertility levels and create distinctions among sub-groups or sub-regions. Normative social structure, social stratification, and economic limitations in the form of socio-economic variables influence fertility through their effect on social psychological processes (Bagozzi and Vanloo 1978).

Bangladesh experienced a significant decline in fertility rates from 1975 to 1994, with the total fertility rate (TFR) dropping from 6.3 to 3.4. However, from 1994 to 2004, the fertility level remained relatively unchanged at 3.3, before seeing a slight decrease to 3.0. Concurrently, the contraceptive prevalence rate notably increased from 44.6% to 58.1%. This stagnation in fertility levels despite improved contraceptive prevalence has raised concerns, given that fertility rates remain higher than the replacement level. Now it is necessary to find: How at present socioeconomic and demographic variables are related to fertility? How do socioeconomic and demographic factors affect regional variations of fertility? How will Bangladesh reach the

M. N. Mahmud (✉)
Department of Statistics, University of Rajshahi, Rajshahi, Bangladesh

K. M. A. Mumin
Rajshahi Science & Technology University, Natore, Bangladesh

M. Pal et al. (eds.), *Public Health and Nutrition*,
https://doi.org/10.1007/978-981-97-7890-4_22

replacement level of fertility? The United Nations projection of a target level of the TFR of Bangladesh is 2.1 (Replacement-level fertility) by 2030 (U.N 1999, 2001).

22.2 Aim

The research seeks to analyze the indirect impact of socioeconomic and demographic factors on fertility differentials in Bangladesh. Additionally, it aims to explore the regional differentials in fertility rates and assess the status of replacement-level fertility in the country.

22.3 Trend in Total Fertility Rate

Since 1975, there has been a consistent decline in the TFR as evident from surveys, with a noteworthy drop from 6.3 births per woman in 1975 to 5.1 in 1989, further decreasing to 3.3 in 1996. Following a plateau at around 3.3 births per woman in the 1990s, there was a subsequent drop to 2.3 births in 2011, where it has since stabilized (Fig. 22.1).

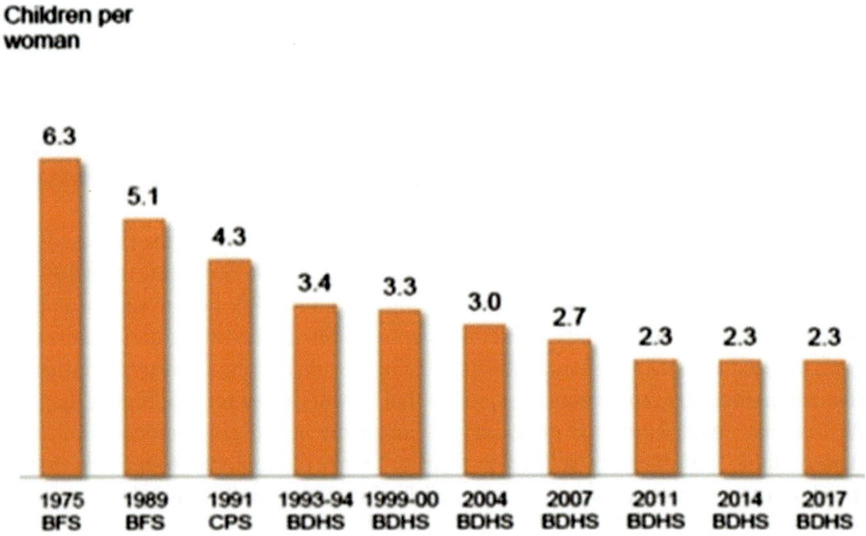

Fig. 22.1 Trend in total fertility rate, 1975–2017

22.4 Variable Selection

Socioeconomic and demographic factors have an indirect impact on fertility disparities. The selection of background variables in this study is based on influential socioeconomic and demographic factors that are reflective of fertility, as supported by related research, key indicators from BDHS data, theory, and hypothesis.

22.4.1 Data and Method

The 2017–18 BDHS sample is representative of the entire population residing in non-institutional dwelling units in Bangladesh, which consists of eight administrative (Barishal, Chittagong, Dhaka, Khulna, Rajshahi, Rangpur, Mymensingh, and Sylhet) divisions. Each division is further divided into zilas, and each zila into upazilas, with urban areas being divided into wards and mohallas and rural areas into union parishads and mouzas. This division allows for the separation of the country into rural and urban areas. The BDHS utilized a carefully chosen dataset to ensure accurate estimations of crucial demographic and health factors across the entire nation, as well as in urban and rural regions individually. Additionally, the survey covered each of the eight divisions. A total of 20,250 residential households were selected, with an anticipated completion of interviews from approximately 20,100 ever-married women aged 15–49 years.

Differentials in fertility are examined by some selected background variables: age at marriage, education, place of residence, religion, region, work status of women, women's participation in nongovernmental organizations (NGOs), husband's education, husband's occupation, and birth status of women in Bangladesh using 2017–18 BDHS data (published October 2020). The average number of children ever-born per ever-married woman of different age groups is used to measure the differentials of the fertility of the selected variables.

22.5 Theory and Background

The widespread belief is that fertility decreases as the age at marriage increases. While marrying early has been linked to increased fertility for women (Osborn 1958), getting married later is believed to decrease fertility (Coale 1975). All else being equal, delayed marriage reduces the time between generations, independently slowing long-term population growth (Davis and Blake 1956). The age at marriage differs (Dahal 1992) from one ethnic group to another which is inversely proportional to fertility.

An enduring result in fertility research is the inverse correlation between education and fertility. Education can influence fertility by delaying marriage, introducing different perspectives and broadening horizons, improving women's understanding and utilization of contraception, and offering enhanced job prospects (Ryder 1967; Janowitz 1976). Higher education influences women's career aspirations, labor market involvement and experiences, familial roles, and fertility (Becker 1981; Rindfuss et al. 1980).

Urban–rural differential in fertility is one of the most widely studied areas in differential fertility. While higher fertility in rural areas than in urban has almost consistently been observed in the present developed countries, results from the developing countries do not show consistent differentials by urban–rural place of residence (U. N. 1965:124–133). Moreover, women in this age group in rural areas may be comparatively suffering more from adolescent sterility resulting from early age at marriage as well as various diseases in the rural areas or may be due to the higher age at menarche (Chowdhury 1977). Recent migration of young couples from rural to urban areas who could not as yet adjust their reproductive behavior to the urban environment might be responsible to some extent for this observed lack of differential. Hill (2011) has shown that fertility levels are the highest in small towns and rural areas and the lowest in the capital city, as expected.

Visaria (1974) found that Muslim women had a marital fertility rate that was approximately 5–9% higher than Hindu women, and these disparities can be attributed not only to differences in contraceptive use but also to the varying social customs and norms practiced within each community.

The examination of regional differences in fertility is crucial because it can reveal any variations in childbearing patterns across different areas. Understanding the factors behind these differences can help create effective strategies and programs for reducing fertility rates. It has been demonstrated that the variations in fertility are the main cause of regional population growth differences in Bangladesh (Sivamurthy and Ahmad 1979). According to Samsik and Hyojin's (2016) study, regional population size and structure changes are directly and/or indirectly influenced by societal structures related to education, employment, and birth control, thereby impacting fertility rates.

Several studies have suggested that women who are part of the workforce tend to have fewer children than those who are not working. The relationship between workforce participation and fertility is not entirely clear, as it is uncertain whether workforce participation is a cause or a result of lower fertility rates (Devanzo 1972; UN 1973). Additionally, David et al. (2007) have revealed a significant negative impact of fertility on female workforce participation, particularly among women aged 20–39 years, with an enduring effect on older women. The study also highlighted the impact of reduced fertility on income per capita, considering changes in female workforce participation, population size, and age demographics.

Abdul and Osamu (2010) have examined the impact of women's status, NGOs, and various demographic factors on declining fertility. Their findings indicate that working women with multiple children aged 2 years and above and involvement in micro-credit-related NGOs have a reduced desire for additional children. Additionally, micro-credit organizations like BRAC and Grameen Bank have proven more effective in lowering fertility rates.

Raphael and Joshua (2018) have found that husbands with higher levels of education had a significant decrease in their fertility by the age of 25 years. This trend was also associated with delayed marriage and increased urbanization, potentially reducing the demand for children. They proposed that policies promoting access to education could lead to a substantial decrease in overall fertility rates in lower-income countries.

Prof. Donald J Bogus has suggested that the occupation of the head of the family has an impact on fertility. He claims that people with better occupations tend to have fewer children, whereas those with lower-paying jobs tend to have more. He also associates income with fertility, stating that as income decreases, fertility increases, and when income reaches a certain level, fertility decreases, but then increases again with a considerable rise in income. He argues against the belief that reaching a certain family size will naturally lead to fewer children. (Bogue 1969). Ayesha and Farasat (2013) have found that husbands engaged in manual labor, such as daily workers, wage-earners, and rickshaw pullers, tend to have low incomes, leading them to desire more children in order to increase their earnings.

Sex preference remains a widespread occurrence globally, particularly in societies like Bangladesh, where the desire for male offspring is prevalent, with sex discrimination often beginning even before birth. Many cultures possess myths and traditions aimed at increasing the likelihood of having boys, and the inability to produce a first male offspring can cause distress among couples, as it is perceived as a significant indicator of individual worth and family status. While women in certain cultures may exhibit less preference for sons, some may desire a male offspring simply to appease their husbands. Jean and Mamta (2000) have found that when parents equally value sons and daughters and are content with having two surviving children irrespective of their sex, there is less pressure for repeated births. The preference for sons is notably higher among rural and Muslim women in Bangladesh, which appears to contribute to an increase in the number of living children per female (BDHS 2018).

22.6 Related Research

In a study conducted by Rashed et al. (2022), the aim was to identify the factors that impact the number of children among working women. The study utilized data from the Bangladesh Demographic and Health Survey (BDHS 2018). The dependent variable in this study was the number of children, while several independent variables were examined, including the education levels of the respondents and their husbands, age at first marriage, wealth index, contraceptive use, place of residence, and religion. The analysis revealed that women's education, age at first marriage, and wealth index had a significant influence on the number of children. Furthermore, it was found that rural women and Muslim respondents had higher fertility rates. The study recommended the promotion of education for women and men, as well as discouraging early marriage, as effective measures to reduce the number of children in families. These findings highlight the importance of considering these factors when addressing fertility among working women.

Islam et al. (2003) found that the Khulna and Rajshahi regions in Bangladesh had the lowest age at first marriage and first birth when examining fertility variation across the six administrative divisions/regions. The reasons behind the low fertility levels in these regions are attributed to the increased utilization of family planning methods, a decreased desire for higher fertility, and longer intervals between non-first births. To effectively decrease fertility levels throughout Bangladesh, program managers and policymakers should take into account the valuable insights gained from the experiences of the Khulna division when planning and implementing future programs.

Shanjida et al. (2023), based on 15 studies involving 212,271 participants in Bangladesh, focused on ever-married women aged 15–49 years utilizing nationally representative Bangladesh Demographic and Health Survey data. The study revealed that Islam (86.8–90.2%) and Hinduism (10–13%) were the predominant religions, with women marrying between the ages of 14 and 20 years and giving birth between 16 and 22 years. Furthermore, the fertility rate in Bangladesh has significantly decreased from 1975 to 2022.

The U.N. (2022) study analyzed the differences in desired and observed fertility among three regions and two socioeconomic groups, using data from the BDHS 1993/94 and 2017/18. The study found that observed and desired fertility varied across regions and socioeconomic groups, with the Western region showing the lowest fertility rates, particularly among the lower wealth quintiles. Notably, observed fertility in the Western region was below replacement level and lower than desired fertility, while poorer women in the Eastern region had observed fertility significantly higher than their desired fertility.

22.7 Categorical Variables with Levels and Hypotheses

General hypothesis: Fertility depends indirectly on socioeconomic and demographic factors	
Variables	Hypotheses
Age at marriage: <15, 15–19, 20–24, 25+	Fertility rates are typically higher within marriage, and delaying the age at which people marry can lead to lower fertility levels
Education: No education; primary; Secondary; higher	Women's education has a significant effect on declining fertility. Higher education is associated with lower fertility
Place of residence: Urban; rural	Urbanization reduces fertility because urban residence would likely increase the costs of raising children
Religion: Muslim; non-Muslim (Hindu, Christian, and Buddhist)	Religious beliefs and personal philosophy may influence people's attitudes to give more births
Regional differentials in fertility: Barisal; Chittagong; Dhaka Khulna; Rajshahi; Sylhet; Mymensingh; Rangpur	Fertility is affected by many different cultural, environmental, and socioeconomic factors
Work status of women: Did not work (home-based work); worked (outside jobs)	Fertility goes down with increasing women employment rates

General hypothesis: Fertility depends indirectly on socioeconomic and demographic factors	
Variables	Hypotheses
Women's participation in NGO's: Yes; no	Women's participation in NGOs enhances empowerment and results in lower fertility
Husband's education: No education; primary Secondary; higher	Parents with higher education levels tend to have fewer children
Husband's occupation: Manual (farmer, agricultural worker, fisherman, laborers, and others); Non-manual (professional worker, businessman, and others)	Research indicates that when husbands take an active role in manual/domestic work, it is linked with higher fertility rates
Birth status of women: Children living with both sexes (i.e., have male and female in a family); Children of living daughters only (i.e., have a female in a family)	The desire for male children boosts both individual and overall fertility rates

22.8 Results and Discussions

22.8.1 Age at Marriage

The average number of children ever-born per ever-married woman is calculated by age groups of women and age at marriage in Table 22.1. It reveals that when the current age is held constant, the average number of children decreases with higher age at marriage. It is observed that fertility increases with an increase in age.

Table 22.1 also presents that the women completing her child bearing period who were married at the age of <15 years have on average produced 2.573, while one who was married at the age of 25+ years has produced an average of 1.660 children which is more than 35% less than those married at <15.

Table 22.1 Average number of children ever-born per ever-married woman by age group and age at marriage in Bangladesh, BDHS 2017–18

	Age at marriage			
Age group of women	<15	15–19	20–24	25+
<20	0.899	0.759	–	–
20–24	1.589	1.124	0.753	–
25–29	2.338	1.783	0.977	0.753
30–34	2.907	2.484	1.754	0.977
35–39	3.187	2.763	2.281	1.754
40–44	3.450	2.919	2.534	2.281
45+	3.642	3.326	2.910	2.534
The average number of children	2.573	2.166	1.868	1.660

It seems that the fertility rate decreases when individuals marry later in life. It is widely acknowledged that countries with early marriage practices tend to have higher fertility rates, in contrast to those who marry at a later stage.

22.8.2 Education

Examination of Table 22.2 presenting the average number of live births per ever-married woman by women's education reveals that women who had no education show the highest completed fertility 3.788. The completed fertility for women with education level secondary and higher is, respectively, 3.305 and 2.447, that is, higher educational level lowers the fertility.

The completed fertility for women who had completed primary education is 3.620, which is less than those with no formal education, although the difference is very small. It can also be seen from Table 22.2 that women with no education tended to have more children in all the groups than those with primary, secondary, and higher levels.

The higher level of fertility for women with no education than educated women may be due to the following reasons.

1. Women with no education are not conscious of having a limited family size.
2. At an age when there are more chances of having fertility, the girls are in colleges and universities and thus do not get children which during this period uneducated girls get.
3. Uneducated women feel very hesitant to use contraceptives to control family size and go on accepting even unnecessary motherhood responsibilities imposed on them.
4. The span of child-producing time in the case of uneducated women is quick, as compared with educated women.
5. In many cases, educated women get employed, and with employment, they cannot afford to have more children.

Table 22.2 Average number of children ever-born per ever-married woman by age group and women's education: Bangladesh, BDHS 2017–18

	Women's education level			
Age group of women	No education	Primary	Secondary	Higher
<20	0.913	0.871	0.802	–
20–24	1.628	1.393	1.1263	0.848
25–29	2.688	2.215	1.638	1.045
30–34	2.725	2.709	2.107	1.373
35–39	3.375	3.121	2.574	1.812
40–44	3.385	3.3175	3.114	2.174
45+	3.788	3.620	3.305	2.447
The average number of children	2.643	2.464	2.095	1.616

Table 22.3 Average number of children ever-born per ever-married woman by age group and urban–rural residence: Bangladesh, BDHS 2017–18

Age group of women	Residence	
	Urban	Rural
<20	0.888	0.868
20–24	1.198	1.919
25–29	1.734	2.567
30–34	2.267	2.747
35–39	2.711	3.212
40–44	2.956	3.414
45+	3.272	3.866
The average number of children	2.147	2.656

22.8.3 Place of Residence

Data on urban–rural fertility in Bangladesh are presented in Table 22.3. Considering the average live births to ever-married women in the age group 45+ (45–49) as completed fertility, it is observed that urban fertility is lower on average by about 0.6 children than the rural one. The lower fertility for urban women is also seen for all age groups except the younger (<20). The reason for higher fertility in the age group (<20) in the urban areas may be the reason that the number of married females in this age group is much less in the urban than in the rural areas due to the higher age at marriage in the urban areas.

When we observe the age differences, higher fertility in the rural area is still apparent, with the overall average number of live births being 2.6 in the rural and 2.1 in the urban areas (Table 22.3). The observed difference in fertility rates between urban and rural areas can be explained by factors such as older age at marriage, higher real income per person, improved health services, access to education, increased employment opportunities for women in urban areas, and other social amenities. In rural areas, children are often viewed as economic assets rather than a burden, leading to higher fertility rates (Caldwell 1978). Additionally, the economic cost of raising children, the lower economic value placed on children in urban settings, and the opportunity cost of mothers' time may have contributed to lower fertility rates in urban women who practice effective birth control methods.

22.8.4 Religion

Religious teachings have a significant impact on fertility rates. Religions that do not impose restrictions on the number of marriages and children tend to have higher fertility rates compared to others. This is because having multiple wives often leads to a larger number of children being born.

Islam is the predominant religion in Bangladesh. Muslims constitute almost 90% of the population of Bangladesh, Hindus about 10%, and others less than 1% (BDHS, 2017–18). Religious value systems, which influence individual values, are different between Muslims and non-Muslims.

Table 22.4 Average number of children ever-born per ever-married woman by age group and religion: Bangladesh BDHS 2017–18

Age group of women	Religion	
	Muslim	Non-Muslim
<20	0.871	0.871
20–24	1.409	1.311
25–29	2.106	1.743
30–34	2.715	2.412
35–39	3.075	2.618
40–44	3.313	3.004
45+	3.633	3.120
The average number of children	2.446	2.154

The average number of children born by religion is presented in Table 22.4. It indicates that Muslims have higher fertility than non-Muslims in each age group. Table 22.4 also depicts standardized age differences, and Muslims have shown the highest average number (2.446) than Non-Muslims women (2.154).

We can see from Table 22.4 that fertility among Muslims is higher as compared with the non-Muslims. The causes of higher fertility may be as follows:

1. Muslims marry at an early stage as compared with non-Muslims.
2. It is presumed that, in Bangladesh, non-Muslims are more inclined toward family planning programs compared with Muslims.
3. Female education among Muslim women is less as compared with non-Muslim women.
4. On the whole literacy among Muslims is less, compared with the non-Muslims with the result that more non-Muslim women go into far employment. Naturally employed women do not prefer to have large families. These wish to limit their family size because there are many problems involved in their upbringing, schooling, and their final settlement in life.

22.8.5 Regional Differentials in Fertility

Table 22.5 shows the average number of children ever-born per ever-married woman by age group among the regions as well as eight administrative divisions of Bangladesh. It can be seen from the table that the variation is prominent in the age group 20–24 and diminishes with increasing age. Figure 22.1 demonstrates the fertility trends among the divisions of Bangladesh. The higher variation in the age groups may be attributed to variations in the proportion of married in these age groups among the regions. The differentials in the level of urbanization, the level of education, and female participation in the labor force might have had varying influences in bringing about the observed variation in fertility. On the contrary, the variation in the higher age groups may be due to the extent of variation in widowhood, divorce, and childlessness in addition to differential behavior toward fertility regulations or family planning practices among the regions which are dependent on socio-cultural differences.

Table 22.5 Average number of children ever-born per ever-married woman by age group and divisions: Bangladesh, BDHS 2017–18

Age group of women	Divisions										
	Barisal	Chittagong	Dhaka	Khulna	Rajshahi	Sylhet	Mymensingh	Rangpur	Mean $\overline{(X)}$	S.D. (σ)	C.V. $\frac{(100\sigma)}{(X)}$
<20	0.963	0.988	0.807	0.622	0.751	1.240	0.909	0.823	0.887	0.185	20.856
20–24	1.429	1.865	1.469	1.093	1.239	2.083	1.865	1.239	1.535	0.359	23.387
25–29	2.170	2.641	1.988	1.549	1.840	2.812	2.641	1.840	2.185	0.461	21.098
30–34	2.813	3.411	2.570	2.336	2.336	3.179	3.411	2.336	2.799	0.476	17.006
35–39	2.444	3.610	2.975	2.498	2.645	3.559	3.610	2.645	2.998	0.516	17.211
40–44	3.513	3.757	3.284	3.108	3.181	3.942	3.757	3.181	3.465	0.321	9.2640
45+	3.738	3.915	3.392	3.322	3.394	3.96	3.915	3.394	3.628	0.279	7.690
The average number of children	2.438 (5)	2.884 (7)	2.355 (3)	2.075 (1)	2.198 (2)	2.968 (8)	2.873 (6)	2.208 (4)	2.499	0.371	16.644

Note: Figures in parentheses indicate ranks of lower to higher fertility in the region

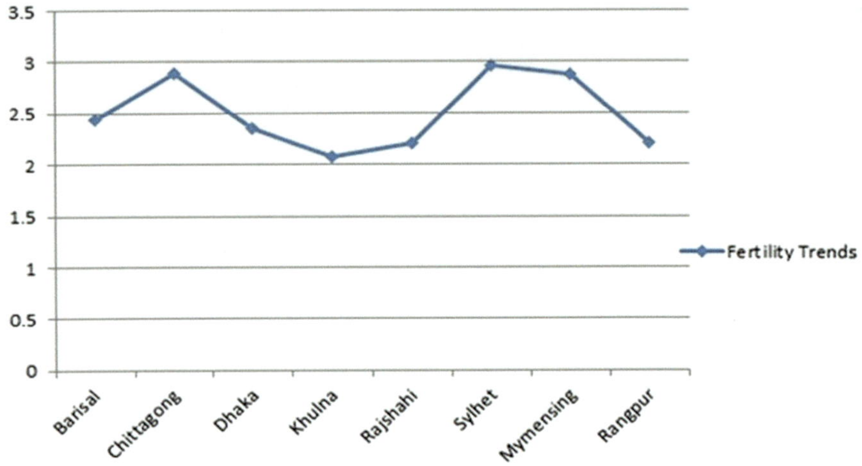

Fig. 22.2 Fertility trends among the divisions of Bangladesh

It appears in Table 22.5 and Fig. 22.2 that fertility is higher in Sylhet, Chittagong, and Mymensingh, with the average number of children ever-born per woman being 2.968, 2.844, and 2.873. Fertility is lowest in Khulna (2.075), Rajshahi (2.198), and Rangpur (2.208). Dhaka and Barisal have intermediate levels of fertility, with average (2.355) and (2.438) children per woman. The following information from BDHS data may be the effect of the regional variation of fertility.

The 2017–18 BDHS data indicate that women in the Barisal division have a higher tendency to be self-employed, less likely to work for relatives, and more likely to receive cash payments compared to women in other divisions. On the contrary, women in Sylhet are less likely to be self-employed and less likely to receive cash payments. Discrepancies in employment type and payment method based on education level are minimal. Additionally, women in Rajshahi division have a higher employment rate compared with women in other divisions. Rural women are more likely to work seasonally, particularly as agricultural laborers, compared to urban women. Women in the Khulna division are more inclined toward agriculture employment, while those in the Dhaka division are less likely to work in agriculture but more likely to have manual jobs. It is observed that women with no education tend to work in the agriculture sector, whereas those with some secondary education are more likely to engage in skilled manual labor.

22.8.6 Work Status of Women

The average number of children born by work status and the current age of women are presented in Table 22.6.

It appears that the number of children born on average is higher for non-working women than working women for each group. The same picture is apparent in the case of an average number of children. Women who are involved with a job are not

Table 22.6 Average number of children ever-born per ever-married woman by age group and women's work status: Bangladesh, BDHS 2017–18

	Women's work status	
Age group of women	Did not work	Worked
<20	1.005	0.884
20–24	1.647	1.450
25–29	2.259	2.036
30–34	2.769	2.451
35–39	3.105	2.735
40–44	3.365	2.944
45+	3.814	3.157
The average number of children	2.566	2.237

dependent on men. Both socially and mentally, these have their rights and absence of dependence, men cannot use women to forcibly increase their fertility. This has also resulted in low fertility. Fertility depends on the social status of the woman. In societies where women are confined only to household jobs, these are considered suitable only for producing children and as such those women who are held in high esteem.

22.8.7 Women's Participation in NGOs

NGOs play a very important role in fertility-reducing effects in Bangladesh. In Bangladesh, NGOs are said to be the alternative institution to promote the national progress of the country. There are data on many NGOs in 2017–18 BDHS such as Grameen Bank, BRAC, BRDP, Mother's Club, and so on.

Bangladesh NGOs are so diverse in terms of activities that it is hard for anybody to find a single sphere where NGOs are not involved directly or individually. Of the NGOs three distinct categories are observable, local, regional, and national. At present, there are a large number of local, regional, and national NGOs working all over Bangladesh to change the socioeconomic through demographic structure of the country.

NGOs are also playing a vital role in human resources development. Human resource development is the pre-condition for economic development and economic conditions are indirectly linked with fertility. The average number of children born by age group and women's participation in NGOs are presented in Table 22.7. Table 22.7 indicates that the average number of children born is lower for women who are concerned with NGOs than others in each age group. The probable causes of lower fertility are as follows:

1. NGOs have implemented numerous programs aimed at improving the quality of life for individuals. By venturing into rural and remote regions, they engage in face-to-face interactions to educate communities on the importance of maintaining good health. Additionally, they offer basic knowledge on medical science, which can have a positive impact on fertility rates.

Table 22.7 Average number of children ever-born per ever-married woman by age group and women's participation in NGOs: Bangladesh, BDHS 2017–18

Age group of women	Member of NGO	
	Yes	No
<20	0.853	1.085
20–24	1.354	1.709
25–29	2.051	2.170
30–34	2.660	2.734
35–39	3.004	3.262
40–44	3.203	3.780
45+	3.537	3.854
The average number of children	2.380	2.656

2. Most of the villagers of our country are poor and illiterate. As a result, they cannot understand properly which thing is bad and which thing is good for them. In this situation, NGOs help the villagers by making proper decisions for their improvement, and that increases their consciousness and, as a result, there creates a tendency in them that family size should be small and population explosion should be checked; otherwise, many economic and social problems are bound to arise.
3. Educational activities taken by the NGOs open a new chapter all over the country. NGOs have taken various educational activities such as formal education, informal education, adult education, mass education, practical education, and many kinds of training. In this way, a large number of villagers are conscious of the family planning system. Many NGOs supply various materials for family planning method that directly affects fertility.

22.8.8 Husband's Education

The level of education attained by husbands plays a significant role in shaping fertility rates. In many societies, husbands' opinions hold considerable weight, influencing decisions related to family planning. Presently, individuals with higher education are increasingly valuing the education of their potential spouses, leading to a more balanced dynamic within families. However, this shift toward prioritizing education in marriages can have adverse effects on fertility rates.

Table 22.8 presents the average number of children ever-born per ever-married woman by husband's education. It reveals those women whose husbands had completed primary education; the average number of children is greater than those, whose husbands had no education although the difference is very small.

Table 22.8 also reveals that women with husbands' secondary educational levels tended to have more children in all age groups than those with higher education. The completed fertility for women whose husbands with primary education is (2.265), which is greater than the higher level that is (1.884). When the average number of children per ever-married woman is calculated, the same picture is visible. That is the higher the education level, the lower the number of children ever-born.

Table 22.8 Average number of children ever-born per ever-married woman by age group and husband's education: Bangladesh, BDHS 2017–18

	Husband's education level			
Age group of women	No education	Primary	Secondary	Higher
<20	0.897	0.867	0.816	0.789
20–24	1.503	1.500	1.205	0.974
25–29	2.204	2.226	1.860	1.439
30–34	2.886	2.783	2.448	1.899
35–39	3.154	3.263	2.857	2.327
40–44	3.356	3.391	3.215	2.709
45+	3.562	3.779	3.452	3.049
The average number of children	2.509	2.544	2.265	1.884

The lower level of fertility for women whose husband's education level is higher than those with secondary may be due to the following reasons:

1. Usually, educated men marry at a late stage, so fewer children are produced, but uneducated men marry at an early age; as a result, they produce more children.
2. Educated men always want to educate their children. As too much money is expended to educate the children, they want to keep their family limited. But an illiterate man never thinks so.
3. An educated man is more conscious about hygiene than an illiterate man and he doesn't take so many children considering the physical condition of his wife.
4. Uneducated men are usually orthodox about religion and they consider family planning as anti-religious and don't use any method. But educated men always think practically and maintain different customs systematically.
5. Educated men are generally involved in different occupations. So, they have to go to different places and they want to maintain a high living standard with other families. But too many children create hindrances to maintain it.

22.8.9 Husband's Occupation

In a country like Bangladesh, the husband's occupation is closely related to fertility. The various occupational categories are included in the 2017–18 BDHS data. For the sake of our analysis, the categories are classified into two major groups, viz., manual and non-manual categories. The average number of children born by current age and husband's occupation are presented in Table 22.9.

Table 22.9 indicates that the average number of children born is higher for manual occupations than for non-manual occupations in each age group. The same scenario is apparent for the average number of children which is higher fertility in manual occupations (2.503) than in non-manual occupations (2.210). It is commonly observed that individuals involved in intellectual pursuits tend to have fewer children in comparison to those engaged in physical labor. Similarly, individuals

Table 22.9 Average number of children ever-born per ever-married woman by age group and husband's occupation: Bangladesh, BDHS 2017–18

	Husband's occupation	
Age group of women	Manual	Non-manual
<20	0.855	0.841
20–24	1.458	1.368
25–29	2.191	1.996
30–34	2.802	2.570
35–39	3.111	2.957
40–44	3.368	3.209
45+	3.596	3.510
The average number of children	2.503	2.210

whose professions involve frequent visits to clubs and other recreational venues also tend to have fewer offspring.

Manual labor is associated with high fertility rates because couples in these occupations often live together and have limited sources of entertainment beyond sexual activity. Additionally, there is a belief that children born into these families will eventually contribute financially from a young age by taking on simple tasks. This perception is reinforced by the low cost of raising children compared with the potential returns they can provide. In our country, agriculture is a predominant occupation, which falls under the category of manual labor. Most of the people depend on agriculture in our country. In this occupation, additional manpower is always welcome. Thus, the addition of a child to the family is considered a matter of joy rather than that of sorrow. When childbirth is a matter of pleasure, obviously fertility rate will considerably increase.

22.8.10 Birth Status of Women

The concept of birth status is a prevalent occurrence worldwide, particularly in societies like Bangladesh. Gender discrimination often starts even before birth in many regions. There is a strong desire for a firstborn son among parents, leading to various cultural beliefs on how to increase the chances of having a male child. Predictions about the gender of the unborn child are common during pregnancy. The inability to produce a first male offspring can cause distress for couples, as it is often seen as a reflection of individual worth and family status. While some cultures show a preference for sons, there are instances where women may want a son solely to please their husbands.

The main focus of this section is to examine the factors encouraging a high rate of growth of human fertility in connection with the aspiration for having male offspring instead of daughters irrespective of religiosity. Birth status is associated with the socio-cultural and economic structure of the society and the needs of the people. Table 22.10 shows differentials in fertility by age and birth status of women.

The data in Table 22.10 indicate that there has been a growing interest to produce more children when women have living daughters only, i.e., have no sons than those

Table 22.10 Average number of children ever-born per ever-married woman by age group with their birth status: Bangladesh, BDHS 2017–18

	Birth status of women	
Age group of women	Children living with both sexes	Children of living daughters only
<20	1.393	1.393
20–24	1.888	2.028
25–29	2.496	2.648
30–34	2.686	3.062
35–39	3.167	3.414
40–44	3.474	3.598
45+	3.629	3.845
The average number of children	2.676	2.855

women who have both living sons and daughters for each age group except (<20). Moreover, the average number of children for living daughters only is greater than living both sexes. Female children are engaged in direct productivities to a lesser extent than combined effect (when male and female are both together). The reasons for these differences are given below:

1. The expectation of old age security is one of the dominant motivations for male sex preference of couples in Bangladesh which directly affects fertility; as a result, fertility has been increasing.
2. Sons play a crucial role in providing old age security, contributing to family income, and sharing parental responsibilities within the family structure.
3. Having sons is highly valued in families, both for their contribution to the overall strength of the family and for the preservation of the family lineage. A larger number of sons are seen as a significant source of strength within the family unit.
4. A large number of parents consider that the daughter is a burden and so are always worried about her marriage expenses.
5. In our society sonless parents feel an inferiority complex in comparison with the parents who have sons.

22.9 Conclusion

The analysis reveals that age at marriage has a reducing effect on fertility; the increase of age at marriage and level of education may effectively reduce the reproductive performance of the women in Bangladesh. The urban–rural differentials of fertility show that the rural fertility is higher than the urban. Besides, labor force participation influences fertility negatively.

The main focus of this study is to consider the regional differential of fertility that the average number of children of Khulna division (2.0 births per woman) and Rajshahi division (2.1 births per woman) have already reached at the replacement level of fertility in Bangladesh. As UN projection of a target level of the TFR of Bangladesh is 2.1 by 2030 (UN 1999, 2001). How is this possible before the target time? Which factors have played a significant role for the two divisions? We have to do more research to find out these socioeconomic and demographic factors. Those may be age at marriage, education, occupation, urbanization, and economic condition of that area. We have to control these factors among other divisions according to Khulna and Rajshahi to reach the desired replacement level of fertility in Bangladesh.

The research shows that we are not far away from reaching the goal of replacement-level fertility all over Bangladesh. If we take proper steps, we will reach the target level before time.

References

Abdul G, Osamu S (2010) Fertility decline and women's status-the role of non-government organizations (NGOs) in Bangladesh: a micro data analysis. Int NGO J 5(1):021–033. http://www.academicjournals.org/INGOJ

Ayesha J, Farasat AS (2013) Fertility differential by husbands' occupational status and income in Dhanbad district, Jharkhand, India. Dev Pract 23(1):79–89. https://doi.org/10.1080/09614524.2012.714352

Bagozzi RP, Vanloo MF (1978) Toward a general. Theory of fertility: a causal modeling approach. Demography 15(3):301

BDHS (2020) Bangladesh demographic and health survey 2017-2018. Institute of Population Research and Training (NIPORT), Dhaka

Becker GSA (1981) Treatise on the family. Harvard University Press, Cambridge, MA

Bogue DJ (1969) Principles of demography. Wiely, New York

Caldwell JC (1978) A general theory of fertility. Mimeo. The Australian National University, Canberra

Chowdhury AKM et al (1977) Malnutrition, menarche and marriage in rural Bangladesh. Soc Biol 24(4):316

Coale AJ (1975) The demographic transition. In: In the population debate—dimensions and perspectives, vol 1. United Nations, New York

Dahal DR (1992) Determinants of fertility in Nepal. In: Bal Kumar KC (ed) Population and development in Nepal, vol 1

David, E. Bloom, David, C., Günther, F. and Jocelyn, E. Finlay (2007) Fertility, female labor force participation, and the demographic dividend. NBER Working Paper No. 13583. http://www.nber.org/papers/w13583

Davis K, Blake J (1956) Social structure and fertility: an analytical frame work. Econ Dev Cult Chang 4(4):211–235

Devanzo J (1972) Cross-sectional arial analysis of factors affecting marital fertility: actual versus relative income. J Marriage Fam 38(4):1

Hill K (2011) Why fertility levels vary between urban and rural areas? Reg Stud 47:895. https://doi.org/10.1080/00343404.2011.581276.hal-00714930

Islam MM, Ubaidur R, Nitai C (2003) Regional variations in fertility in Bangladesh. Genus 59(3–4):103–145

Janowitz BS (1976) An analysis of the impact of education on family size. Demography 13(2):189

Jean D, Mamta M (2000) Fertility, education and development. discussion paper, No. DEDPS 20, January 2000. London School of Economics and Political Science, London. https://eprints.lse.ac.uk/6663/1/Fertility%2C_Education_and_Development.pdf

Osborn F (1958) Population: an international dilemma. The Population Council, New York

Raphael G, Joshua L (2018) Does male education affect fertility? Evidence from Mali. Econ Lett 172(2018):118–122. https://doi.org/10.1016/j.econlet.2018.08.028

Rashed A, Aminur R, Yothin S (2022) Factors influencing the number of children born to working women in Bangladesh: a population-based study. Journal of pediatrics. Perinatol Child Health 6:484–494

Rindfuss RR, Bumpass L, St. John, C. (1980) Education and fertility: implications for the roles women occupy. Am Sociol Rev 1980(45):431–447

Ryder NB (1967) The character of modern fertility. In: Peterson W (ed) Readings in population, vol 369. The Macmillan Company, New York, p 26

Samsik L, Hyojin C (2016) Social structural determinants of regional variations in fertility. Adv Sci Technol Lett 131:60–63. https://doi.org/10.14257/astl.2016.131.12

Shanjida C, Meshbahur MR, Aminul H (2023) Role of women's empowerment in determining fertility and reproductive health in Bangladesh: a systematic literature review. AJOG Glob Rep 3(3):100239. https://doi.org/10.1016/j.xagr.2023.10023

Sivamurthy M, Ahmad S (1979) Regional disparities in population change and Department in Bangladesh. In: Paper presented at the seminar on population change and development in some African and Asiatic countries. Cairo Demographic Centre, Cairo

United Nations (1965) Population Bulleting, No. 7, 1963. United Nations, New York

United Nations (1973) The determinant and consequences of population trends. In: Population Studies No. 50, vol 1. United Nations, New York

United Nations (1999) United Nations: world population prospects: the 1998 revision. United Nations, New York

United Nations (2001) United Nations world population prospects, the 2000 Revision. In: Comprehensive Tables (United Nations publication, Sales No. E.01.XIII.8), vol 1. United Nations, New York

United Nations (2022) Department of Economic and Social Affairs, Population Division. World population prospects. https://population.un.org/wpp/Download/Standard/Population/. United Nations, New York

Visaria L (1974) Religious differentials in fertility. In: Ashish Bose PB, Desai AM, Sharma JN (eds) Population in India's development 1947–2000. Vikas Publishing House Pvt. Ltd., Delhi

Index

M. Pal et al. (eds.), *Public Health and Nutrition*,
https://doi.org/10.1007/978-981-97-7890-4

GPSR Compliance

The European Union's (EU) General Product Safety Regulation (GPSR) is a set of rules that requires consumer products to be safe and our obligations to ensure this.

If you have any concerns about our products, you can contact us on ProductSafety@springernature.com

In case Publisher is established outside the EU, the EU authorized representative is:

Springer Nature Customer Service Center GmbH
Europaplatz 3
69115 Heidelberg, Germany

Batch number: 07935681

Printed by Printforce, the Netherlands